# Kinanthropometry VIII

T0227526

The International Society for the Advancement of Kinanthropometry held its 8th International Conference in Manchester in July 2002. This volume contains a selection of papers presented to the Conference, where the meeting was held in conjunction with the 12th Commonwealth International Sport Conference, immediately prior to the XVII Commonwealth Games.

The book is structured into five parts:

* methodological issues in kinanthropometry
* paediatric science
* applications of kinanthropometry
* women and exercise
* health relations.

The collation of the chapters into an edited book provides readers with an outline of the current state of knowledge in kinanthropometry.

**Thomas Reilly** is President of the World Commission of Science and Sports and Director of the Research Institute for Sport and Exercise Sciences at Liverpool John Moores University. **Mike Marfell-Jones** is Chair of Health Science, Universal College of Learning, Wellington, New Zealand, and President of the International Society for the Advancement of Kinanthropometry.

# Kinanthropometry VIII

Proceedings of the 8th International
Conference of the International
Society for the Advancement
of Kinanthropometry (ISAK)

Edited by

## Thomas Reilly

and

## Mike Marfell-Jones

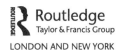

Routledge
Taylor & Francis Group
LONDON AND NEW YORK

First published 2003
by Routledge
2 Park Square, Milton Park, Abingdon, Oxfordshire OX14 4RN

Simultaneously published in the USA and Canada
by Routledge
711 Third Avenue, New York, NY 10017

First issued in paperback 2014

*Routledge is an imprint of the Taylor and Francis Group, an informa business*

© 2003 Taylor & Francis

*Publisher's Note*
This book was prepared from camera-ready-copy supplied
by the authors

*British Library Cataloguing in Publication Data*
A catalogue record for this book is available from the British Library

*Library of Congress Cataloging in Publication Data*
A catalog record for this book has been requested

ISBN 13: 978-1-138-88046-7 (pbk)
ISBN 13: 978-0-415-28969-6 (hbk)

# Contents

## PART II
Paediatric Science

## PART III
Anthropometry in Sports

# Preface

The study and practice of anthropometry have been with us for centuries, but its umbrella discipline, kinanthropometry – the study of human size, shape, proportion, composition, maturation and gross function, in order to better understand growth, exercise, performance and nutrition – is a virtual neonate in the scientific world. This new discipline, whose name is a neologism derived from the Greek root words kinein (to move), anthropos (man) and metrein (to measure), has enjoyed a rapid growth in recognition and participation in its thirty years of existence. The International Society for the Advancement of Kinanthropometry (ISAK) is an international group that has made its role the stewardship of kinanthropometry and is dedicated (as its name indicates) to its advancement. As major components of that advancement, ISAK offers on-going anthropometric training courses in all five continents and encourages its members to publish and present quality work in international fora.

ISAK has made a practice of holding its Biennial General Meetings in association with major conferences prior to either the Olympic or Commonwealth Games. In the past decade that has occurred in Victoria, Canada, in 1994 (prior to the XV Commonwealth Games); in Dallas in 1996 (prior to the Atlanta Olympics); in Adelaide in 1998 (prior to the XVI Commonwealth Games in Kuala Lumpur); and in Brisbane in 2000 (prior to the Sydney Olympics). At each of these conferences, kinanthropometrists have made an increasing contribution to the success of the scientific gathering by presenting quality papers of their research and findings.

In July 2002, the tradition continued in Manchester, England where ISAK's meeting was held in conjunction with the 12th Commonwealth International Sport Conference, immediately prior to the XVII Commonwealth Games. These proceedings, which contain a refereed selection of the best kinanthropometry papers presented in Manchester, have been compiled so that their contents may be of benefit to a far wider audience than those few privileged enough to attend the conference itself. ISAK thanks the editors most sincerely for their efforts in compiling this volume and congratulates the authors on their work and its dissemination.

Mike Marfell-Jones
President
International Society for the Advancement of Kinanthropometry

# Introduction

Thomas Reilly[1] and Mike Marfell-Jones[2]
[1]Research Institute for Sport and Exercise Sciences, Liverpool John
Moores University, Henry Cotton Campus, 15-21 Webster Street,
Liverpool, L3 2ET, UK
[2]UCOL, Private Bag 11 022, Palmerston North, New Zealand

The contents of this volume represent the Proceedings of Kinanthropometry VIII, the 8th International Conference on the subject area of kinanthropometry. The conference was incorporated within the Twelfth Commonwealth and International Sport Conference held at Manchester on 19-23 July 2002, the week immediately preceding the Commonwealth Games and was supported by the Association of Commonwealth Universities. The kinanthropometry strand of the conference was organised on behalf of the International Society for Advancement of Kinanthropometry (ISAK) which was itself formed at a previous Commonwealth Conference – in Glasgow 1986.

During the conference at Manchester there were workshops and specific scientific sessions held jointly with the British Association for Sport and Exercise Sciences (BASES). Not all communications were worked up into manuscripts for the Proceedings and not all of those that were written up succeeded in satisfying peer reviewers. Whilst the conference programme covered a whole range of topics under the umbrella of kinanthropometry, only those that fitted into a series of coherent themes were selected for inclusion in this book.

The content is structured into five parts, the first of which is focused on methodological issues in kinanthropometry. Topics range from research design to contemporary investigative techniques, and novel technologies in particular. Manuscripts dealing with ergometry were included in this section of the book. Part II is devoted to paediatric science, including topics on growth and maturation. Part III is focused on applications of kinanthropometry to sports. The material here yields new insights into factors influencing performance in contemporary sports. The theme of elite performance is extended into the next Part which is devoted to women and exercise. This extension highlights the partial overlap in content between the different parts, the editorial choice of location being based on the best fit with the main themes. Finally, manuscripts with health-related impact are clustered together, even if measurements were on adolescent populations or sports participants.

The collation of the chapters into an edited book provides readers with an outline of the current state of knowledge in kinanthropometry. The contents also give a flavour of the different creative approaches used by researchers in the area to address contemporary questions. The international contributions reflect a broad interest in the subject area world wide and therefore the book should have a large appeal across a number of countries.

The editors are grateful to contributors for their punctuality in meeting deadlines and in responding to the comments from the review process. We also acknowledge the invaluable technical assistance of Ms Lesley Roberts at the Research Institute for Sport and Exercise Sciences at Liverpool John Moores University for putting the camera-ready-copy of the text together.

Thomas Reilly
Mike Marfell-Jones

# Part I
# METHODOLOGY

# 1 What is this Thing called Measurement Error?

Greg Atkinson
School of Sport and Exercise Sciences, Loughborough University,
Leicestershire, LE11 3TU, UK

## 1. INTRODUCTION

An anthropometrist wishes to establish whether a certain method of measuring adipose tissue is sufficiently reliable to be used in future research work. The anthropometrist recruits 20 subjects and obtains two repeated measurements under the same conditions. The researcher is not an expert in statistics and, therefore, refers to the literature for what are perceived to be the most appropriate statistical analyses and to see how such analyses are interpreted. Consequently, the researcher employs (i) a paired t-test, to check that there has been no change in the sample mean measurement over the two weeks, (ii) the intraclass correlation coefficient (ICC) to check that the degree of relationship between test and retest is above 0.8, and (iii) the technical error of measurement (TEM) to check that the "absolute variability" between test and retest is below 5%.

The above scenario will be familiar to most sport and exercise scientists and the statistical analyses that are mentioned above are the most commonly chosen procedures (Atkinson and Nevill, 1998). Unfortunately, researchers have rarely considered such questions as: What does an ICC or TEM represent in terms of exactly how much error is present? Why does an ICC above 0.8 or a TEM below 5% denote an *"acceptable"* level of error? How can an ICC and TEM appear *"acceptable"*, even though a significant difference between test and retest may have been found with the paired t-test? Is a sample size of twenty sufficient for arriving at conclusions in a reliability study?

The aim of the present review is to answer the above questions by identifying the most appropriate statistics for analysing measurement error, by outlining exactly what these measurement error statistics describe, and by discussing how these statistics are used to judge whether a particular measurement tool is reliable or not.

## 2. WHAT IS MEASUREMENT ERROR?

Measurement error is generally thought of as being the variability associated with two or more observations made under controlled conditions. The most important investigation of measurement error is where the *only* variable that is "allowed" to alter is time (i.e. test-retest error). The choice of time period (*s, min or days*) in a study that investigates test-retest error should be governed by how the measurement tool will be used in future practice. Some variables can be measured frequently over a relatively short period of time without complications. For example, it is possible to measure body temperature and heart rate every second (Edwards *et al.*, 2002). For other variables, the researcher might need to ensure that enough time is allowed between repeated measurements for serial effects of testing to dissipate (e.g. when physical performance is measured). If the act of taking a measurement has effects on a subsequent observation, *systematic error* is present.

If systematic errors can be discounted, there can still be random variation present in measurements (i.e. sometimes test > retest and sometimes test < retest). It should be noted that the paired t-test, chosen by the researcher in the above hypothetical scenario, can *only* test whether the average systematic difference between test and retest is significantly different from zero, and can provide no information on the degree of random error that is present (Atkinson and Nevill, 1998). In effect, the judgement of adequate agreement between test and retest on the basis of a non-significant hypothesis test such as the paired t-test is synonymous with the scenario of individuals concluding that they are, on average, "comfortably warm" when they have one arm in a bucket of water at 1 °C and the other arm in water at 50 °C!

Random test-retest measurement error for which time is the only non-constant factor, and which is linked to the concept of reliability, is my present concern. Issues related to reliability are when error is investigated between different measurement tools (i.e. *validity*; Nevill, 1996) or between different observers (i.e. *objectivity;* Morrow, 1989). Investigations into validity and objectivity could be considered as secondary in importance to a basic reliability check. If there is too much error between measurements made under the simplest conditions of the same observer and measurement tool being involved, then examination of additional sources of error due to method and observer is superfluous. In other words, if a measurement tool is deemed unreliable, it will neither be valid nor objective.

In section 4, more details are provided on how researchers can quantitatively measure the implications of measurement error. In general, measurement error impacts on all sub-disciplines of sport and exercise science (Hopkins, 2000, Atkinson and Nevill, 2001) by:-

(i)   Helping to make choices between different measurement tools, equipment and protocols that are purported to measure the same characteristic. Kinanthropometrists, through accreditation procedures, might also be familiar with the appraisal of an individual's ability to make adequate measurements.

(ii)  Affecting the chances of making a type II (false negative) error in empirical investigations involving samples of subjects, e.g. concluding that a particular ergogenic aid did not improve the mean performance of a sample of athletes when, in reality (i.e. in the population), there *was* an improvement in performance that was "swamped" by the presence of too much measurement error. Similarly, if one is interested in the precision of estimate through the use of confidence intervals, too much error makes confidence intervals wide and, therefore, research conclusions ambiguous (Hopkins, 2002).

(iii) Influencing the categorical decisions that are made on whether individual athletes are above or below certain "cut-off" values, e.g. for drug controls or team selection, and whether an improvement in performance of an individual athlete, due to some intervention, is real or can be attributable to measurement error.

## 3. WHAT IS RELIABILITY?

Despite the above influences of error on the practical uses of a measurement tool for sports science support work or research, it is surprising how rarely the definitions of reliability encompass such relationships. For example, reliability has been defined as the *"repeatability of measurements"* (Vincent, 1995) or *"consistency of test scores"* (Baumgartner *et al.*, 2002). Such definitions do not seem to distinguish between the description of measurement error and the concept of reliability. Reliability has also been considered to be *"the absence of measurement error"* (Safrit and Wood, 1989) or *"test scores [that] are not changing over a short period of time"* (Baumgartner *et al.*, 2002). These definitions are surprising given that almost every human measurement on a quantitative scale (ratio or interval data) would be expected to show at least *some* random error between test and retest. Morrow *et al.* (1995) acknowledged that some amount of error is unavoidable when they stated that, *"a test is said to be reliable if one obtains the same (or nearly the same) score each time a test is administered"*. Nevertheless, the definition of *"nearly the same"* is still open to interpretation. Baumgartner *et al.* (2002) hinted at a more informative interpretation of reliability when they said that error is *"tolerated"* when it *"does not change the interpretation of data"*.

Ideally, a definition of reliability should encompass exactly how a measurement tool is designated as being reliable or not. As Baumgartner *et al.* (2002) suggested, a decision should be made based on a practical (not necessarily statistical) consideration of how the error impacts on the performance of the measurement tool (Bland and Altman, 1999). Atkinson and Nevill (1998) defined reliability as *"the amount of measurement error that has been deemed acceptable for the effective practical use of a measurement tool"*. This definition denotes that reliability is *not* the same as measurement error description, but involves an informed decision based on consideration of the *implications* of measurement error description. Therefore, in order to incorporate a consideration of the impact of measurement error into a reliability study, it is important to understand what a particular measurement error statistic represents in reality.

## 4. STATISTICAL DESCRIPTION OF ERROR

The description of measurement error conventionally involves calculation of a standard deviation statistic, as long as the population from which the data are sampled is normally distributed. For example, the standard deviation for the repeated measurements of a skinfold thickness obtained from a hypothetical subject and presented below is 1.9 mm:-

|    |    |    |    |    |    |    |    |
|----|----|----|----|----|----|----|----|
| 8  | 9  | 10 | 12 | 11 | 14 | 10 | 12 |

This standard deviation should not simply be interpreted as representing the general "variability" in the data. In line with the thinking above, such an interpretation of the standard deviation cannot be used to judge reliability fully in a meaningful manner. Inspection of the raw data shows that the range of values is from 8 to 14 mm, a difference of 6 mm, which, as another representation of general "variability", is somewhat larger than 1.9 mm. Like all standard deviations, the described variability is related to a central tendency statistic, which in this case, is the mean ($\bar{x}$) of all the repeated measurements. In classical measurement theory, the $\bar{x}$ of all possible repeated measurements is termed the hypothetical "true score". The true score is hypothetical, because it is extremely difficult to obtain thousands of repeated measurements on individuals in research (Atkinson and Nevill, 2000). The standard deviation that relates to the true score was given the name "*standard error of measurement*" (SEM) by the famous statistician Charles Spearman (Spearman, 1904).

The $\bar{x}$, or the best estimate of the "true score" of the above data is 10.8 mm. Again, it would be a mistake to think that the SEM of 1.91 mm represents the *maximum* possible variability from the "true score", since there are data (e.g. 8 mm) that are more than 1.9 mm away from $\bar{x}$. The exact meaning of the SEM is related to the known relationship between any standard deviation statistic and coverage percentiles of data. For example, a range can be calculated based on $\bar{x}$ –SEM to $\bar{x}$ +SEM (8.9 to 12.7 mm in our example). This range would encompass the central 68% of all repeated measurements. The range of $\bar{x}$ –1.96SEM to $\bar{x}$ +1.96SEM (7.0 to 14.5 mm), would cover the central 95% of all repeated measurements. A probability of 0.95 happens to be the accepted definition of "reasonably certain" by statisticians, i.e. it would be reasonably certain that any measurement taken from the subject above would fall within the range 7.0 to 14.5 mm.

In order for a SEM to be useful, a researcher would want to know how far away a true score could be from a particular observation, and not *vice versa* as the above calculations suggest. In other words, a researcher wishes to make inferences about the unobtainable true score from the measurement that is obtained. This "reverse" inference from measurement to true score when using the SEM has been criticised (for a recent discussion see Charter and Feldt, 2001), but most researchers would generally view a SEM of 1.9 mm to mean that there is a 68%

(p=0.68) chance that the true score lies within ± 1.9 mm of the observation that has been made. A researcher could be "reasonably certain" (p=0.95) that the true score would lie between ± 1.96 SEM of the observed value (Harvill, 1991).

The scenario above is not very common in the sport and exercise sciences. A researcher is usually interested in describing the measurement error for a population of interest, which might include individuals of different ability or score levels. Consequently, a *sample* of individuals is usually assessed on a test-retest basis. A SEM can still be described for a sample by calculating the standard deviation of all the subject test-retest differences ($SD_{diff}$), and dividing this statistic by the square root of 2, as illustrated in Table 1. The SEM in this situation represents the maximum expected difference between hypothetical true score and observed score for 68% of all individuals in the population of interest (Harvill, 1991). If a researcher multiplies the SEM by 1.96, then he/she would be reasonably certain that this value would represent the maximal difference between true score and observation for any individual drawn from the population of interest.

Several other measurement error statistics are based on the SEM (Table 1). The coefficient of variation statistic for example is basically the SEM expressed as a percentage of the observed score. Therefore, a CV of 10% means that there is a 68% chance of the true score being within 10% of an observed score. The CV is useful for describing error when there is a positive relationship between error and the size of the measured value. Such "proportional error" has been found to be common in the Sport and Exercise Sciences, and is most precisely controlled for by calculating a coefficient of variation or other ratio-based statistic from logarithmically-transformed data (Nevill and Atkinson, 1997). The use of CV for describing error with some measurements (e.g. joint angles) is erroneous, since such variables are interval or circular, i.e. it is possible to observe values less than one.

The ICC is basically the SEM expressed relative to the between-subjects variability that is present, the closer the ICC being to 1, the smaller the measurement error is relative to between-subject variability. This latter concept is termed "relative reliability" (Baumgartner, 1989). Therefore, an ICC of 0.8 means that the measurement error is relatively "small" compared to the inter-subject variability that is present. Note that the ICC does not describe error in the units of measurement, which can make judgements on reliability difficult. For a full discussion of the many types of ICC statistic, readers are directed to Muller and Buttner (1994) and Atkinson and Nevill (1998). One has to be careful in the choice of ICC (there are at least eight), since some types of ICC do not distinguish between systematic and random errors. The TEM statistic, which would be familiar to kinanthropometrists (Nevill and Atkinson, 2000), also considers random and systematic errors together as "total error" (Table 1). In my view, the total error ICCs and the TEM should be employed only if one is certain that there can be no significant sources of systematic error from subjects or researcher. Use of the TEM to help assess the reliability of a performance test for example could hinder the identification and control of important systematic errors such as

Table 1. Formulae and definitions for common reliability statistics. $Sd_{diff}$ = standard deviation of individual test-retest differences (d) in sample, n = sample size in reliability study, $\bar{x}$ = grand mean of all absolute scores for test and retest in sample, $MS_{subjects}$ = mean squared error for subjects. Note that formulae are shown for a simple test-retest study. For reliability studies having multiple retests, formulae are provided by Atkinson and Nevill (1998; 2001).

| Statistic | Formula | Meaning | Assumptions |
|---|---|---|---|
| Standard error of measurement (SEM) | $$SEM = \frac{SD_{diff}}{\sqrt{2}}$$ | The maximum difference (in units) between observed value and true score with a certainty of 68%. | 1. The population of errors is normally distributed. 2. There is no relationship between error and size of measured value. |
| Technical error of measurement (TEM) | $$TEM = \sqrt{\frac{\sum d^2}{2n}}$$ | The maximum difference (in units) between observed value and true score with a certainty of 68%. | 1. The population of errors is normally distributed. 2. There is no relationship between error and size of measured value. 3. There is no systematic learning or fatigue effect between measurements |
| Coefficient of variation (CV) | $$CV = \frac{SEM}{\bar{x}} \times 100$$ | The maximum difference (as a percentage) between the observed value and true score with a certainty of 68% | 1. The population of logged errors is normally distributed. 2. The error is proportional to the size of the measured value |
| Intraclass correlation coefficient (ICC) | $$ICC = \frac{MS_{subjects} - SEM^2}{MS_{subjects}}$$ Simplest form of ICC shown | Measurement error expressed relative to the between-subject variability | 1. The population of errors is normally distributed. 2. There is no relationship between error and size of measured value. |
| 95% limits of agreement (LOA) | $$LOA = 1.96 \times SD_{diff}$$ | The maximum difference (in units) between any two repeated observations with a certainty of 95% | 1. The population of errors is normally distributed. 2. There is no relationship between error and size of measured value |

learning effects. A statistic, which is commonly used by biologists to describe error, and is in fact the type of ICC that also does not distinguish between systematic and random error, is the coefficient of concordance (Lin, 1989). Caution should also be exerted when interpreting this statistic (Atkinson and Nevill, 1997).

## 5. JUDGEMENT OF RELIABILITY

As mentioned above, most definitions of reliability have not adequately acknowledged that error is inevitable in quantitative data. Because error is likely, what becomes important is the judgement of how much error is acceptable for the situations in which the measurement tool is employed. It follows that "acceptance" is an operational definition totally dependent on practical relevance, rather than any generalised criteria such as a correlation coefficient being greater than 0.8 or a coefficient of variation being less than 10% for example. Measurement error may be deemed acceptable on the basis of it being less than that associated with another measurement tool, or whether the error affects the interpretation of data collected in research or on individuals (Hopkins, 2000).

### 5.1 Comparison of measurement tools, laboratories and individuals

The SEM can be a useful statistic for comparing error between different measurement tools and laboratories, and it is in fact the statistic advised for these purposes by the International Standards Organisation (ISO, 1994). Used in this way, it is stressed that the meaning of the SEM is arbitrary as long as it is used consistently for judging which measurement method is associated with the smallest SEM. In other words, one could just as easily use the $Sd_{diff}$ or the LOA for these purposes. For example, Edwards *et al.* (2002) compared LOA between different methods of measuring body temperature. Researchers should be wary of employing the ICC to compare measurement error between different laboratories using different samples (even drawn from the same population), since the ICC is particularly sensitive to the range of measurements in the sample (Atkinson, 1995; Atkinson and Nevill, 1997). Ideally, one should formally examine whether error differs between measurement tools or laboratories via a hypothesis test (e.g. a paired t-test on the squared differences), or by comparing the confidence intervals for the error statistic between different measurement methods.

### 5.2 Reliability and research conclusions

In research, as outlined in 2 (i) above, measurement error is important in interpreting conclusions from a study performed on a sample of subjects. A finding of no statistically significant difference or relationship in a study might just mean that the error was too large for the difference to be detected (a "type II" error).

Such a scenario will be familiar to readers who have performed a statistical power calculation prior to an investigation, and indeed measurement error does impact on statistical power (Atkinson *et al.*, 2001). Therefore, the researchers question here becomes: Is the measurement error small enough to detect practically meaningful differences or relationships under typical research conditions of using the measurement tool with realistic sample sizes? Such a question can be answered by converting a measurement error statistic to the denominator error term in a statistical power test. For example, the limits of agreement can be converted back to the $Sd_{diff}$ and used in a power calculation involving a paired t-test. Atkinson and Nevill (1999) provided a worked example of using the LOA to estimate statistical power and supplied a nomogram for use with different sample sizes, LOA and effect sizes. Such power calculations can also be performed using the ICC and SEM statistics (Hopkins, 2002).

In adopting the concept of relating measurement error to its impact on research conclusions through statistical power, it should be remembered that measurement error has *not* been an issue for any analysis that has had sufficient power for the null hypothesis to be rejected in a study. If a researcher has found that an effect of a particular treatment is significant, it is meaningless for a peer reviewer to be concerned about the influence of random measurement error on results. The peer reviewer could be concerned that the null hypothesis has been incorrectly rejected (a type I error), but such a concern involves consideration of sampling bias and an incorrect choice of analysis, rather than how much random error is present. It is also clear that the use of "cut-off" values of acceptable error statistics (e.g. ICC > 0.9) should be discouraged, since "acceptance" is a research-specific concept. For example, Hofstra *et al.* (1997) found that methods for measuring exercise-induced bronchospasm in children were reliable, even though ICCs were found to be less than 0.6. Such a conclusion was reached on the basis that the effect size of this particular phenomenon (i.e. the difference between bronchospasm being present and absent) is large and easily detected.

### 5.3 Reliability and individual assessment

It was illustrated above that the SEM can be used to estimate a range in which the true score could lie, given a measurement being obtained on an individual. Nevertheless, how can this information be used to confirm or reject acceptable reliability? The answer to this question revolves around the instructions of Baumgartner *et al.* (2001) that consideration of the SEM should not alter the interpretation of conclusions on individuals. In this respect, several proponents of the SEM have provided calculations, which apply the SEM to a particular question involving an individual subject (e.g. How certain is it that the measurements of two individuals are really different or merely due to measurement error? or Is the difference between repeated measurements made on an individual real or due to error?). Interested readers are directed towards Harvill (1991) and Beckerman *et al.* (2002) for details of these applications of SEM. Interestingly, when the SEM is applied to the examination of whether a change in measurement has occurred with probability of 0.95, the calculation is synonymous with that of the LOA (Harvill, 1991; Eliasziw *et al.*, 1994; Atkinson and Nevill, 1998; Wyrwich and Wolinsky, 2000; Beckerman *et al.*, 2001).

The 95% LOA is a statistic, which does not involve consideration of a true score at all, but is fully in line with how the International Standards Association advises scientists to make decisions about error on individuals. The advice of ISO (1994) is that it is important to describe with reasonable certainty (usually p=0.95) what the maximal unexplained difference between any two observations could be. Such advice seems sensible, since a true score can rarely be obtained from hundreds of repeated measurements in the real world. For some variables, the conceptualisation of a true score might not be logical. For example, sports competitions are not usually won on the basis of the average of hundreds of individual performances; it is the individual performance itself that usually governs an outcome. Therefore, a LOA (or *"repeatability coefficient"*) of ± 5 units means that it is reasonably certain that the difference between any two repeated measurements on an individual will be no more than 5 units. The researcher's task is then to judge whether such a difference would impact on conclusions regarding individuals (e.g. would the difference lead to an athlete being designated as reaching a certain standard consistently with repeated observations?).

It may well be that a measurement tool is designated as being reliable enough for research, but not for making judgements on individuals. Several researchers have indicated to me that they are surprised by the amount of error suggested when they calculate LOA for a particular variable. It is stressed that LOA are statistics designed to be applied to decisions on individual people. Increased uncertainty is often the "price" one has to pay when working with individuals rather than the multiple observations from a sample of subjects in research. In this respect, a researcher should be quite clear in stating whether the reliability of a measurement tool is examined for research purposes or for assessing individuals. It is stressed, again, that "acceptable reliability" is an operational definition.

## 6. PRECISION OF ERROR STATISTICS

Examination of measurement error involves parameter estimation. In other words, all error statistics are merely estimates of the error present in the population of interest. In this respect, there can be error in the estimation of measurement error itself. Statisticians have shown that precision of error estimate is adequate as long as the sample size in a test-retest reliability study is at least 40 subjects (Morrow, 1989; Morrow *et al.*, 1995; Bland and Altman, 1999). This sample size could be smaller if one takes multiple retest measures in the reliability study (Nevill and Atkinson, 1998; Hopkins, 2000), but one would need to be wary of any differences in error between pairs of test-retests. For example, the error between the second test and the third test might be smaller than the error between the first test and the second test. This problem with repeated measurements, called *"sphericity"*, is discussed in more detail by Atkinson (2001; 2002) and Atkinson and Nevill (2001).

Often it is not possible to recruit as many as 40 subjects for a reliability study, especially if the measurement is invasive or complicated. In such situations, it becomes even more important to quote confidence intervals for a measurement error statistic. A confidence interval would provide information on the likely range of values within which the error parameter for the population could be (Morrow and Jackson, 1993; Bland and Altman, 1999). Very small sample sizes (<10) in a reliability study may mean that the error statistic is also *biased* small relative to the population parameter. Even the so called *"unbiased"* SD is in reality biased small when derived from a small sample. Correction factors for such a bias are available in the literature (Royston and Matthews, 1991). Several authors have provided an argument that the correction of this bias should not involve the t-statistic (Royston and Matthews, 1991; Charter and Feldt, 2001).

## 7. SUMMARY

Measurement error and reliability are not the same. Examination of reliability involves the researcher making an informed decision on the acceptability of measurement error that has been unambiguously described. The informed decision should be based on the error being lower than another measurement tool, or the error having little impact on intended uses of the measurement tool. Such uses could be in answering questions in research or on individuals. Researchers should aim for 40 subjects in a reliability study. Irrespective of sample size, confidence intervals should be presented in a reliability study in order for the precision of error statistics to be estimated.

## REFERENCES

Atkinson, G., 1995, A comparison of statistical methods to assess measurement repeatability in ergonomics research. In *Sport, Leisure and Ergonomics*, edited by Atkinson, G. and Reilly, T. (London: E. and F.N. Spon) pp. 218-222.

Atkinson, G., 2001, Analysis of repeated measurements in physical therapy research. *Physical Therapy in Sport*, **2**, 194-208.

Atkinson, G., 2002, Sport performance: variable or construct? *Journal of Sports Sciences*, **20**, 291-292.

Atkinson, G. and Nevill, A.M., 1997, Comment on the use of concordance correlation to assess the agreement between two variables. *Biometrics*, **53**, (2), 775-777.

Atkinson, G. and Nevill, A.M., 1998, Statistical methods in assessing measurement error (reliability) in variables relevant to sports medicine. *Sports Medicine*, **26**, 217-238.

Atkinson, G. and Nevill, A.M., 2000, Typical error versus limits of agreement. *Sports Medicine*, **30**, 375-377.

Atkinson G. and Nevill A.M., 2001, Selected issues in the design and analysis of sport performance research. *Journal of Sports Sciences*, **19**, 811-827.

Atkinson, G., Nevill, A.M. and Edwards, B., 1999, What is an acceptable amount of measurement error? The application of meaningful 'analytical goals' to the reliability analysis of sports science measurements made on a ratio scale. *Journal of Sports Sciences*, **17**, 18.

Baumgartner, T.A., 1989, Norm-referenced measurement: reliability. In *Measurement Concepts in Physical Education and Exercise Science* edited by Safrit, M.J. and Wood, T.M., (Champaign: Human Kinetics), pp. 45-72.

Baumgartner, T.A., Strong, C.H. and Hensley, L.D., 2002, *Conducting and Reading Research in Health and Human Performance* (New York: McGraw-Hill).

Beckerman, H., Roebroeck, M.E., Lankhorst, G.J. *et al.*, 2001, Smallest real difference, a link between reproducibility and responsiveness. *Quality of Life Research*, **10**, 571-578.

Bland, J.M. and Altman, D.G., 1999, Measuring agreement in method comparison studies. *Statistical Methods in Medical Research*, **8**, 135-160.

Charter, R.A. and Feldt, L.S., 2001, Confidence intervals for true scores: is there a correct approach? *Journal of Psychoeducational Assessment* 19, 350-364.

Edwards, B., Waterhouse, J., Reilly, T. and Atkinson, G., 2002, A comparison of the suitabilities of rectal, gut, and insulated axilla temperatures for measurement of the circadian rhythm of core temperature in field studies. *Chronobiology International*, **19**, 579-597.

Eliasziw, M., Young, S.L., Woodbury M.G. and Fryday-Field, K., 1994, Statistical methodology for the concurrent assessment of interrater and intrarater reliability: using goniometric measurements as an example. *Physical Therapy*, **74**, 777-788.

Harvill, L.M., 1991, An NCME instructional module on standard error of measurement. *Educational Measurement: Issues and Practice*, **10**, 33-41.

Hofstra, W.B., Sont, J.K., Serk, P.J., Neijens, H.J., Kuethe, M.C. and Duiverman, E.J., 1997, Sample size estimation in studies monitoring exercise-induced bronchoconstriction in asthmatic children. *Thorax*, **52**, 739-741.

Hopkins, W., 2002, *A new view of statistics.* Internet site, http://www.sportsci.org/resource/stats/index.html.

Hopkins, W., 2000, Measures of reliability in sports medicine and science. *Sports Medicine*, **30**, 1-15.

ISO, 1994, Accuracy (trueness and precision) of measurement methods and results. Use in practice of accuracy values. *International Standards Publication*, ISO 5725-4.

Lin, L.I-K., 1989, A concordance correlation coefficient to evaluate reproducibility. *Biometrics*, **45**, 255-268.

Morrow, J.R., 1989, Generalizability theory. In *Measurement Concepts in Physical Education and Exercise Science*, edited by Safrit M.J. and Wood T.M., (Champaign: Human Kinetics), pp. 73-96.

Morrow, J.R. and Jackson, A.W., 1993, How "significant" is your reliability? *Research Quarterly for Exercise and Sport*, **64**: 3, 352-355.

Morrow, J.R, Jackson, A.W, Disch, J.G and Mood, D.P., 1995, *Measurement and Evaluation in Human Performance.* (Champaign: Human Kinetics).

Muller, R. and Buttner, P., 1994, A critical discussion of intraclass correlation coefficients. *Statistics in Medicine*, **13**, 2465-2476.

Nevill, A., 1996, Validity and measurement agreement in sports performance. *Journal of Sports Sciences*, **14**, 199.

Nevill, A.M. and Atkinson, G., 1997, Assessing agreement between measurements recorded on a ratio scale in sports medicine and sports science. *British Journal of Sports Medicine*, **31**, 314-318.

Nevill, A.M. and Atkinson, G., 1998, Assessing measurement agreement (repeatability) between 3 or more trials. *Journal of Sports Sciences*, **16**, 29.

Nevill, A.M. and Atkinson, G., 2000, Statistical methods for exercise physiology and kinanthropometry. In *Exercise Physiology and Kinanthropometry Laboratory Manual*, edited by Eston, R.G. and Reilly, T. (London: E. and F.N. Spon), pp. 237-274.

Royston, P. and Matthews, J.N.S., 1991, Estimation of reference ranges from normal samples. *Statistics in Medicine*, **10**, 691-695.

Safrit, M.J. and Wood, T.M., 1989, editors. *Measurement Concepts in Physical Education and Exercise Science.* (Champaign: Human Kinetics).

Spearman, C., 1904, General intelligence: objectively determined and measured. *American Journal of Psychology*, **15**, 201-293.

Vincent, J., 1995, *Statistics in Kinesiology.* (Champaign, Illinois: Human Kinetics Books).

Wyrwich, K.W. and Wollinsky, F.D., 2000, Identifying meaningful intra-individual change standards for health-related quality of life measures. *Journal of Evaluation in Clinical Practice*, **6**, 39-49.

# 2    Measurement of Energy Expenditure in Sports and Occupational Health

Philip N. Ainslie and Thomas Reilly
Research Institute for Sport and Exercise Sciences, Liverpool John
Moores University, 15-21 Webster Street, Liverpool, L3 2ET, UK

## 1. INTRODUCTION

This brief overview includes a historical review of the methods used for measuring energy expenditure. For this overview, the 'gold standard' method of measuring energy expenditure (EE), the doubly-labelled water technique, is emphasised. Other methods, such as direct calorimetry, indirect calorimetry systems, heart rate and energy expenditure relationships, questionnaires and activity recall, work-rate analysis, motion sensors, combined heart rate and motion sensors for the estimation of EE are then highlighted in relation to their validation against the doubly-labelled water method. The major advantages and disadvantages of each method are then considered. Finally, recommendations are made for the most useful practical measurement tool, after consideration of factors such as the type and duration of activity, expense, and sample size.

## 2. THE MEASUREMENT OF ENERGY EXPENDITURE TECHNIQUES: A HISTORICAL OVERVIEW

The scientific study of animal respiration was first recorded in the 1600s. In 1660, Robert Boyle observed that mice that had been sealed in bell jars, expired at the same time as a burning flame was extinguished. Thus Boyle established two important principles, namely the equivalence of fire and life as combustion processes and the requirement of air to support these processes (West, 1998). Of greater significance was the work of John Mayrow in 1668 (Speakman, 2001). Mayrow observed that mice died when they had consumed about one-fourteenth of the air in a bell jar. Mayrow accordingly established the idea that air consists of different parts, only some of which are usable for the process of respiration. This idea led to the invention of a chamber that allowed the quantification of the consumed portion; this chamber was the first respirometer.

A century after the innovative work of Boyle and Mayrow, the French chemists Lavoisier and Seguin started systematic studies of respiration as a process analogous to combustion. The procedures used by Lavoisier and Seguin mimicked closely those developed by Mayrow, the key difference being the framework within which the observations were interpreted (Speakman, 2001). Lavoisier and

Seguin made several important discoveries about oxygen consumption. Firstly, they found that larger people consume more oxygen than smaller people, an observation relevant to kinanthropometry. Secondly, people sitting quietly at rest were found to consume less oxygen than those standing up or moving around, a finding relevant to ergonomics. Finally, they discovered that oxygen consumption was elevated after a meal. Perhaps most importantly, Lavoisier and Seguin established the methodology of indirect calorimetry that has remained the benchmark for quantifying animal and human energy expenditure to this day.

The chambers within which animals and humans are confined have become increasingly sophisticated since the end of the 18th century. Moreover, sealed systems have been replaced with open-flow systems linked to advanced gas analysis equipment, so subjects no longer need die in the course of providing measurements! Nevertheless, such chambers will never be able to reproduce the complexity of activities in which people are engaged as they go about their daily lives. The inadequacy of traditional calorimetry has been recognised for some time, and there have been many attempts to develop methods, such as heart rate and motion monitoring, that enable energy demands associated with free-living activities to be determined (Westerterp, 1999; Speakman, 2001). The doubly-labelled water (DLW) technique allows the energy demands of free-living subjects to be measured. The success of this method prompted Prentice (1990) to remark that its development was as significant an event in the history of animal and human nutrition, as the work of Lavoiser and Sequin had been earlier. The DLW method subsequently became the 'gold standard' for the measurement of energy expenditure and forms a method against which other approaches may be validated.

## 3. METHODS FOR THE MEASUREMENT OF ENERGY EXPENDITURE

*3.1 Direct versus indirect calorimetry:* Direct calorimetry measures total heat loss from the body; indirect calorimetry measures total energy production by the body. With the former, the subject is placed in a thermally-isolated chamber, and the heat he/she dissipates (by evaporation, radiation, conduction and convection) is recorded accurately and measured precisely (Jequier, 1985). In indirect calorimetry, on the other hand, oxygen consumption and carbon dioxide production are what are really measured. Assuming that all the oxygen is used to oxidise degradable fuels and all the $CO_2$ thereby evolved is recovered, it is possible to calculate the total amount of energy produced (Ferrannini, 1988). In this review, only indirect calorimetry and its extensions will be considered, as direct calorimetry is of limited practical interest in the present context of total energy output by free-living populations.

*3.2 Doubly-labelled water (free-living indirect calorimetry):* The use of DLW for the assessment of free-living EE in humans was first reported by Schoeller and van Santen (1982), and the technique has been evaluated subsequently (Prentice, 1990; Speakman and Roberts, 1995; Schoeller and Delany, 1998). This method provides information on the total energy expended by a free-living subject for a period of

4-20 days, a period likely to reflect the normal energy requirement of the subject. The subject takes an oral dose of water containing a known amount of stable (non-radioactive) isotopes of both hydrogen and oxygen. The isotopes, $^2$H (deuterium) and $^{18}$O, mix with the normal hydrogen and oxygen in the body water within a few hours. As energy is expended in the body, $CO_2$ and water are produced. The $CO_2$ is lost from the body in breath, whilst the water is lost in breath, urine, sweat and other evaporations. As $^{18}$O is contained in both $CO_2$ and water, it is lost from the body more rapidly than $^2$H, which is contained in water but not in $CO_2$.

The difference between the rate of loss of $^{18}$O and $^2$H reflects the rate at which $CO_2$ is produced, which in turn can be used to estimate energy expenditure, if a value for the respiratory quotient is assumed (Westerterp, 1999). A plot of the change in concentrations of the two isotopes in body fluids, from which the rate of loss of these isotopes from the body fluid can be calculated, is shown in Figure 1.

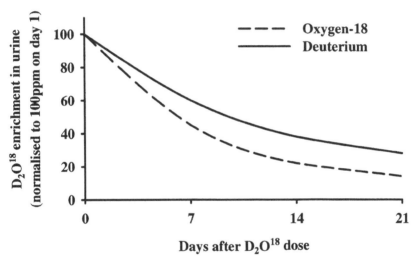

**Figure 1.** Decline of $^2$H (deuterium, D) and $^{18}$O in body fluids (urine, plasma or saliva) during a hypothetical doubly-labelled water experiment [from Westerterp, 1999, with permission].

An example of what has been learnt by using the technique is the level of total EE in all age-groups, including premature infants, hospitalised patients, children, obese people, pregnant and lactating women and elderly, for whom other methods might have serious problems. Applications of DLW include the validation of techniques for assessing dietary intake and physical activity, assessment of energy requirement, and the assessment of the effect of dietary and physical activity interventions, including its use with endurance athletes competing at elite level.

The DLW method is not without some disadvantages, despite its clear advantages. These include; a) the high cost of the $^{18}$O, and the specialised expertise required for the analysis of the isotope concentrations in body fluids by mass spectrometry [the present cost for a) $^{18}O$ and subsequent EE measurements is around \$600-\$900 for a 70-kg subject], b) total EE is measured over about 4 to 21 days, so no knowledge is obtained about brief periods of peak expenditure, c) in field studies, because $CO_2$ production and not $O_2$ utilisation is being measured, some error is introduced if the respiratory quotient is not known. Nevertheless, the fact that the results provide the closest measure of free-living EE, makes the DLW method an extremely valuable reference technique for validating estimates of energy requirements obtained by other methods.

*3.3 Indirect calorimetry systems:* There are two main indirect calorimetry systems for the measurement of oxygen uptake and hence EE. Firstly, the *closed-circuit method* requires the subject to be isolated from the outside air. The respirometer originally contains pure oxygen, and as the subject breathes in this closed system the $CO_2$ is continuously removed as it passes through soda lime. The gas volume gradually decreases, and the rate of decrease is a measure of the rate of oxygen consumption. This method works reasonably well for measuring resting or basal metabolic rate, but absorbing the large volume of $CO_2$ produced during prolonged, strenuous exercise becomes a problem.

Secondly, the *open-circuit method* is more suited to measuring exercise metabolism. Two main procedures in the open-circuit method have been developed. In one, the flow-through technique (Kinney, 1980), a large volume equivalent to the outside air passes through a hood worn by the subject. The subject inspires and expires into the air stream flowing through the hood. Airflow and percentage of $O_2$ and $CO_2$ are measured precisely to calculate $\dot{V}O_2$ and $\dot{V}CO_2$ and hence RER. This method is particularly useful for long-term measurements with the subject at rest or performing only mild exercise.

The second procedure, the time-honoured Douglas bag method (although a meteorological balloon is commonly used), is accurate and theoretically sound. With this procedure, the subject wears a nose clip and mouthpiece or a facemask. Outside air or its equivalent is inhaled through the mouthpiece or mask containing a one-way valve and exhaled into a Douglas bag or Tissot tank. The volume of air in the bag or tank is measured to calculate minute ventilation. A sample of air is obtained to measure the $O_2$ and $CO_2$ concentrations. The method of measurement and appropriate formula to calculate $\dot{V}O_2$, $\dot{V}CO_2$ and hence EE are important, and have been described in detail by Elia and Livesey (1992).

In the laboratory, modern on-line electronic equipment usually replaces the Douglas bag method, whereby ventilation, $O_2$ and $CO_2$ percentages are determined instantaneously and continuously. The electronic equipment confines the procedure to the laboratory. The Douglas bag method is not as restrictive because a bag can be carried on the back or by an assistant close by, permitting its use in the field.

*Indirect calorimetry systems (portable):* Nathan Zuntz (1847–1920) recognised the advantage of having the subject carry a self-contained unit, if oxygen consumption is to be measured during exercise. He developed what was probably the first such unit, which resembles a large rucksack. This was a forerunner of the portable calorimeter designed by Kofranyi and Michaelis (1940), which was subsequently improved by Wolff (1958) and later modified by

Humphrey and Wolff (1977). The system designed by Humphrey and Wolff (1977), called the Oxylog, was a battery-operated, self-contained, portable instrument, weighing about 3 kg, but is engineered for on-line measurement of oxygen consumption. Carbon dioxide was not measured and so an RER value was assumed. It has been found to be reasonably accurate in field measurements during rest and up to moderately strenuous exercise (Harrison *et al.*, 1982; McNeill *et al.*, 1987).

Advances in technology have produced a range of portable systems which can also measure $CO_2$ production and breath-by-breath pulmonary gas exchange. These systems, namely the Metamax (Borsdorf Germany) and, latterly, the Cosmed K4 b² (Rome, Italy), are the most recent on the market. The K4 b² device is the new portable system designed by Cosmed to measure gas exchange on a true breath-by-breath basis during any kind of activity. The system is fully portable whilst also allowing breath-by-breath pulmonary gas exchange measurements, direct field assessment of human performance and cardio-pulmonary limitations during any kind of activity. The K4 machine has the same facilities as a laboratory station and is light in weight (600 grams), which helps to ensure subject comfort as well as portability. However, measurements using these portable systems are normally limited to 1–5 hours. In addition, the expense of the systems would normally only allow subjects to be monitored on an individual basis.

[The Oxylog is available from P.K. Morgan Ltd, Rainham, Kent, UK. The Metamax system is obtainable from Cortex Biophsik GmbH, Borsdorf Germany. The K4 b² apparatus is available from Cosmed Ltd, Rome, Italy. The price of each system varies, but currently ranges from $20 000 for the Oxylog system to almost $60 000 for the new K4 b² system from Cosmed.]

*3.4 Heart rate and energy expenditure relationships:* During exercise, there is a fairly close relationship between heart rate and EE, so records of heart rate allow an estimate of EE to be made. In order to allow for the variation in fitness between individuals, a calibration curve based on simultaneous measurements of heart rate and oxygen consumption, using indirect calorimetry, in a variety of activities, must be made for each subject (Montoye *et al.*, 1996).

A typical human response curve, illustrated in Figure 2, shows how at low levels of EE, heart rate does not increase as steeply for a given change in EE, probably due to changes in stroke volume between lying, sitting and standing. This may be one reason why 24-h estimates of EE from heart rate may have errors of up to 30% in individuals, although the average for a group of subjects is likely to be within 10% of the true value (Davidson *et al.*, 1997).

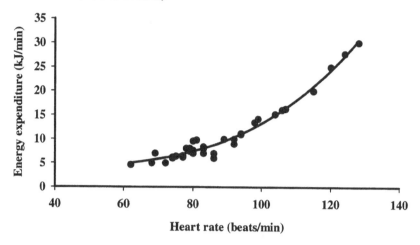

**Figure 2.** The relationship between heart rate and EE in a healthy male subject.

Monitoring of heart rate also provides information on the amount of time spent in high-intensity activity, which may be useful for assessment of physical activity rather than EE. Furthermore, it provides a relatively cheap method of estimating EE. However, heart rate is affected by factors other than physical activity. Data conversion needs individual measurements of heart rate in combination with oxygen consumption, and heart rate monitors are not well tolerated by subjects for time periods representative of daily life for one week or more. [The present cost for a heart rate monitor and the equipment to down-load the data ranges from $100-$300.]

*3.5 Questionnaires and activity recall:* There is a range of questionnaires and activity recall methods available for the assessment of energy expenditure in humans. Only the questionnaires which have been validated against DLW will be described and considered, in this review. A literature search has yielded four different methods which have been used in combination against the DLW method. These questionnaires include a) activity and recall questionnaires, b) Baecke questionnaire, c) Five-City questionnaire, and d) the Tecumseh questionnaire.

Studies on activity questionnaires incorporated a 1-week (Bratterby *et al.*, 1997) or 2-week activity diary (Schulz *et al.*, 1989), three 7-day activity recall questionnaires (Racette *et al.*, 1995; Bonnefoy *et al.*, 2001), the physical activity scale for the elderly (Schuit *et al.*, 1997), the Baecke questionnaire, the Five-City questionnaire, and the adapted version of the Tecumseh Community Health study questionnaire (Philippaerts *et al.*, 1999).

The activity diary method has been described by Bouchard *et al.* (1983). Subjects record at every 15 min of the waking day a number corresponding to one of a group of categories (Bratteby *et al.*, 1997) or 12 activity categories (Schulz *et al.*, 1989), according to their average physical activity during that time period. Numbers are converted to the average daily metabolic rate by multiplying the integrated mean 24-h activity score with the measured BMR. The 'activity recall' method includes a standard questionnaire that categorizes activities by their intensity, using the compendium of Ainsworth *et al.* (1993). Energy expenditure is then calculated by multiplying the amount of time spent in each activity by the corresponding metabolic equivalent. Reilly and Thomas (1979) used diary cards for monitoring habitual activities of professional footballers outside training and competition. The energy expenditure in training and competition was estimated using heart rate and work-rate data, respectively. The daily energy expenditure values of 14.442 MJ correspond with more recent estimates based on DLW. The physical activity scale for the elderly (PASE) is a brief questionnaire designed by Washburn *et al.* (1993). It comprises activities commonly engaged in by elderly persons, and the reference period is one week. The PASE-score is the sum of the time spent in each activity, multiplied by an item weight factor.

Baecke's inventory is a brief questionnaire with three categories, work, sport and leisure, adding up to give a total activity index (Baecke *et al.*, 1982). The Five-City questionnaire requires the time spent in vigorous activities, moderate activities, light activities, and sleeping to be recorded. Each category is multiplied by the reported hours and a weight factor to calculate an activity index. The Tecumseh questionnaire is an adapted version of that designed by Reiff *et al.* (1967). Subjects are interviewed on the estimated hours per week of sports participation, home repair and maintainace activities, sleeping and eating, quiet leisure time and remaining activities. The hours per week are multiplied by the PAL values listed by Ainsworth *et al.* (1993) to obtain a figure for total activity.

**Table 1.** Correlation between the activity score of questionnaires and the DLW assessed physical activity level.

| Questionnaire | Subject No. | Correlation | Reference |
|---|---|---|---|
| Activity diary | 6 | 0.72** | Schulz *et al.*, 1989 |
| Activity diary | 50 | Not presented | Bratteby *et al.*, 1997 |
| Activity recall | 13 | 0.67* | Racette *et al.*, 1995 |
| Activity recall | 19 | 0.52* | Bonnefoy *et al.*, 2001 |
| PASE | 21 | 0.68** | Schuit *et al.*, 1997 |
| Baecke questionnaire | 19 | 0.69*** | Philippaerts *et al.*, 1999 |
| Five-City questionnaire | 19 | 0.42 | Philippaerts *et al.*, 1999 |
| Tecumseh questionnaire | 19 | 0.64** | Philippaerts *et al.*, 1999 |

* ($p < 0.05$), ** ($p < 0.01$), *** ($p < 0.001$)

Most of the studies on activity questionnaires have shown an association between the derived activity score and the DLW assessment of EE (Table 1). Baecke's questionnaire tended to show the highest correlation, and the next best were the physical activity scale for the elderly and the Tecumseh questionnaire.

The index of the Five-City questionnaire was not significantly related to the DLW method. As expected, an activity diary was superior to activity recall. The cost is minimal.

*3.6 Work-rate analysis:* As EE is a function of work-rate, various forms of monitoring physical activity have been developed and employed. These have been used in occupational, playground and sports contexts. Measurements of activity are made typically by means of video analysis, film analysis or monitoring of movements. Movement variables are calibrated to allow EE to be estimated. For a review of motion analysis methods see Reilly (1996).

*3.7 Motion sensors:* There are several types of motion sensors available to measure walking and estimate energy expenditure in free-living subjects. Pedometers typically detect the displacement of physical objects with each stride. They tend to lack sensitivity as they do not quantify stride length or total body displacement (Levine *et al.*, 2001). Accelerometers detect total body displacement electronically with varying degrees of sensitivity:- uniaxial accelerometers in one axis and triaxial in three axes. Portable uniaxial accelerometer units, such as the Caltrac accelerometer, have been widely used to detect walking (Haymes and Byrnes, 1993). Careful evaluation demonstrates that these instruments are not sufficiently sensitive to quantify walking in free-living individuals, but rather they are more valuable for comparing activity levels between groups of subjects (Pambianco *et al.*, 1990; Swan *et al.*, 1997; Johnson *et al.*, 1998; Basset *et al.*, 2000).

Triaxial accelerometers have provided increased precision in application to walking. Of these, the Tracmor triaxial accelerometer (Maastrict, The Netherlands) has been most widely validated (Pannemans *et al.*, 1995; Bouten *et al.*, 1996; Bouten *et al.*, 1997). This unit has several advantages besides being lightweight and portable (Bouten *et al.*, 1997). First, the units have been validated against a motor-driven rotating arm where test-to-test repeatability is within ~0.5% (Bouten *et al.*, 1997). Second, conditions for optimum usage have been defined (e.g., site of attachment of accelerometer unit) (Bouten *et al.*, 1997). Third, on a treadmill, Tracmor output has been demonstrated to correlate well with EE ($r = 0.95$) (Bouten *et al.*, 1994). Finally with respect to detecting body motion, Tracmor output correlates well with daily EE (measured using DLW) divided by basal metabolic rate in free-living subjects ($r = 0.73$; $p < 0.001$) (Bouten *et al.*, 1996; Westerterp and Bouten, 1997).

Levine *et al.* (2001) recently validated the Tracmor triaxial accelerometer system for walking. The results showed that the Tracmor can be used to predict the energetic cost of walking, provided that separate regression equations are derived for each subject to convert Tracmor output to EE. Similar to the use of heart rate, a calibration curve based on simultaneous measurements of Tracmor output and oxygen consumption, measured using indirect calorimetry, is required to increase its accuracy in estimating EE. When tested on an increased gradient, the Tracmor failed to detect the increased energetic cost of walking on an steep incline. The Tracmor unit is soon to be on the market. [The Tracmor accelerometers will cost approximately $100 and are reusable. The software costs $800-$1000.]

*3.8 Combined heart rate and motion sensors:* To date, there is a limited amount of research on the combination of both heart-rate and motion sensors. To our knowledge, only one group (Rennie *et al.*, 2000) has used a one-piece instrument that is able to measure both heart rate and movement. In previous studies, separate instruments have been employed to record these two measurements (Meijer *et al.*, 1989; Haskell *et al.*, 1993; Moon and Butte, 1996). The results of this preliminary study by Rennie and co-workers showed near perfect agreement in the calculation of energy expenditure, when compared with direct measurement of room calorimetry, highlighting its ability to estimate EE and the pattern of EE activity throughout the day. Further validations in free-living individuals, against DLW, are necessary. At present, systems are not yet available.

## 4. EVALUATION AND PRACTICAL RECOMMENDATIONS ON THE MEASUREMENT OF ENERGY EXPENDITURE FOR EXERCISE AND OCCUPATIONAL HEALTH

Of all the methods for the assessment of energy expenditure reviewed, each has a number of positive and negative aspects. Although, the DLW is considered the 'gold standard' method against which other methods are to be validated, the price of the DLW and the sophisticated analysis involved make it impractical for use with large groups.

Indirect calorimetry provides an accurate method of measurement of both EE and respiratory gas exchange both in the laboratory and in the field. However, the nature of the equipment limits useage to less than 8 hours. In addition, the expense of such portable systems limits the measurement to the individual level.

Heart-rate monitoring is an objective method of estimating EE. However, heart rate is affected by more factors than physical activity. Data conversion needs individual measurements of heart rate in combination with oxygen consumption, and heart rate monitors are not well tolerated by subjects for time intervals representative of daily life for one week or more. Heart-rate monitoring remains a proxy measure for physical activity (Livingstone, 1997).

Positive aspects of questionnaires, like the Baecke questionnaire, are the short time needed for a subject to complete the 21 questions, the simple scoring system for the calculation of an activity index, and the coverage of the subject's normal daily pattern. A disadvantage of questionnaires is the fact that subjects can easily overestimate or underestimate the time spent in activity, and most questionnaires are not applicable for all subject categories from children, people with and without jobs, to the elderly (Westerterp, 1999).

Motion sensors yield objective data, but have only recently become available on the market. The majority of the recent research seems to show how effective they are becoming in the measurement of physical activity and energy expenditure. Perhaps the future in estimating EE lies in the use of a combination of both motion sensors and heart rate monitoring. At present, the information about, and validation of, such techniques are lacking. Future research needs to target the design of such a combined device.

In conclusion, the preferred method to determine EE is likely to depend principally on factors such as the number of subjects to be monitored, the time period of measurements and the finances available. Small subject numbers over a short period may be measured accurately by means of indirect calorimetric methods (stationary and portable systems). For periods over 3-4 days, ideally EE should be measured using the DLW method. However, the use of motion sensors is very promising in the measurement of EE, and has a number of advantages over the DLW technique. Furthermore, if used correctly, both heart rate and questionnaire methods may provide valuable estimates of EE. Additional studies are needed to examine the possibility of improving the accuracy of measurement by combining two or more techniques. The accurate measurement of physical activity and energy expenditure is critical for determining current levels of physical activity, monitoring compliance with physical activity guidelines, understanding the dose-response relationship between physical activity and health and determining the effectiveness of intervention programmes designed to improve physical activity levels.

**Acknowledgements**

P. Ainslie was supported by a grant from Mars Incorporated.

**REFERENCES**

Ainsworth, B.E., Haskell, W.L., Leaon, A.S., Jacobs, D.R., Montoye, H.J., Sallis, J.F. and Paffenbarger, R.S., 1993, Compendium of physical activities: classification of energy costs of human physical activities. *Medicine and Science in Sports and Exercise*, **25**, 71-80.

Baecke, J.A., Burema, H.J. and Frijters, J.E.R., 1982, A short questionnaire for the measurement of habitual physical activity in epidemiological studies. *American Journal of Clinical Nutrition*, **36**, 936-942.

Basset, D.R., Ainsworth, B.E., Swartz, A.M., Strath, S.J., O'Brien, W.L. and King, G.A., 2000, Validity of four motion sensors in measuring moderate intensity physical activity. *Medicine and Science in Sports and Exercise*, **32**, S471-S480.

Bonnefoy, M., Normand, S., Pachiaudi, C., Lacour, J.R., Laville, M. and Kostka, T., 2001, Simultaneous validation of ten physical activity questionnaires in older men: a doubly labeled water study. *Journal of American Geriatric Society*, **49**, 28-35.

Bouchard, C.A., Tremblay, A., Leblanc, C., Lortie, G., Savard, R. and Theriault, G., 1983, A method to assess energy expenditure in children and adults. *American Journal of Clinical Nutrition*, **37**, 461-467.

Bouten, C.V., Koekkoek, K.T., Verduin, M., Kodde, R. and Janssen, J.D., 1997, A triaxial accelerometer and portable data processing unit for the assessment of daily physical activity. *IEEE Trans Biomedical Engineering*, **44**, 136-147.

Bouten, C.V., Verboeket-Van De Venne, P., Westerterp, K.R., Verduin, M. and Janssesn, J.D., 1996, Daily physical activity assessment: comparison between movement registration and doubly labeled water. *Journal of Applied Physiology*, **81**, 1019-1026, 1996.

Bouten, C.V., Westerterp, K.R., Verduin, M. and Janssesn, J.D., 1994, Assessment of energy expenditure for physical activity using a triaxial accelerometer. *Medicine and Science in Sports and Exercise*, **26**, 1516-1523.

Bratterby, L.-E., Sandhagen, B., Fan, H. and Samuelson, G., 1997, A 7-day activity dairy for the assessment of daily energy expenditure validated by the doubly labelled water methods in adolescents. *European Journal of Clinical Nutrition*, **51**, 585-591.

Davidson, L., McNeill, G., Haggart, P., Smith, J.S. and Franklin, M.F., 1997, Free-living energy expenditure of adult men assessed by continuous heart rate monitoring and doubly labelled water. *British Journal of Nutrition*, **78**, 696-708.

Elia, M. and Livesey, G., 1992, Energy expenditure and fuel selections in biological systems: the theory and practice of calculations based on indirect calorimetry and tracer methods. In: *Metabolic Control of Eating, Energy Expenditure and the Bioenergetics of Obesity*. World Review of Nutrition and Dietetics Vol. 70, edited by Simopoulos, A.P. (Basel, Karger), pp. 68-131.

Ferrannini, E., 1988, The theoretical bases of indirect calorimetry: A review. *Metabolism*, **37**, 287-301.

Harrison, M.H., Brown, G.A. and Belyasin, A.J., 1982, The Oxylog: an evaluation. *Ergonomics*, **25**, 809-820.

Haskell, W.L., Yee, M.C., Evans, A. and Irby, P.J., 1993, Simultaneous measurements of heart rate and body motion to quantify physical activity. *Medicine and Science in Sports and Exercise*, **25**, 109-115.

Haymes, E.M. and Byrnes, W.C., 1993, Walking and running energy expenditure estimated by Caltrac and indirect calorimetry. *Medicine and Science in Sports and Exercise*, **25**, 1365-1369.

Humphrey, S.J.E. and Wolff, H.S., 1977, The Oxylog (Abstract) *Journal of Applied Physiology*, **267**, 120.

Jequier, E., 1985, Direct and indirect calorimetry in man. In *Substrate and Energy Metabolism*, edited by Garrow, J.S. and Halliday, D. (Libbey, London), pp. 82-91.

Johnson, R.K., Russ, J. and Goran, M.I., 1998, Physical activity related energy expenditure in children by doubly labeled water as compared with the Caltrac accelerometer. *International Journal of Obesity*, **22**, 1046-1052.

Kinney, J.M., 1980, The application of indirect calorimetry to clinical studies. In *Assessment of Energy Metabolism in Health and Disease*, (Columbus, OH: Ross Laboratories), pp. 42-48.

Kofranyi, E. and Michaelis, H.F., 1940, Ein tragbarer Apparnt zur Bestimmung des Gasstoffwechsels [A portable apparatus to determine metabolism]. *Arbeitsphyiololgie*, **11**, 148-150.

Levine, J.A., Baukol, P.A. and Westerterp, K.R., 2001, Validation of the Tracmor triaxial accelerometer system for walking. *Medicine and Science in Sports and Exercise*, **33**, 1593-7.

Livingstone, M.B.E., 1997, Heart-rate monitoring: the answer for assessing energy expenditure and physical activity in population studies? *British Journal of Nutrition*, **78**, 869-871.

McNeill, G., Cox, M.D. and Rivers, J.P.W., 1987, The Oxylog oxygen consumption meter: a portable device for measurement of energy expenditure. *American Journal of Clinical Nutrition*, **45**, 1415-1419.

Meijer, G., Westerterp, K., Koper, H. and Ten Hoor, F., 1989, Assessment of energy expenditure by recording heart rate and body acceleration. *Medicine and Science in Sports and Exercise*, **21**, 343-347.

Montoye, H.J., Kemper, H.C.G., Saris, W.H.M. and Washburn, R.A., 1996, *Measuring Physical Activity and Energy Expenditure*. (Champaign, IL: Human Kinetics).

Moon, J.K. and Butte, N.F., 1996, Combined heart rate and activity improve estimates of oxygen consumption and carbon dioxide production rates. *Journal of Applied Physiology*, **81**, 1754-1761.

Pambianco, G., Wing, R.R. and Robertson, R., 1990, Accuracy and reliability of the Caltrac accelerometer for estimated energy expenditure. *Medicine and Science in Sports and Exercise*, **22**, 858-862.

Pannemans, D.L., Bouten, C.V. and Westerterp, K.R., 1995, 24 h energy expenditure during a standardised activity protocol in young and elderly men. *European Journal of Clinical Nutrition*, **49**, 49-56.

Philippaerts, R.M., Westerterp, K.R. and Lefevre, J., 1999, Doubly labeled water validation of three physical activity questionnaires. *International Journal of Sports Medicine*, **20**, 284-289.

Prentice, A.M., 1990, The doubly-labelled water method for measuring energy expenditure, technical recommendations for use in humans. Nahre-4, (Vienna: International Atomic Energy Agency).

Racette, S.B., Schoeller, D.A. and Kushner, R.F., 1995, Comparison of heart rate and physical activity recall with doubly labeled water in obese women. *Medicine and Science in Sports and Exercise*, **27**, 126-133.

Reiff, G.G., Montoye, H.J., Remmington, R.D., Napier, J.A., Metzner, H.L. and Epstein, F.H., 1967, Assessment of physical activity by questionnaire and interview. *Journal of Sports Medicine and Physical Fitness,* **7**, 135-142.

Reilly, T., 1996, Motion analysis and physiological demands. In: Science and Soccer, edited by Reilly, T. (London: E and F.N Spon), pp. 65-81.

Reilly, T. and Thomas, V., 1979, Estimated daily energy expenditures of professional association footballers. *Ergonomics*, **22**, 541-548.

Rennie, K., Rowsell, T., Jebb, S.A., Holburn, D. and Wareham, N.J., 2000, A combined heart rate and movement sensor: proof of concept and preliminary testing study. *European Journal of Clinical Nutrition,* **54**, 409-414.

Schoeller, D.A. and Delany, J.P., 1998, Human energy balance: what have be learned from the doubly labeled water method? *American Journal of Clinical Nutrition,* **68**, 927S-979S.

Schoeller, D.A. and van Santen, E., 1982, Measurement of energy expenditure in humans by doubly labelled water method. *Journal of Applied Physiology,* **53**, 955-959.

Schuit, A.J., Schouten, E.G., Westerterp, K.R. and Saris, W.H.M., 1997, Validity of the physical activity scale (PASE) for the elderly according to energy expenditure assessed by the doubly labeled water method. *Journal of Clinical Epidemiology,* **50**, 541-546.

Schulz, S., Westerterp, K.R. and Bruck, K., 1989, Comparison of energy expenditure by the doubly labeled water technique with energy intake, heart rate and activity recording in man. *American Journal of Clinical Nutrition,* **49**, 1146-1154.

Speakman, J.R., 2001, The history and theory of the doubly labeled water technique. *American Journal of Clinical Nutrition,* **68**, 932S-938S.

Speakman, J.R. and Roberts, S.B., 1995, Recent advances in the doubly labeled water technique. *Obesity Research,* **3**, 1S-74S.

Swan, P.D., Byrnes, W.C. and Haymes, E.M., 1997, Energy expenditure estimates for the Caltrac accelerometer for running, race walking, and stepping. *British Journal of Sports Medicine,* **31**, 235-239.

Washburn, R.A., Smith, K.W., Jettee, A.M. and Janney, C.A., 1993, The physical activity scale for the elderly (PASE): development and evaluation. *Journal of Clinical Epidemiology,* **46**, 163-172, 1993.

West, J.B., 1998, *High Life: A History of High-Altitude Physiology and Medicine.* (Oxford, England: Oxford University Press).

Westerterp, K.R., 1999, Assessment of physical activity level in relation to obesity: current evidence and research issues. *Medicine and Science in Sports and Exercise,* **31**, S522-S525.

Westerterp, K.R. and Bouten, C.V., 1997, Physical activity assessment: comparison between movement registration and doubly labeled water method. *Z Ernahrungswiss,* **36**, 263-267.

Wolff, H.S., 1958, The integrating pneumotacograph: a new instrument for the measurement of energy expenditure by indirect calorimetry. *Quarterly Journal of Exercise and Physiology,* **43**, 270-283.

# 3 Prediction of Bone, Lean and Fat Tissue Mass Using Dual X-ray Absorptiometry as the Reference Method

Alexandra Mavroeidi and Arthur D. Stewart
University of Aberdeen, Kings College, Aberdeen,
AB24 3FX, UK

## 1. INTRODUCTION

Physical activity and exercise training programmes confer considerable adaptation on the morphology of the human body affecting bone, lean tissue and fat. Training may induce specific development of muscle groups for certain sports affecting muscle mass (Spenst *et al.*, 1993), while physical activity is known to influence the amount and distribution of overlying fat (Nindl *et al.*, 1996). On the other hand, recent research has associated certain forms of exercise with an increase in bone mineral content and bone mineral density of the participants (ACSM, 1995).

The use of anthropometry has been very popular over the years in estimating human body composition outside the laboratory (Lukaski, 1989) providing an inexpensive and convenient way of obtaining data. Skinfold thickness at various sites, and bone breadths, heights and corrected limb circumferences, have been used to describe body size, in various ratios and indices, and in multiple regression equations to predict body density and to calculate body fat and fat-free mass. More recently, one of the most important and exciting developments in human composition studies has been the introduction of atomic absorptiometry, which is based on proton attenuation in vivo as a function of tissue composition (Pietrobelli *et al.*, 1996). Dual x-ray absorptiometry (DXA) is based on the fact that the components of the body can be grouped into three classes (bone mineral, fat (lipid), and fat-free soft tissue) according to their attenuation properties. The x-ray properties of these compartments are disparate, primarily due to their different proportions of high atomic number elements. Thus, for example bone mineral contains a large amount of calcium and phosphorus, whereas soft tissue is composed mainly of hydrogen, carbon and oxygen.

The purpose of this study was to predict bone, lean and fat tissue mass as assessed by anthropometric measurements, using DXA as the reference method. With a total of 20 male subjects (10 lightweight rowers and 10 sedentary controls) this study aimed to explore if there are any distinct anthropometric differences between rowers and controls, whether there is a difference in fat distribution between the two groups, and how well existing equations for predicting body fat correspond with the results obtained by DXA.

## 2. METHODS

Volunteers were drawn from the University of Aberdeen community. The subjects were young, non-smoking, Caucasian males, aged between 18 and 30 years. The control group comprised of 10 relatively sedentary male adults with a mean exercising time (±SD) of 1.3 (±1.7) hours per week. The lightweight competitive rowers group was recruited from the University of Aberdeen Boat Club, and consisted of 10 athletes, who exercised on average 8.7 (±3.2) hours per week.

All measurements were carried out at the Osteoporosis Research Unit at Woolmanhill NHS Trust Hospital, Aberdeen, Scotland, UK. Subjects wore a pair of shorts and a t-shirt, were fully hydrated, having not exercised for 24 hours prior to the measurement day and having not eaten within 3 hours of the scan. The study had the approval of the Grampian Research Ethics Committee and written, informed consent, was obtained from all subjects prior to any measurements.

The whole-body composition scan was carried out using a LUNAR PRODIGY™ X-ray scanner (Lunar Corporation, GE Medical Systems). Scans were analysed in the same systematic way according to the manufacturers' protocol, using the enCORE software (version 3.50.176), by dividing the anatomical sub-regions of the body into left and right arms, legs, torso and pelvis. For each of the subdivided anatomical sections, regional fat, fat free soft tissue, and BMC tissue (g) values were obtained as well as total data for arms, legs, and trunk and whole body.

All anthropometric measurements of the limbs were made on the right side of the body in all cases, according to procedures outlined in Norton and Olds (1996). Subjects were measured wearing shorts and loose fitting t-shirts. Body weight was measured using the Seca weighing scales (L5761, Seca Heavy Duty Analogue Flour Scales, Body Care, Hamburg, Germany). Skeletal heights, such as total and sitting height, were measured using a permanently wall-mounted stadiometer (Holtain, Ltd, Crymych, UK) and iliospinale height was measured using a segmometer (Rosscraft, Canada). Skeletal breadths including biacromial, bicristal and chest depth were measured using the portable Campbell Calliper 20 (Rosscraft, Canada) bone caliper, while biepicondylar humerus, bistyloidus, biepicondylar femur, and biomalleolar breadth were measured using a Tommy 2 (Rosscraft, Canada) bone caliper. Body girths, which included maximum upper arm, maximum forearm, mid thigh, maximum calf, chest, flexed biceps, waist, abdominal, and hip girth, were measured using a Body Care (Hoechstmass, Germany) flexible anthropometric tape. Triple skinfold thickness measurements were made using the same pair of calipers (Harpenden Ltd, British Indicators, UK) on a total of 14 anatomical sites (pectoral, triceps, subscapular, supraspinale, abdominal, thigh, biceps, forearm (mid and radial), calf (medial and mid) suprailium, suprailiac and axilla skinfold). The medians of these measurements were used for subsequent analysis.

The median values of the triplicate skinfolds along with the rest of the antropometric measurements were inserted into *Anthropometric Definer* software version 1.5 (Hawes and Soucie, 1993). Using existing prediction equations, percentage fat, muscle, and skeletal muscle mass were estimated. In addition, the same data were also analysed using LifeSize Software (release 1.0) (Olds and Norton, 2000) to obtain additional percent fat estimates using an array of equations. Moreover, Stewart and Hannan's (2000a) prediction equations were used to give supplementary estimates of percentage fat tissue.

Statistical analysis was carried out using the Statistical Package for Social Sciences (SPSS version 9.0 for Windows). Statistical significance was set at $p<0.05$ to describe the relationships between the variables.

## 3. RESULTS

The physical characteristics of the subjects from both groups (rowers and controls) are summarised in Table 1.

**Table 1.** Physical characteristics of subjects.

|  | Rowers | Controls | $p^*$ |
|---|---|---|---|
| Age (years) | 21 (2.6) | 26 (2.8) | <0.01 |
| Height (m) | 1.801 (0.038) | 1.783 (0.052) | NS |
| Mass (kg) | 70.3 (5.3) | 74.8 (11.0) | NS |
| BMI (kg.m$^{-2}$) | 21.7 (1.3) | 23.4 (2.5) | NS |

Mean values (± SD) reported for the two groups, NS: not significant ($p>0.05$), *Independent $t$-test

Intra-tester percent Technical Error of Measurement (%TEM) for skinfolds averaged 4.9% (±1.3 (SD)) in controls and 5.2% (±1.1) in rowers. The lowest value was observed at the axilla (3.7±1.8%) and the highest at the thigh (6.0±4.6%) measurement.

Anthropometric data revealed that there were no statistically significant differences between the two groups for the skeletal dimensions although the abdominal and waist girth (cm) were found to be statistically significant ($p<0.01$), after adjusting for the age difference between the groups (76.9 (±3.1) (SD)) and 86.4 (±9.4), 73.9 (±2.2) and 81.9 (±8.2) in rowers and controls, respectively).

In order to investigate the differences in regional subcutaneous fat distribution within the two groups, the subscapular to triceps (Malina, 1996) and abdominal to medial calf (Stewart, 1999) skinfold ratios (median values used) and the waist to hip circumferences ratio (Malina, 1996), were calculated and compared. All showed significant differences, as illustrated in Table 2.

**Table 2.** Fat distribution indices in rowers and controls.

| Ratio | Rowers | Controls | Mean differ. | SE of differ. | $p*$ |
|-------|--------|----------|--------------|---------------|------|
| ST | 1.22(±0.20) | 1.60(±0.47) | 0.38 | 0.16 | 0.030 |
| AMC | 1.01 (±0.35) | 1.94 (±0.69) | 0.93 | 0.24 | 0.001 |
| WH | 0.80(±0.04) | 0.84(±0.02) | 0.04 | 0.01 | 0.004 |

Mean values (± SD) reported for the two groups, ST: subscapular/triceps ratio;
AMC: abdominal/medial calf ratio; WH: waist/hip ratio, *Independent samples *t*-test

Dual X-ray absorptiometry revealed that both total and regional (arms, legs and trunk) amount of fat (g) were different between the rowers and controls. Fat free soft tissue (g) was significantly different only in the arms (Table 3).

**Table 3.** Total and regional fat and FFST of the two groups.

| | Fat (g) | | | FFST (g) | | |
|---|---|---|---|---|---|---|
| | Rowers | Controls | $p*$ | Rowers | Controls | $p*$ |
| Arms | 475 | 1237 | 0.003 | 7053 | 6253 | 0.043 |
| | (±182) | (±685) | | (±798) | (±840) | |
| Legs | 2762 | 5127 | 0.004 | 21742 | 20220 | NS |
| | (±1186) | (±1854) | | (±1724) | (±2426) | |
| Trunk | 3092 | 8439 | 0.002 | 28755 | 26780 | NS |
| | (±1225) | (±4620) | | (±2641) | (±2378) | |
| Total | 6685 | 15257 | 0.004 | 61708 | 57425 | 0.090 |
| | (±2589) | (±7141) | | (±5120) | (±5556) | |

Mean values (± SD) reported for the two groups, *Independent samples *t*-test

In order to investigate the differences in regional fat distribution within the two groups, the arms: legs and torso: legs fat (as assessed by DXA) ratios were computed (Table 4).

**Table 4.** Regional fat distribution in rowers and controls as assessed by DXA.

| DXA fat ratio | Rowers | Controls | Mean difference | SE of difference | $p*$ |
|-------|--------|----------|-----------------|------------------|------|
| Arms/Legs | 0.18(±0.05) | 0.23(±0.06) | 0.05 | 0.02 | 0.06 |
| Torso/Legs | 1.16(±0.23) | 1.58(±0.40) | 0.42 | 0.15 | 0.01 |

Mean values (± SD) reported for the two groups, *Independent samples *t*-test

As can be seen from Table 4, both the ratios were smaller for the rowers suggesting a different fat patterning, although only the torso: legs ratio was found to be significantly different (the arms: legs ratio was borderline significant). On the other hand, total and regional BMC did not differ between the groups.

Additionally, the difference between the fat percentages as predicted by a number of fat prediction equations and as assessed by DXA can be seen in Figures 1 and 2. The positive differences indicate that the prediction equation underestimated percentage fat, while the negative differences indicate an overestimation of percentage fat by a particular equation, when compared to percentage DXA fat.

For the rowers, these differences were statistically significant for the Wilmore and Behnke (1969), Durnin and Womersley (1974), Jackson and Pollock (1978) 3- and 7-site prediction equations ($p<0.01$), when compared to fat measured by DXA. The graph also indicates that the best (most close to % fat as measured by DXA) prediction equation was Stewart and Hannan's 2-site prediction equation (overestimating rowers fat by an average percentage of 0.2 ± 1.1 (SD)), while the poorest was the equation of Durnin and Womersley (overestimating fat by a mean percentage of 5.6 (±2.3)).

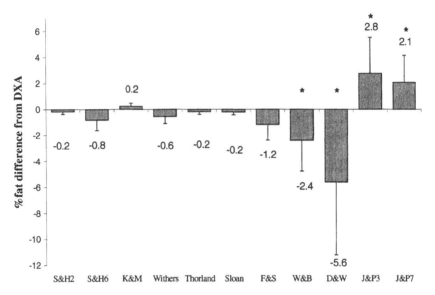

**Figure 1**. Percentage fat difference in rowers as predicted by different equations using DXA as the reference method.

For the control group, a different pattern resulted (Figure 2). The statistically significant differences were evident for the equations of Stewart and Hannan using 6-site equation ($p<0.05$), Katch and McArdle (1973) ($p<0.01$), Thorland *et al.* (1984) ($p<0.05$), Forsyth and Sinning, Durnin and Womersley and Jackson and Pollock's 3- and 7-site equations ($p<0.01$), when compared to the percentage fat obtained by means of DXA.

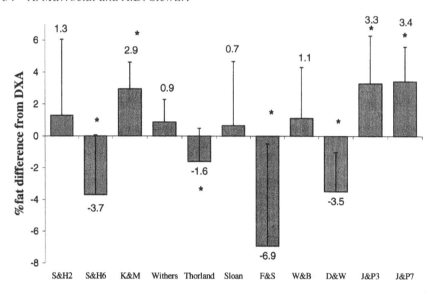

**Figure 2**. Percentage fat difference in controls as predicted by different equations using DXA as the reference method.

## 4. DISCUSSION

During this present investigation, distinct differences regarding body composition were revealed between lightweight rowers and controls. Despite not having definite differences in the skeletal dimensions, total fat and fat distribution differences were apparent between the two groups, as revealed by both the anthropometric measurements and the DXA results.

The absence of differences in skeletal dimensions between the rowers and controls, is in contrast to the findings of Rodriguez (1986), whose study of 144 male lightweight rowers revealed that on average these athletes were taller (2.09 cm), lighter (–2.22 kg), had longer upper and lower extremities, smaller sitting height, narrower shoulders and wider hips than their control peers. Upper arm flexed and tensed girth was higher, but forearm, thigh and calf girths were all smaller. Paradoxically, comparison between medallists and non-medallists revealed that the winners had wider shoulders and higher forearm girth. In our study sample, these distinct morphological differences were not observed suggesting that probably the process of self-selection was not apparent at this university team level of rowing, which may be of a lower competitive standard.

As far as FFST is concerned, in absolute terms it did not differ between the two groups (Table 3), but as a percentage of total mass the rowers had on average 10.1 (±2.3) % (mean ± SE) more FFST than the controls ($p<0.01$). This concurs with the findings of Spenst *et al.* (1993), who estimated percent muscle mass, using the prediction equation of Martin *et al.* (1990), in participants from several sporting disciplines (62 male athletes from six sporting activities namely: basketball, body building, gymnastics, sprinting, distance running and power athletes). A significant difference between athletes' and controls' muscle mass was demonstrated, but no differences were found between athletes of the different sporting activities in relation to total mass, indicating that sport-specific training appears to result in a 'generalised component' of muscularity.

Total fat (assessed by DXA) was found to be significantly lower in rowers with a simultaneous higher amount of FFST in the group. Indeed, it is well documented that rowers are amongst those athletes with a very low total body fat. Rodriguez (1986) reported that the level of adiposity of lightweight rowers was significantly lower than of their control peers, with male medallists having less adipose tissue and greater muscle mass than non-medallists.

In addition, the present data suggest a fat centralisation pattern amongst the control subjects and a peripheral fat distribution in rowers, which may be attributed to the difference of exercise levels between the two groups (since all of the above differences were adjusted for the age difference between the two groups). The regional subcutaneous fat distribution indices (Table 2) demonstrated that rowers had a lower ratio of fat on the abdominal and subscapular regions to fat on their calves and triceps, than controls. Similar conclusions can be drawn from the DXA-derived indices of fat distribution (arms-to-legs and torso-to-legs fat mass ratios seen in Table 4). Several factors have been identified to influence total fat and its distribution including sex, age, maturation, ethnicity, dietary habits and exercise (Malina, 1996). It has been shown that physical activity has an influence on fat quantity (Rognum *et al.*, 1982) and is associated with reduced upper-body adiposity and increased relative fat storage on the arms and legs (Nindl *et al.*, 1996). The findings of this present investigation are also in agreement with the ones of Stewart and Hannan (2000b) who investigated 121 male athletes of 9 different disciplines (including rowers) and controls, and concluded that exercise was an important determinant of relative fat distribution, even though the type of exercise was unimportant.

Although one would expect subcutaneous fat, which is the largest component (Lohman, 1981) to be representative of total body fat, increasing the understanding of the proportional distribution of fat between compartments has made the concept less plausible (Hawes, 1996). In an investigation by Nindl *et al.* (1996), 165 U.S. soldiers were studied while undergoing heavy physical training and semi-starvation. A hierarchy in fat mobilisation, as assessed by DXA, was observed with fat primarily being displaced by the abdomen, followed by the arms and then legs, as a consequence of weight loss. This was, though, not supported by the skinfold data in the arms and legs, a finding which could be explained by a change in partitioning between subcutaneous and internal fat with weight loss. In the present study, DXA results (Table 3) showed that both total and regional fat were lower amongst rowers, when compared to controls ($p<0.01$). It would seem that in athletes, a high proportion of fat situated in the subcutaneous compartment would explain why skinfolds are a relatively good predictor of total fat (Stewart and Hannan, 2000a).

This investigation also revealed that some of the prediction equations, grossly miscalculated percentage fat in both groups. Indeed, the most commonly used equations of Durnin and Womersley (1974) and Jackson and Pollock (1978), were the most inappropriate for calculating percentage fat in rowers, as well as within the control subjects. On the other hand, other equations developed for more specific populations, showed a better agreement with DXA fat (e.g. Stewart and Hannan's (2000a) equations for predicting percentage fat in athletic populations including rowers).

This is probably because for athletes, the adaptation of the body composition to exercise may threaten the validity of generalized prediction equations. The findings of Sinning *et al.* (1985) indicated that using the two compartment (fat and fat-free mass) method as the reference criterion, the majority of generalised prediction equations were not valid for predicting the fat content of athletes. The researchers stated that Durnin and Womersley's (1974) equation overestimated fat to an extreme degree, while those of Jackson and Pollock were the most accurate and suitable for body composition screening in male athletes. When the raw data in both these studies were more closely inspected, it was revealed that the participants in the study of Jackson and Pollock were taller and leaner (and thus closer to the athletic morphology) than those studied by Durnin and Womersley. In addition, it is also possible that Jackson and Pollock used a greater proportion of athletic or physically active individuals than Durnin and Womersley.

The present study agrees in part with the review of Sinning *et al.* (1985). The equation of Durnin and Womersley was consistently overestimating athletes' body fat by an average of 5.6 ($\pm$2.3)% (Figure 1), the difference from DXA fat being highly significant ($p<0.01$). Wilmore and Behnke's (1969) equation also overestimated fat ($p = 0.004$). On the other hand, the 3- and 7-site equations of Jackson and Pollock (1978) significantly underestimated percentage fat in this group ($p = 0.005$ and $0.012$, respectively).

The rest of the equations varied slightly and non-significantly in their predictions of fat, when compared to DXA (ranged from an underestimation of 0.2% (Katch and McArdle, 1973) to an overestimation of 1.2% fat (Forsyth and Sinning, 1973)). Of them, Stewart and Hannan's 2-site equation (2000a) had the best agreement with DXA fat (mean overestimation of 0.2% fat with the smallest SD of 1.1%). This is probably because their equation was derived from a recent and purely athletic population (82 male athletes, including 13 rowers). Thus, the regression analysis from which the prediction equation originated was based on anthropometric data of today's athletes. Some of the equations commonly used to predict body fat were derived from regression analysis of data obtained by athletes going back as far as the 1960s. Since then the duration, intensity and variety of training involved in most sports have changed in line with elevated competitive standards. This, combined with the secular trend for increasing height, may also have conferred a commensurate change in body morphology and body composition.

For the controls, a strikingly different pattern resulted, as viewed in Figure 2. Assuming DXA results to be accurate, seven out of the eleven equations significantly miscalculated percentage fat in this group. The difference from DXA fat was significant for Stewart and Hannan's 6-site equation (2000a) and that of Thorland *et al.* (1984) ($p<0.05$) and highly significant for the equations of Katch and McArdle (1973), Forsyth and Sinning (1973), Durnin and Womersley (1974) and Jackson and Pollock's (1978) 3- and 7-site equations ($p<0.01$).

In conclusion, while self-selection into rowing equations of subjects whose physiques may be genotypically advantageous cannot be ruled out, the exercise involved in rowing could explain the observed differences on total adiposity, fat distribution and muscle mass between the two groups. These differences seem to affect the optimal skinfold selection to predict total adiposity in each category and thus the accuracy of prediction equations developed. Therefore, caution is imperative in selecting appropriate equations for predicting adiposity, especially in athletes.

## REFERENCES

American College of Sports Medicine, 1995, Position stand on osteoporosis and exercise. *Medicine and Science in Sports and Exercise*, **27**, i-vii.

Durnin, J.V.G.A. and Womersley, J., 1974, Body fat assessed from total body density and its estimation from skinfold thickness: measurements on 481 men and women aged from 16 to 72 years. *British Journal of Nutrition*, **32**, 77-97.

Forsyth, H.L. and Sinning, W.E., 1973, The anthropometric estimation of body density and lean body weight of male athletes. *Medicine and Science in Sports*, 5174-5180.

Hawes, M.R., 1996, Human body composition. In *Kinanthropometry and Exercise Physiology Manual*, edited by Eston, R. and Reilly, T. (London, E. & F. N. Spon), pp. 5-33.

Hawes, M.R. and Soucie, A., 1993, *Anthropometric Definer* software, Athletic Computer Systems, Calgary, Canada.

Jackson, A.S. and Pollock, M.L., 1978, Generalized equations for predicting body density in men. *British Journal of Nutrition*, **40**, 497-504.

Katch, F.I. and McArdle, W.D., 1973, Prediction of body density from simple anthropometric measurements in college-age men and women. *Human Biology*, **45**, 445-454.

Lohman, T.G., 1981, Skinfolds and body density and their relation to body fatness: A review. *Human Biology*, **53**, 181-225.

Lukaski, H.C., 1987, Methods for the assessment of human body composition: traditional and new. *American Journal Clinical Nutrition*, **46**, 537-556.

Malina, R.M., 1996, Regional body composition: Age, sex and ethnic variation. In *Human Body Composition*, edited by Roche, A.F., Heymsfield, S.B. and Lohman, T.G. (Champaign, IL: Human Kinetics), pp. 217–255.

Martin, A.D., Spenst, L.F., Drinkwater, D.T. and Clarys, J.P., 1990, Anthropometric estimation of muscle mass in men. *Medicine and Science in Sports and Exercise*, **22**, 729-733.

Nindl, B.C., Friedl, K.E., Marchitelli, L.J., Shippee, R.L., Thomas, C.D. and Patton, J.F., 1996, Regional fat placement in physically fit males and changes with weight loss. *Medicine and Science in Sports and Exercise*, **28**, 786-793.

Norton, K. and Olds, T., 1996, *Anthropometrica: A Textbook of Body Measurements for Sport and Health Courses*, (Sydney: UNSW Press).

Olds, T. and Norton, K. 2000, LifeSize Release 1.0, Educational Software for Body Composition Analysis, Human Kinetics Software, Australia.

Pietrobelli, A., Formica, C., Wang, Z. and Heymsfield, S.B., 1996, Dual-energy X-ray absorptiometry body composition model: review of physical concepts. *American Journal of Physiology*, **271**, E941-51.

Rodriguez, F.A., 1986, Physical structure of international lightweight rowers. In *Kinanthropometry III*, edited by Reilly, T., Watkins, J. and Borms, J. (London, E & F.N. Spon), pp. 255-61.

Rognum, T.O., Rodahl, K. and Opstad, P.K., 1982, Regional differences in the lipolytic response of the subcutaneous fat depots to prolonged exercise and severe energy deficiency. *European Journal of Applied Physiology*, **49**, 401-8.

Sinning, W.E., Donly, D.G., Little, K.D., Cunningham, L.N., Racaniello, A., Siconolfi, S.F., and Sholes, J.L., 1985. Validity of 'generalized' equations for body composition analysis in male athletes. *Medicine and Science in Sports and Exercise*, **28**, 17124-30.

Sloan, A.W., 1967, Estimation of body fat in young men, *Journal of Applied Physiology*, **23**, 311-15.

Spenst, L.F., Martin, A.D. and Drinkwater, D.T., 1993, Muscle mass of competitive male athletes. *Journal of Sports Sciences*, **11**, 3-8.

Stewart, A.D., 1999, *Body composition of athletes assessed by Dual X-ray Absorptiomerty and other methods*, University of Edinburgh, Doctor of Philosophy Thesis.

Stewart, A.D. and Hannan, W.J., 2000a, Body composition prediction in male athletes using dual X-ray absorptiometry as the reference method. *Journal of Sports Sciences*, **18**, 263-274.

Stewart, A.D. and Hannan, J., 2000b, Sub-regional tissue morphometry in male athletes and controls using DXA. *International Journal of Sport Nutrition and Exercise Metabolism*, **11**, 157-169.

Thorland, W.G., Johnson, G.O., Tharp, G.D., Housh, T.J. and Cisar, C.J., 1984, Estimation of body density in adolescent athletes, *Human Biology*, **56**, 439-48.

Wilmore, J.H. and Behnke, A.R., 1969, An anthropometric estimation of body density and lean body weight in young men. *Journal of Applied Physiology*, 2725-31.

Withers, R.T., Craig, N.P., Bourdon, P.C. and Norton, K.I., 1987, Relative body fat and anthropometric prediction of body density of male athletes. *European Journal of Applied Physiology*, **56**, 191-200.

# 4 The Relationship Between Flexibility Measurements and Length of Body Segments

M. Hossein Alizadeh[1] and A. Majid Masiha[2]
[1]Faculty of PE & Sport Sciences, Tehran University,
Enghelab Ave., 16 Azar Street, Iran
[2]Iran University Sport Organization

## 1. INTRODUCTION

Flexibility is recognized as an important component of physical fitness, and some tests of flexibility are included in most physical fitness batteries. The inclusion of a test of flexibility is due to the belief that a lack of flexibility may contribute to an athlete's performance or perhaps be the cause of injury.

During the past decades many clinical techniques have been described for measuring the flexibility of trunk and hip (Kippes and Parker, 1987; Shephard *et al.*, 1990; Shaulis *et al.*, 1994). These include the use of radiographs, inclinometers, spondylometers, goniometers and plum lines. Each of these techniques has disadvantages, such as cost, exposure to radiation, needs for specialized equipment, and questionable reliability. Probably because there are many techniques for measuring trunk and hip motion, no one method has been developed fully (i.e. its reliability and validity demonstrated) for clinical use. Moreover, in most reliability studies of trunk and hip motion unhealthy subjects have been used rather than focusing on the subjects whom physical educationists examine most often. The sit-and-reach and toe-touch tests are most often employed to assess hamstring and low-back flexibility. These are widely used in many fitness centres, schools, and universities. In some countries such as America and Iran the sit-and-reach test, therefore, has been incorporated in almost every national fitness test battery. The use of the sit-and-reach flexibility test emanated from Wells and Dillon (1952) who compared scores on the sit-and-reach test to those from a standing and bobbing test (toe-touch test) in 100 college-age women. This is because the sit-and-reach score provides a simple measure of flexibility in the trunk, hip, and hamstring muscles (Wells and Dillon, 1952). This test is the sole test of flexibility adopted in a number of large-scale representative population surveys such as the Canada fitness survey (Shephard, 1986). The results of this particular test seem relatively independent of body build (Wear, 1963).

Despite the use of this test in many centres, it is a crucial question whether differences in limb length may be influential when measuring flexibility of leg and lumbar muscles. Extensive cross-sectional data on sit-and-reach scores at various ages have now been obtained through the Canada Fitness Survey but it is unclear to what extent the changes in score for this test reflect the general loss of flexibility with length of body limbs. Wilmore and Costill (1988) suggested that limb length might be an additional limitation to the sit-and-reach test; therefore, its role must be investigated. Many years ago some other investigators such as Wear (1963) and Broer and Galles (1958) found similar results in their investigations. Wear showed that sit-and-reach test is significantly related to excess of trunk and arm length over leg length in college-age males. Similar results were found by Broer and Galles (1958) when they used toe-touch-test to measure the flexibility of college women.

The most common assumption when interpreting sit-and-reach and toe-touch tests is that individuals with better scores possess a higher degree of trunk and hip flexibility than subjects with lower scores (Gajdosik and Lusin, 1983). Testing of flexibility remains one of the most perplexing challenges to physical educators and the effects of length of upper and lower extremities on the scores of sit-and-reach and toe-touch tests are poorly understood (Simoneau, 1998). Hence controversy exists regarding the effect of limb length on the sit-and-reach and toe-touch.

The purpose of this study was to examine the relationship between length of body segments and the scores in sit-and-reach and toe-touch tests.


## 2. METHODS

One hundred male students ranging in age from 19-25 years volunteered to be subjects in the study. All subjects gave written informed consent. The height and the lengths of subjects' limbs (arm and leg) were measured in a relaxed standing position by means of a tape measure to the nearest centimetre. The height of the trunk was measured while the subjects were in a sitting position and the distance between the acromion process and the surface of the chair was measured in centimetres. The length of the arms was also measured from acromion process to the tip of the middle finger in centimetres. In the lower extremity, the length of the femur was measured from the great tuberosity of the femur to the lateral epicondyle of the femur with the subject in a standing position. After measurements the subjects completed a 3-min period of stretching. Subjects were then given three trials of the sit-and-reach and toe-touch tests. The sit-and-reach test was administered using a sit-and-reach box and described in Hoeger and Hopkins (1992). In demonstrating the sit-and-reach procedure, it was emphasized that the subjects assumed a sitting position on the floor while their knees were kept straight without bending. The feet were placed together without any distance between them. In the starting position, the subjects were asked to place the feet against the box and slowly reach forward as far as possible. The fingertips of both hands were to be placed on the box, moving together along the scores on the box;

no jerking or bouncing was permitted. The test was performed in bare feet. The final position was typically held for a minimum of 2 s.

The criterion score was the distance reached during the test. Three trials were taken and the average was used for analysis. The toe-touch test was administrated while the subjects were positioned on a step; then they were asked to bend forward and push the moveable scale with straight knees as far as possible. No jerking or bouncing was permitted. Three trials were all recorded and the average was used for analysis.

## 3. RESULTS

The mean age, height, mass and flexibility data for the entire sample (N=100) are presented in Table 1.

There was a significant relationship between the height and the subjects' scores of flexibility in the sit-and-reach and the toe-touch tests. Hence it seems that the results of these tests are influenced by height. In recognizing the effect of upper or lower extremity flexibility on the tests, the results indicated that the muscle flexibility of the lower extremity was more affected by the length of the lower extremity than the trunk and arms length. The results also indicated no significant relationship between the length of arm, trunk and the scores for sit-and-reach and toe-touch tests. Table 2 presents the correlations between body segments length and toe-touch and sit-and-reach tests.

**Table 1**. Descriptive and flexibility characteristics of subjects.

| Characteristic | M | SD | Range |
|---|---|---|---|
| Age | 21.00 | 1.50 | 19-25 |
| Height (m) | 1.746 | ±0.060 | 1.60-1.915 |
| Mass (kg) | 66.9 | ±10.6 | 48-96 |
| Trunk length (cm) | 64.2 | ±2.7 | 59-71 |
| Arm length (cm) | 78.9 | ±3.8 | 69-90 |
| Thigh length (cm) | 44.7 | ±2.4 | 40-51 |
| Leg length | 138.6 | ±3.05 | 133-138 |
| Sit-and-reach (cm) | 34.2 | ±9.6 | 5-55 |
| Toe touch (cm) | 31.6 | ±9.15 | 6.6-53.8 |

**Table 2.** Correlation between some characteristics of anthropometry measurements, sit-and-reach and toe-touch tests.

|                 | Sit-and-reach | Toe touch |
| --------------- | ------------- | --------- |
| Height          | -0.196        | -0.202*   |
| Length of trunk | -0.023        | 0.012     |
| Length of arm   | -0.122        | -0.135    |
| Length of leg   | -0.215        | -0.263*   |

## 4. DISCUSSION

Two flexibility tests used in health-related fitness are the sit-and-reach and toe-touch tests. The importance of these tests is based on trunk and hip flexibility measurements. According to the findings of this study, subjects' height influences flexibility of hamstring and lower back muscles as indicated by the sit-and-reach and toe-touch test. In recognizing the effect of upper and lower extremity flexibility and limb length, the results indicated that the flexibility of the lower extremity was affected more by the length of this extremity than the length of trunk and arms.

The findings of this research agree with those of Hoeger and Hopkins (1992) who reported a bias for individuals of extreme proportional arm/leg length differences. They suggested a modified sit-and-reach test to negate the effects of shoulder girdle mobility and proportional differences between arms and legs. They stated that "the sit-and-reach test as it is presently administrated has inherent limitations in that it does not allow for proportional differences between arm and leg length". They also stated that individuals with long legs and/or short arms have a structural disadvantage in performing the test. They, therefore, will receive lower scores than individuals with short legs and/or long arms who achieve the same degree of hip flexion.

Minkler and Patterson (1994) also showed that the modified sit-and-reach test was moderately related to hamstring flexibility (r=0.66 and r=0.40) in females and males respectively, but its relation to low-back flexibility was quite low (r=0.25 and r=0.40). It seems that an accurate and reliable method of assessing hamstring flexibility is of utmost importance. Jackson and Langford (1989) investigated the validity of the sit-and-reach test in 52 males and 52 females ranging in age from 20 to 45 years. They found good support (r=0.89 for males and r=0.70 for females) for the test as a measure of hamstring flexibility but less support (r=0.59 and r=0.12) for the test as a measure of low-back flexibility.

In addition, the effect of previous exercise on test results and the effect of practice on skill performance cannot be totally ignored. When the reliability of sit-and-reach and toe-touch tests which are field tests of physical ability are determined, the effect of previous exercise or skill performance should be considered as influential factors. More investigations should be carried out to show the role of skill performance on sit-and-reach and toe-touch results.

## Acknowledgments

We thank Tehran University students for their assistance in this study.

## REFERENCES

Beattie, P., Rothstein, J.M. and Lamb, R.L., 1987, Reliability of the attraction method for measuring lumbar spine backward bending. *Physical Therapy*, **67**, 364-369.

Broer, M.R. and Galles, N.R., 1958, Importance of relationship between various body measurements in the performance of the toe-touch test. *Research Quarterly*, **29**, 253-263.

Gajdosik, R. and Lusin, G., 1983, Hamstring muscle tightness. *Physical Therapy*, **63**, 1085-1088.

Hoeger, W.W.K. and Hopkins, D.R., 1992, A comparison of the sit and reach and the modified sit-and-reach in the measure of flexibility in women. *Research Quarterly for Exercise and Sport*, **63**, 191-195.

Kippes, V. and Parker, W.A., 1987, Toe-touch test, A measure of its validity, *Physical Therapy*, **67**, 1680-1684.

Minkler, S. and Patterson, P., 1994, The validity of the modified sit-and-reach test in college-age students. *Research Quarterly for Exercise and Sport*, **65**,189-192.

Shaulis, D., Golding, L.A. and Tandy, R.D., 1994, Reliability of the AAHPERD functional fitness assessment across multiple practice sessions in older men and women. *Journal of Aging and Physical Activity*, **2**, 273-279.

Shephard, R.J., 1986, *Fitness of a Nation: Lessons form the Canada Fitness Survey*. (Basel: Karger Publishing).

Shephard, R.J., Berridge, M. and Montelpare, W., 1990, On the generality of the sit-and-reach test: An analysis of flexibility data for an aging population. *Research Quarterly for Exercise and Sport*, **61**, 326-330.

Simoneau, G.G., 1998, The impact of various anthropometric and flexibility measurements of the sit-and-reach test. *Research Quarterly for Exercise and Sport*, **12**, 232-237.

Wear, C.L., 1963, Relationship of flexibility measurements to length of body segments. *Research Quarterly*, **23**, 115-118.

Wells, K.F. and Dillon, E.K., 1952, The sit and reach test: A test of back and leg flexibility. *Research Quarterly*, **23**, 115-118.

Wilmore, J. H. and Costill, D.L., 1988, *Athletic Training for Sport and Activity*. (Dubuque, IA: W. C. Brown).

# 5 Effect of Testing Protocol on the Determination of Lactate Threshold in Competitive Cyclists

R.C. Richard Davison[1], James Balmer[2] and Steve R. Bird[3]
[1]Department of Sport, Exercise and Biomedical Sciences, University of Luton, Luton, LU1 3JU, UK
[2]Department of Sport and Health, Liverpool Hope University, Liverpool, L16 9JD, UK
[3]Centre for Rehabilitation, Exercise and Sport Science, Victoria University, Melbourne, Australia

## 1. INTRODUCTION

In addition to the wide range of terminology and determination methods for the lactate threshold (Tlac) (Weltman, 1995), there is also a range of possible protocols to elicit the characteristic increase blood lactate concentrations with increasing exercise intensity. Ramp, incremental and discontinuous protocols have all been used, but, to date, very few studies have directly investigated the effect of testing protocol on the determination of Tlac. Yoshida (1984) reported that the Tlac or Onset of Blood Lactate Accumulation (OBLA, 4 mmol·l⁻¹) was at a significantly higher workload for a 1-min vs 4-min incremental protocol. Interestingly there was no difference in the $\dot{V}O_2$ at Tlac and OBLA for the two protocols when the thresholds were determined from arterial blood, but there was a difference when venous blood lactate was measured. This suggested that a longer increment was required when measuring venous blood lactate. Weltman et al. (1990) compared a continuous (3-min) incremental running protocol to a 10-min discontinuous protocol and found no difference in Tlac expressed as $\dot{V}O_2$, running speed or heart rate. A short (30-s) pause in an incremental treadmill protocol has also been shown not to affect the determination of Tlac (Weltman et al., 1990). To date, no study has directly compared the three commonly used protocols. Therefore the aim of this study was to compare the Tlac derived from ramp, incremental and discontinuous incremental protocols in a group of highly trained cyclists.

## 2. METHODS

### 2.1 Subjects

Twelve male trained competitive cyclists of varying age (43±16 years) and ability (RMP$_{max}$, 391±59 W; $\dot{V}O_{2peak}$, 4.73±0.6 l·min⁻¹) volunteered for this study. All subjects were well-trained cyclists who regularly competed in local cycling races. Subjects gave written informed consent according to institutional ethical regulations prior to participation in the study.

## 2.2 Procedures

Subjects undertook the following four tests, in random order, on their own bicycle (fitted with an SRM Powermeter, Julich, Germany) mounted on a Kingcycle ergometer. The power meter was calibrated using the appropriate system software and calibration was checked before and after each test. During the tests, power output (W) and pedal cadence (rev·min$^{-1}$) were recorded at 1-s intervals and mean values were calculated for each minute of the test. Each test was performed using a Kingcycle test rig and subjects were required to maintain the power output displayed on a computer screen using version 5.5 Kingcycle computer software. Heart rate (beats·min$^{-1}$) was recorded at 5-s intervals (Polar, Kempele, Finland) throughout each test and mean values were calculated for each min. During LT$_{ramp}$, Tlac$_{inc}$ and Tlac$_{dis,}$ tests expired air was measured over 1-min intervals using the Covox on-line gas analysis system. Values for $\dot{V}O_2$ were recorded at 1-min intervals during the warm-up period and throughout the test. Tests for each subject were conducted at the same time of day over a 4-week period. No attempt was made in this study to correct for body mass as the focus of the investigation was a comparison between the different protocols.

### Kingcycle Ramp Minute Power Test (RMP$_{max}$)

On arrival at the laboratory, the bicycle's rear tyre pressure was standardised using a track pump with tyre pressure gauge (Silca, Italy), SRM Training System (SRM, Germany) was fitted to the bicycle and both the SRM and Kingcycle were calibrated according to the manufacturers' instructions. For each RMP$_{max}$ test, subjects were instructed to warm-up at a self-selected intensity. On completion of their warm-up, each subject completed 5 min of continuous cycling, maintaining the starting power calculated for the RMP$_{max}$ test. During the RMP$_{max}$ test, work rate increased per minute by 5.0 ± 0.2% (mean ± SD) of peak power achieved during an habituation test. Ramp rate during the tests ranged from 15 to 25 W·min$^{-1}$. dependent on each individual cyclist's predicted peak power. Starting power output for the test was calculated for subjects to reach volitional exhaustion between 9-11 min. During tests, gear ratio and pedal cadence (rev·min$^{-1}$) were self-selected. Maximal power (RMP$_{max}$) was calculated as the highest average power measured with the SRM Training System during any 60-s period of the test.

### Threshold test using a ramped protocol (Tlac$_{ramp}$)

Following a 5-min warm-up at a power output equivalent to about 45% of RMP$_{max}$, subjects completed a continuous ramped exercise protocol as described by Bird and Davison (1997). Starting power was ~ 45% RMP$_{max}$ and ramp rate was 6 W·min$^{-1}$. During the test, subjects selected their own pedal cadence (rev·min$^{-1}$) and were allowed to change gear *ad libitum*. The test was completed when subjects reached volitional exhaustion.

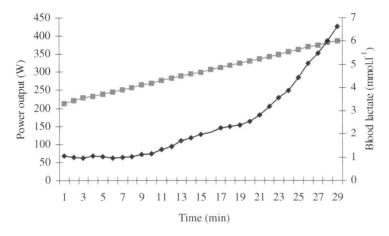

**Figure 1**. A schematic representation of power output and blood lactate response recorded for one individual during a Tlac$_{ramp}$ test (with power recorded using Kingcycle).

## Threshold test using a continuous incremental protocol (Tlac$_{inc}$)

Following a 5-min warm-up at a power output of about 45% of RMP$_{max}$, subjects completed a continuous incremental exercise test. Starting power was ~45% RMP$_{max}$ and workload increased by 24 W at the end of each 4-min stage. Subjects self-selected pedal cadence (rev·min$^{-1}$) and changed gear ratio *ad libitum*. The test was completed when subjects reached volitional exhaustion.

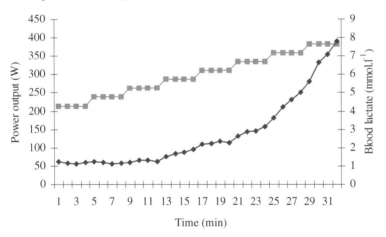

**Figure 2**. A schematic illustration of power output and blood lactate response recorded for one individual during a Tlac$_{inc}$ test (with power recorded using Kingcycle).

*Threshold test using a discontinuous incremental protocol (Tlac$_{dis}$)*

Following a 5-min warm-up at a power output equivalent to about 45% of RMP$_{max}$, subjects completed a discontinuous incremental exercise protocol. Starting power was ~ 45% RMP$_{max}$ and workload was increased by 24 W at the end of each 4-min stage. Between stages, subjects were required to stop pedalling for 15 s until power output had dropped to ~ 75 W; this power was maintained for a further 30 s at which point subjects had 15 s to accelerate to the required power of the next stage. Subjects selected their own pedal cadence (rev·min$^{-1}$) and were allowed to change gear *ad libitum*. The test was completed when subjects reached volitional exhaustion.

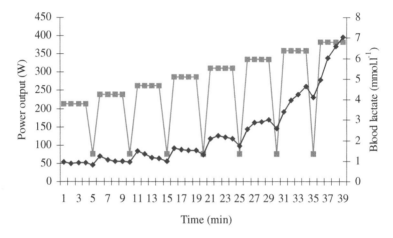

**Figure 3**.   A schematic illustration of power output and blood lactate response recorded for one individual during a Tlac$_{dis}$ test (with power recorded using Kingcycle).

## Blood lactate during Tlac$_{ramp}$, Tlac$_{inc}$ and Tlac$_{dis}$

For the Tlac$_{ramp}$, Tlac$_{inc}$ and Tlac$_{dis}$, tests fingertip capillary blood samples (20 ul) were collected at 1-min intervals from the start of the warm-up to completion of the test. Each sample of fingertip capillary whole blood was assayed for blood lactate (Biosen 5030L, EKF Industrie, Electronik GmbH, Barleben, Germany). Each blood sample was assayed (in duplicate) for the concentration of blood lactate (mmol·l$^{-1}$) and the average value of the duplicate samples was used in all subsequent analyses.

### Determination of threshold intensity

Individual values for power output (W), heart rate (beats·min$^{-1}$) and oxygen uptake ($\dot{V}O_2$ l·min$^{-1}$) were determined at designated lactate thresholds. Blood lactate threshold (Tlac) was identified as the first abrupt increase in lactate concentration above the baseline blood lactate level (as previously defined by Farrell *et al.*, 1993. The point of OBLA was identified as the fixed blood lactate concentration of 4 mmol·l⁻¹. Values for blood lactate were plotted against time and Tlac and OBLA were determined by three investigators using visual inspection of the blood lactate response during each test. The mean selection of the three reviewers was used in the subsequent analyses.

**Statistical analyses**

Results are expressed as mean ± SD. Power output (W), heart rate (HR), oxygen uptake ($\dot{V}O_2$), blood lactate concentration (BLa) and pedal cadence (Rev) for each threshold were expressed as absolute values (W, b·min⁻¹, l·min⁻¹, mmol·l⁻¹ and rev·min⁻¹ respectively) and relative values (%$RMP_{max}$, %$HR_{peak}$ and % $\dot{V}O_{2peak}$ respectively). After checks for violations of the assumptions for using parametric statistics, data were analysed using a one way repeated measures ANOVA. Level of significance was p<0.05 and post hoc comparisons were completed using Tukey HSD tests.

## 3. RESULTS

### 3.1 Absolute values at Tlac

Mean values (n = 12) for power output (W), heart rate (beats·min⁻¹), oxygen uptake (l·min⁻¹) and blood lactate concentration (mmol·l⁻¹) at Tlac determined from the three Tlac tests are shown in Table 1. Power output at Tlac ($SRM_w$@Tlac) and heart rate at Tlac (HR@Tlac) for $Tlac_{ramp}$ was higher (p<0.05) when compared with $Tlac_{inc}$ and $Tlac_{dis}$. Oxygen uptake ($\dot{V}O_2$ @Tlac) was higher for $Tlac_{ramp}$ when compared with $Tlac_{inc}$ but not $Tlac_{dis}$. There was no difference (p>0.05) for blood lactate concentration (BLa@Tlac) and pedal cadence (Rev@Tlac) between tests.

**Table 1.** Mean ± SD values for power output (W), heart rate (beats·min⁻¹), $\dot{V}O_2$ (l·min⁻¹), blood lactate concentration (mmol·l⁻¹) and pedal cadence (rev·min⁻¹) at Tlac (n = 12).

| | $Tlac_{ramp}$ | | $Tlac_{inc}$ | | $Tlac_{dis}$ | |
|---|---|---|---|---|---|---|
| | Mean ± SD | Range | Mean ± SD | Range | Mean ± SD | Range |
| $SRM_w$@Tlac | 224 ± 29 *# | 174-260 | 207 ± 30 | 168-252 | 206 ± 21 | 174-235 |
| HR@Tlac | 135 ± 13 *# | 109-152 | 128 ± 14 | 106-151 | 127 ± 11 | 110-146 |
| $\dot{V}O_2$ @Tlac | 2.97 ± 0.46 * | 2.11-3.91 | 2.76 ± 0.46 | 1.94-3.54 | 2.81 ± 0.30 | 2.31-3.31 |
| BLa@Tlac | 1.66 ± 0.55 | 1.02-2.85 | 1.53 ± 0.38 | 0.90-2.3 | 1.58 ± 0.41 | 1.01-2.42 |
| Rev@Tlac | 94 ± 8 | 79-105 | 91 ± 7 | 79-105 | 91 ± 6 | 81-105 |

\* denotes significantly higher than $Tlac_{inc}$ (p<0.05)
\# denotes significantly higher than $Tlac_{dis}$ (p<0.05)

## 3.2 Absolute values at OBLA

Mean values (n = 12) for power output (W), HR (beats·min[-1]) and oxygen uptake (l·min[-1]) determined at OBLA for the three Tlac tests are shown in Table 2. Values for power at OBLA ($SRM_w$@OBLA) were higher (p<0.05) for the $Tlac_{ramp}$ and $Tlac_{dis}$ tests when compared with $Tlac_{inc}$ and heart rate at OBLA (HR@OBLA) was higher (p<0.05) for $Tlac_{ramp}$ than $Tlac_{inc}$ and $Tlac_{dis}$. Oxygen uptake ($\dot{V}O_2$ @OBLA) was higher (p<0.05) for $Tlac_{dis}$ than $Tlac_{ramp}$ and $Tlac_{inc}$ and $\dot{V}O_2$ @OBLA for $Tlac_{ramp}$ was higher than $Tlac_{inc}$. There was no difference between tests (p = 0.13) for pedal cadence (Rev@OBLA).

**Table 2.** Mean ± SD values for power output (W), heart rate (beats·min[-1]), oxygen uptake (l·min[-1]) and pedal cadence (rev·min[-1]) at OBLA (n = 12).

|  | $Tlac_{ramp}$ | | $Tlac_{inc}$ | | $Tlac_{dis}$ | |
|---|---|---|---|---|---|---|
|  | Mean ± SD | Range | Mean ± SD | Range | Mean ± SD | Range |
| $SRM_w$@OBLA | 283 ± 40 * | 225-354 | 274 ± 37 | 219-348 | 285 ± 42 * | 229-351 |
| HR@OBLA | 156 ± 13 *# | 135-179 | 152 ± 13 | 134-172 | 151 ± 14 | 128-171 |
| $\dot{V}O_2$ @OBLA | 3.85 ±0.62* | 2.80-4.80 | 3.73 ± 0.55 | 2.80-4.63 | 3.94 ± 0.55*$ | 3.20-4.90 |
| Rev@OBLA | 95 ± 6 | 83-105 | 96 ± 7 | 86-111 | 93 ± 8 | 81-104 |

\* denotes significantly higher than $Tlac_{inc}$ (p<0.05)
\# denotes significantly higher than $Tlac_{dis}$ (p<0.05)
\$ denotes significantly higher than $Tlac_{ramp}$ (p<0.05)

## 3.3 Relative values at Tlac

Mean values (n = 12) for power output ($\%RMP_{max}$), heart rate ($\%HR_{peak}$) and oxygen uptake ($\%\dot{V}O_{2peak}$) at Tlac for the three Tlac tests are shown in Table 3. Power at Tlac ($\%RMP_{max}$) and heart rate at Tlac ($\%HR_{peak}$) were higher (p<0.05) for $Tlac_{ramp}$ when compared with $Tlac_{inc}$ and $Tlac_{dis}$ and $\%\dot{V}O_{2peak}$ was higher (p<0.05) for $Tlac_{ramp}$ when compared with $Tlac_{inc}$ but not $Tlac_{dis}$.

**Table 3.** Mean ± SD values for power output ($\%RMP_{max}$), heart rate ($\%HR_{peak}$), oxygen uptake ($\%VO_{2peak}$) at TLac (n = 12).

|  | $Tlac_{ramp}$ | | $Tlac_{inc}$ | | $Tlac_{dis}$ | |
|---|---|---|---|---|---|---|
|  | Mean ± SD | Range | Mean ± SD | Range | Mean ± SD | Range |
| % $RMP_{max}$ @Tlac | 57.5 ± 4.3 *# | 50.0-63.4 | 53.1 ± 5.2 | 48.4-66.4 | 53.2 ± 4.5 | 46.6-61.8 |
| %$HR_{peak}$@Tlac | 74.9 ± 5.0 *# | 64.1-83.0 | 70.8 ± 4.5 | 62.4-77.8 | 70.5 ± 3.3 | 66.5-79.0 |
| % $\dot{V}O_{2peak}$ @Tlac | 62.9 ± 7.6 * | 51.6-73.3 | 58.3 ± 5.8 | 47.4-65.8 | 59.7 ± 5.8 | 47.8-69.1 |

\*denotes significantly higher than $Tlac_{inc}$ (p<0.05)
\# denotes significantly higher than $Tlac_{dis}$ (p<0.05)

## 3.4 Relative values at OBLA

Mean values (n = 12) for power output ($\%RMP_{max}$), heart rate ($\%HR_{peak}$) and oxygen uptake ($\% \dot{V}O_{2\,peak}$) at OBLA for the three Tlac tests are shown in Table 4. Power ($\% RMP_{max}$) was higher (p<0.05) for $Tlac_{ramp}$ and $Tlac_{dis}$ when compared with $Tlac_{inc}$ however $\% RMP_{max}$ for $Tlac_{ramp}$ and $Tlac_{dis}$ were similar (p>0.05). Heart rate ($\%HR_{peak}$) was higher (p<0.05) for $Tlac_{ramp}$ when compared with $Tlac_{inc}$ and $Tlac_{dis}$. Values for oxygen uptake ($\% \dot{V}O_{2\,peak}$) for $Tlac_{ramp}$ and $Tlac_{dis}$ were higher (p<0.05) when compared with $Tlac_{inc}$ and $Tlac_{dis}$ was higher (p<0.05) than $Tlac_{ramp}$.

**Table 4**. Mean ± SD values for power output ($\%RMP_{max}$), heart rate ($\%HR_{peak}$), oxygen uptake ($\%VO_{2peak}$) at OBLA (n = 12).

| | $Tlac_{ramp}$ | | $Tlac_{inc}$ | | $Tlac_{dis}$ | |
|---|---|---|---|---|---|---|
| | Mean ± SD | Range | Mean ± SD | Range | Mean ± SD | Range |
| $\%RMP_{max}$ @OBLA | 72.7± 6.1 * | 65.3-82.9 | 70.4± 6.0 | 59.8-81.9 | 73.1± 4.9 * | 64.3-80.3 |
| $\%HR_{peak}$ @OBLA | 86.3± 4.6 *# | 79.4-98.1 | 84.6± 3.9 | 78.8-93.6 | 83.5± 4.0 | 75.3-92.4 |
| $\% \dot{V}O_{2\,peak}$ @OBLA | 81.5± 9.4 * | 66.0-99.0 | 79.0± 8.5 | 65.8-96.7 | 83.5± 8.6*$ | 65.2-100 |

\* denotes significantly higher than $Tlac_{inc}$ (p<0.05)
\# denotes significantly higher than $Tlac_{dis}$ (p<0.05)
\$ denotes significantly higher than $Tlac_{ramp}$ (p<0.05)

## 4. DISCUSSION

There has been and continues to be considerable debate in the literature over the whole concept of lactate threshold (Antonutto and Di Prampero, 1995; Weltman, 1995; Myers and Ashley, 1997). Most of this debate has focussed on the determination of Tlac from the relationship between blood lactate concentrations and increasing exercise intensity (Stegmann *et al.*, 1981; Yeh *et al.*, 1983; Beaver *et al.*, 1985; Cheng *et al.*, 1992; Coyle, 1995); there has been much less investigation into the effect of different protocols on the determination of Tlac. Therefore the aim of this study was to compare the exercise intensity associated with lactate threshold derived from three different protocols – continuous incremental, discontinuous incremental and ramp.

Exercise intensity associated with a blood lactate threshold has been used by numerous investigators to predict the performance ability of endurance cyclists (for review see Coyle, 1995). In the present study Tlac occurred at approximately $55\%RMP_{max}$ which is lower than that found for professional cyclists (Mujika and Padilla, 200; Lucia *et al.*, 2002) but equivalent to amateur racing cyclists (Lucia *et al.*, 2002). The $\%HR_{peak}$ at Tlac was higher than the value reported by Yoshida (1984) for eight healthy male students (72 vs 58% respectively) but lower than that reported for elite male on- and off road cyclists (86 %, 85%; Wilber *et al.*, 1997) and professional cyclists (84%, Padilla *et al.*, 2000). In the present investigation, Tlac occurred at about 60% $\dot{V}O_{2\,max}$. This was markedly higher than values reported by Massé-Biron *et al.* (1992), Yoshida (1984) and Yoshida *et al.* (1987) for non-cyclists (49, 36 and 40%, respectively), but slightly lower than recorded for professional cyclists (77%, Mujika and Padilla, 2001) or elite on- and off-road cyclists (77%, 80%; Wilber *et al.*, 1977). Although we have made comparisons here with several other studies, there should be some caution in interpreting the results of these comparisons, as none of these studies used exactly the same protocol or method of determination of Tlac. For example Yoshida *et al.* (1987) used a 25 W·min$^{-1}$ incremental test with arterial blood sampled at 1-min intervals compared to the 4-min discontinuous (1-min rest) incremental used by Padilla *et al.* (2000).

The ramp rate chosen in this study was much lower than that for most other ramp studies (15-50 W·min$^{-1}$) (Heck *et al.*, 1985; Hughson *et al.*, 1987; Campbell *et al.*, 1989) except for Campbell *et al.* (1989) who used a 8 W·min$^{-1}$ ramp in one of their protocols. To the authors' knowledge Campbell *et al.* (1989) are the only group that has examined the effect of different ramp rates on blood lactate concentration. They did not make any comparison of Tlac across protocols as the principal focus of that study was to demonstrate that there was no threshold, rather a continuous increase in lactate. However, examination of Figure 1 of their results reveals that for a fixed 4 mmol·l$^{-1}$ lactate concentration the steeper ramp (50 W·min$^{-1}$) resulted in a higher $\dot{V}O_2$ (~4.4 l·min$^{-1}$) compared to the 8 W·min$^{-1}$ (~3.9 l·min$^{-1}$) step. The overall rate of increase in the workload was similar for the ramp and continuous incremental protocols in this study (6 W·min$^{-1}$), yet we found significantly higher absolute and relative power, HR and $\dot{V}O_2$ at both Tlac and OBLA. With the inclusion of the rest period the overall rate of increase in workload for the discontinuous protocol was lower (4.8 W·min$^{-1}$) than the other two protocols, thereby increasing the total test duration. Comparing incremental and discontinuous protocols, this did not affect absolute power and HR at Tlac, agreeing with Weltman *et al.* (1990). In contrast, the inclusion of the 1-min rest in the incremental resulted in a higher absolute and relative power and $\dot{V}O_2$ at OBLA, which somewhat disagrees with Heck *et al.* (1989), who found no differences in treadmill velocity at OBLA for 0.5, 1 and 1.5 min rest periods during an incremental protocol.

A unique aspect of this study was the frequent (every minute) sampling for lactate, affording greater detail in the blood lactate concentrations from each protocol. Previous studies using incremental protocols only measured lactate at the end of each stage and the only other authors that have used ramp protocols have only measured every 2 or 3 min (Lucia *et al.*, 2002b). Figures 1 and 2 from the ramp and continuous incremental protocols protocol show a relatively smooth exponential curve with very little indication of an inflection beyond a shift from baseline values. The discontinuous protocol (Figure 3) shows a radically different profile where in the early workloads the lactate concentration falls during the 4-min stage and then for the final workloads rises all the way through the stage. This has major implications for the method of determination and may explain the slightly different inter-protocol trends between the Tlac and OBLA determination. Previous studies have shown that stages of a longer duration tend to result in lower workloads at Tlac (Yoshida, 1984; Heck *et al.*, 1985; Bentley *et al.*, 2001). Obviously, a longer stage would result in a greater rise in lactate in these final stages and result in a steeper rise in values measured at the end of each stage, possibly exaggerating any deflection in the curve or causing the fixed 4 mmol·l$^{-1}$

concentration to be reached at an earlier workload. This is the first study reporting this pattern of lactate concentration during a discontinuous test and this would indirectly support the view (Hughson *et al.*, 1987; Campbell *et al.*, 1989) that during a ramp protocol there is a continuous rise in blood lactate whereas a clear Tlac inflection may be a consequence of an incremental protocol.

In conclusion, this study has demonstrated differences in both absolute and relative power, HR and $\dot{V}O_2$ at Tlac and OBLA across three different protocols. Therefore great care must be taken when comparing lactate threshold values produced from different protocols. The relationship between performance and lactate thresholds determined from different protocols is an important factor that warrants further investigation.

## REFERENCES

Antonutto, G. and Di Prampero, P.E., 1995, The concept of lactate threshold. *Journal of Sports Medicine and Physical Fitness*, **35**, 6-12.

Beaver, W.L., Wasserman, K. and Whipp, B.J., 1985, Improved detection of lactate threshold during exercise using a log-log transformation. *Journal of Applied Physiology*, **59**, 1936-1940.

Bentley, D.J., McNaughton, L.R. and Batterham, A.M., 2001, Prolonged stage duration during incremental cycle exercise: effects on the lactate threshold and onset of blood lactate accumulation. *European Journal of Applied Physiology*, **85**, 351-357.

Bird, S.R. and Davison, R.C.R., 1997, *BASES Guidelines for the Physiological Testing of Athletes*, (Leeds: BASES).

Campbell, M.E., Hughson, R.L. and Green, H.J., 1989, Continuous increase in blood lactate concentration during different ramp exercise protocols. *Journal of Applied Physiology*, **66**, 1104-1107.

Cheng, B., Kuipers, H., Snyder, A.C., Keizer, H.A., Jeukendrup, A. and Hesselink, M., 1992, A new approach for the determination of ventilatory and lactate thresholds. *International Journal of Sports Medicine*, **13**, 518-522.

Coyle, E.F., 1995, Integration of the physiological factors determining endurance performance ability. In *Exercise and Sport Sciences Reviews*, edited by Holloszy, J.O. (Baltimore: Williams & Wilkins), pp. 25-64.

Farrell, P.A., Wilmore, J.H., Coyle, E.F., Billing, J.E. and Costill, D.L., 1993, Plasma lactate accumulation and distance running performance. *Medicine and Science in Sports and Exercise*, **25**, 1091-1097.

Heck, H., Mader, A., Hess, G., Mucke, S., Muller, R. and Hollmann, W., 1985, Justification of the 4-mmol/l lactate threshold. *International Journal of Sports Medicine*, **6**, 117-130.

Hughson, R.L., Weisiger, K.H. and Swanson, G.D., 1987, Blood lactate concentration increases as a continuous function in progressive exercise. *Journal of Applied Physiology*, **62**, 1975-1981.

Lucia, A., Hoyos, J., Santalla, A., Perez, M. and Chicharro, J.L., 2002a, Kinetics of $\dot{V}O_2$ in professional cyclists. *Medicine and Science in Sports and Exercise*, **34**, 320-325.

Lucia, A., Rivero, J.L., Perez, M., Serrano, A.L., Calbet, J.A., Santalla, A. and Chicharro, J.L., 2002b, Determinants of $\dot{V}O_2$ kinetics at high power outputs during a ramp exercise protocol. *Medicine and Science in Sports and Exercise*, **34**, 326-331.

Masse-Biron, J., Mercier, J., Collomp, K., Hardy, J.M. and Prefaut, C., 1992, Age and training effects on the lactate kinetics of master athletes during maximal exercise. *European Journal of Applied Physiology*, **65**, 311-315.

Mujika, I. and Padilla, S., 2001, Physiological and performance characteristics of male professional road cyclists. *Sports Medicine*, **31**, 479-487.

Myers, J. and Ashley, E., 1997, Dangerous curves. A perspective on exercise, lactate, and the anaerobic threshold. *Chest*, **111**, 787-795.

Padilla, S., Mujika, I., Orbananos, J. and Angulo, F., 2000, Exercise intensity during competition time trials in professional road cycling. *Medicine and Science in Sports and Exercise*, **32**, 850-856.

Stegmann, H., Kindermann, W. and Schnabel, A., 1981, Lactate kinetics and individual lactate threshold. *International Journal of Sports Medicine*, **2**, 160-165.

Weltman, A., 1995, *The Blood Lactate Response to Exercise*, (Champaign: Human Kinetics).

Weltman, A., Snead, D., Stein, P., Seip, R., Schurrer, R., Rutt, R. and Weltman, J., 1990, Reliability and validity of a continuous incremental treadmill protocol for the determination of lactate threshold, fixed blood lactate concentrations, and $\dot{V}O_2$max. *International Journal of Sports Medicine*, **11**, 26-32.

Wilber, R.L., Zawadzki, K.M., Kearney, J.T., Shannon, M.P. and Disalvo, D., 1997, Physiological profiles of elite off-road and road cyclists. *Medicine and Science in Sports and Exercise*, **29**, 1090-1094.

Yeh, M.P., Gardner, R.M., Adams, T.D., Ynowitz, F.G. and Crapo, R.O., 1983, "Anaerobic threshold": problems of determination and validation. *Journal of Applied Physiology*, **55**, 1178-1186.

Yoshida, T., 1984, Effect of exercise duration during incremental exercise on the determination of anaerobic threshold and onset of blood lactate accumulation. *European Journal of Applied Physiology*, **53**, 196-199.

Yoshida, T., Chida, M., Ichioka, M. and Suda, Y., 1987, Blood lactate parameters related to aerobic capacity and endurance performance. *European Journal of Applied Physiology*, **56**, 7-11.

# 6 A Rowing Protocol to Determine Lactate Threshold

J.J. Forsyth[1] and T. Reilly[2]
[1]Sport and Exercise Sciences, North East Wales Institute
of Higher Education, Plas Coch, Mold Road, Wrexham, LL11,
2AW, North Wales
[2]Research Institute for Sport and Exercise Sciences, Liverpool John
Moores University, Henry Cotton Campus, 15-21 Webster Street,
Liverpool, L3 2ET, UK

## 1. INTRODUCTION

Lactate parameters have been successfully used to assess and predict endurance performance (Farrell *et al.,* 1979; Bishop *et al.,* 1998), to prescribe specific training intensities (Londeree, 1997), and to measure adaptations to training (McLellan and Cheung, 1992). Variables that could influence the validity and reliability of a test to measure blood lactate concentration include protocol, mode of exercise, and methods of detecting a "threshold".

A common protocol to predict endurance performance, and to estimate a maximal lactate steady state (MLSS), defined as the point at which lactate production exceeds lactate clearance (e.g. Heck *et al.,* 1985), is a 3-min, multi-stage, incremental test (Yoshida, 1984; Weltman *et al.,* 1990; Bishop *et al.,* 1998; Jones and Doust, 1998). A stage duration of only 3 min appears to be appropriate, if the lactate threshold ($T_{lac}$) or MLSS is determined by changes in lactate when plotted against exercise intensity, rather than by fixed blood lactate concentrations (Heck *et al.,* 1985; Smith *et al.,* 1997; Bourgois and Vrijens, 1998). A protocol of this nature has the advantage that it can be carried out in a relatively short amount of time on a single testing occasion.

Few protocols have been used to ascertain lactate variables using rowing ergometers such as the Concept II (Nottingham, UK). Womack *et al.* (1989) used a discontinuous protocol with a starting intensity equivalent to a 500-m split time of 2:30 (min:s) with a reduction of 5 s every 3 min to measure the exercise intensity at a fixed blood lactate concentration of 4 mmol.l[-1]. However, a decrease in 500-m split time by 5 s does not produce equal increments in power output (measured in watts) since resistance on the rowing ergometer varies indirectly with speed to the power 1.95 (Calentano *et al.,* 1974), designed to reflect the action of normal rowing. Since other protocols for assessing lactate variables during cycle ergometry and treadmill exercise use proportional increases in power output (e.g. Weltman *et al.,* 1990), this should also be the case when using a rowing ergometer. It seems that the reliability and suitability of a protocol using the Concept II rowing ergometer to measure blood lactate concentration are yet to be established.

The most conventional method of determining $T_{lac}$ is to plot blood lactate concentration against a variable such as power output or oxygen consumption

($\dot{V}O_2$), and to determine visually the point at which lactate increases in a curvilinear or exponential fashion above resting levels (Green *et al.*, 1983; Yoshida *et al.*, 1987). Several mathematical models have been proposed to assist in the visual determination of the "threshold", the most common being a plot of the log $\dot{V}O_2$ against log lactate (Beaver *et al.*, 1985; Myers *et al.*, 1994; Smith *et al.*, 1997), and the $D_{max}$ method described by Cheng *et al.* (1992) and supported by Bishop *et al.* (1998). Fixed blood lactate concentrations of 2.0 and 4.0 mmol·l⁻¹ (Mader *et al.*, 1976; Heck *et al.*, 1985), or the onset of blood lactate accumulation (OBLA) (Sjödin and Jacobs, 1981) are also commonly used. Although using fixed blood lactate concentrations to determine $T_{lac}$ might be suitable for measuring adaptations to training (Londeree, 1997), concern has been expressed over their usefulness for representing MLSS (Bourgois and Vrijens, 1998; Jones and Doust, 1998), or distinguishing differences between individuals (Stegmann *et al.*, 1981). Furthermore, there is potential for errors due to alterations in nutritional and training status (Hughes *et al.*, 1982; Yoshida, 1984), and as previously stated, due to changes in stage duration (Smith *et al.*, 1997).

The aim of this investigation was, therefore, to establish the reliability of a continuous, multi-stage, 3-min, incremental test protocol on the Concept II rowing ergometer for assessing $T_{lac}$, as detected by a variety of commonly used methods. A protocol needs to be reliable, so that changes occurring with training, or diet, for instance, can be assessed.

## 2. METHODS

Eight subjects volunteered and gave their informed consent to take part in the study. All subjects were male, with a mean (±SD) age of 26.1 (±4.3) years, height of 1.79 (±0.04) m and body mass of 84.7 (±12.8) kg. Subjects were trained athletes, who were accustomed to using the Concept II rowing ergometer (Model C, Nottingham, UK). The study was approved by the Human Ethics Committee at Liverpool John Moores University.

Subjects were tested on 3 separate occasions at the same time of day within a 2-week period, under the same experimental conditions. A minimum of three days separated trials to allow for adequate recovery. An additional testing session was carried out, in order to familiarise the subjects fully with the procedures, and to determine the protocol that would be used on the three occasions. Subjects were required to refrain from strenuous physical activity, to avoid alcohol and to ensure adequate food intake and hydration prior to testing. Physical activity 48 h and dietary intake in the 24 h prior to each session were recorded, and replicated on the 3 occasions.

Subjects warmed up for 5 min at an intensity equivalent to between 50% and 60% of maximum oxygen consumption ($\dot{V}O_{2max}$). This intensity and the initial intensity of the protocol were determined on an individual basis during the familiarisation visit, and selection was based on protocols described by others (Weltman *et al.*, 1990; Jones and Doust, 1998). After the warm-up, subjects rested for 5 min, remaining seated. The mean initial intensity for the protocol was 113.5±11.5 (range 120–153) W, which equated to 55.1±6.3% $\dot{V}O_{2max}$, relative to body mass. The intensity was then increased by 18.4±1.2 W (corresponding to an increase in mean $\dot{V}O_2$ of 4.03±0.98 ml.kg$^{-1}$min$^{-1}$) every 3 min, until subjects reached volitional exhaustion or were unable to maintain the required power output. Subjects were encouraged to keep stroke rate between 24 and 32 strokes.min$^{-1}$. The lever was set according to recommendations by Hahn *et al.* (2000), with the setting for lightweight males being 3, and heavyweight males being 4. Therefore, both resistance and oxygen uptake were related to body size.

Capillary blood (20 µl) was removed from the toe tip during the last 20 s of each increment, as well as prior to exercise, and at 1, 5 and 10 min post-exercise. Removing blood from the toe enables the subject to carry on rowing, without interruption to the protocol (Forsyth and Farrally, 2000). Samples were assessed immediately from whole-blood using an Accusport lactate analyser (Boehringer Mannheim GmbH), reported as being highly reliable for both intra and inter-day assessments (Bosquet *et al.*, 1998).

Ventilatory variables were assessed using an on-line, open-circuit gas analyser (Aerosport TEEM 100, Ann Arbor, Mich, USA), calibrated prior to exercise with known concentrations of gas, and by a 3-l syringe (GDX Corporation). The medium flow pneumotachograph was used. Heart rate (HR) was monitored throughout via short-range telemetry (Cardiosport Excel Sport PC), and perceived exertion (RPE) (Borg, 1970) was rated at the end of each increment.

Methods used to detect $T_{lac}$ included a) the log–log model ($T_{lac-log}$) reported by Beaver *et al.* (1985); b) the $D_{max}$ method (Cheng *et al.*, 1992); c) visual method ($T_{lac-vis}$) and d) the fixed blood lactate concentration of 4.0 mmol.l$^{-1}$ ($T_{lac}$-4 mM). The $T_{lac-log}$ method requires plots of log lactate against the log of the variable assessed, in this instance log power output, log $\dot{V}O_2$, log HR and log RPE. The data points were divided into two segments, and the division point between them was determined visually as the point where the steep portion of the curve begins. Each segment, below and above the division point, was fitted using a linear regression equation (1.1),

$$\log Y = a + b \log X \qquad (1.1)$$

where $Y$ is blood lactate concentration and $X$ is the selected variable (VO$_2$, HR, power output and RPE). The solution for the threshold was determined by the intersection of the two lines, hence

$$\log (X) = (a_1 - a_2)/(b_2 - b_1) \qquad (1.2)$$

where $a_1$ and $a_2$ is the intercept, and $b_1$ and $b_2$ is the slope of the linear segments below and above the division point.

For the $D_{max}$ method, third order polynomial regressions of the variables used ($\dot{V}O_2$, HR, power output and RPE) against blood lactate concentration were determined. The slope of the straight line formed by the two endpoints of each curve was calculated, and $D_{max}$ was defined as the maximal perpendicular distance from the curve to the straight line.

The $T_{lac-vis}$ method involved plotting blood lactate concentration against power output, and was defined as the highest exercise intensity before a curvilinear increase in blood lactate concentration occurred. Since an error in the lactate assay using Accusport was found by Bosquet *et al.* (1998) to be ±0.34 mmol.l$^{-1}$, an increase of more than this was required for $T_{lac-vis}$ determination. Two independent observers were consulted, with a third observer used, if the initial two observers were not in agreement as to where $T_{lac-vis}$ occurred. Plots were coded to avoid investigator bias. This threshold was also described according to $\dot{V}O_2$, HR, RPE and blood lactate concentration. For $T_{lac}$-4 mM determination, plots of blood lactate concentration against all variables were drawn and values were extrapolated from the curve. Ventilatory threshold ($T_{vent}$) was also determined and defined as the exercise intensity at which there was an increase in the ventilatory equivalent for oxygen ($\dot{V}E/\dot{V}O_2$) without a corresponding increase in $\dot{V}E/\dot{V}CO_2$ (Caiozzo *et al.*, 1982), assessed visually when plotted against time.

Test–retest reliability of the lactate thresholds using the four different methods ($T_{lac-log}$, $D_{max}$, $T_{lac-vis}$, $T_{lac}$-4 mM) and $T_{vent}$ were assessed independently using a repeated measures ANOVA, and a Pearson product moment correlation analysis. Limits of agreement for repeated measures (Bland and Altman, 1986) were also determined between trials 1 and 2, 2 and 3, and 1 and 3. All methods of analysis for determining a threshold were compared using a repeated measured ANOVA and paired t-tests. The level of significance was set at $p=0.05$.

## 3. RESULTS

Subjects completed between 5 to 10 stages of the protocol, with mean test duration being 20.0±4.21 min. Mean $\dot{V}O_{2\,max}$ for all trials was 4.01±0.58 (range 2.97–5.00) l.min$^{-1}$, which equated to relative values of 48.2±9.0 (range 36.1–63.2) ml.kg$^{-1}$.min$^{-1}$. Mean maximum HR (HR$_{max}$) was 181±11 (range 164–204) beats.min$^{-1}$ and mean maximum power output was 235.5±36.9 (range 173.2–304.4) W. Final stage blood lactate concentration was 6.7±1.7 mmol.l$^{-1}$ with a range of 3.8 to 10.6 mmol.l$^{-1}$. Values for $\dot{V}O_{2\,max}$, HR$_{max}$, maximum power output and end-stage and post-exercise blood lactate concentration did not differ significantly between the three trials.

Analysis of variance revealed no significant differences ($p>0.05$) between the 3 trials for any of the 4 methods used to detect $T_{lac}$, when the threshold was described using power output, $\dot{V}O_2$ and RPE. There were also no significant differences between trials when using $T_{vent}$. When using HR to describe $T_{lac}$, the $T_{lac-vis}$ method showed significant differences between trials ($p=0.008$). Mean HR at $T_{lac-vis}$ was lowest on the third trial, compared to the first and second trials (Table 1.1). Other methods ($T_{lac}$-4 mM, $D_{max}$, $T_{lac-log}$ and $T_{vent}$) showed no significant differences when using HR as the variable (Table 1).

Generally, correlations between trials were strongest when power output was the variable used to describe the threshold. For instance, the $D_{max}$ method showed significant correlations between the 3 trials ranging from $r=0.88$ to $r=0.99$. Correlations were also high and significant for the $T_{lac}$-4 mM method, ranging from $r=0.82$ to $r=0.94$, and for $T_{vent}$ ($r=0.80$ to $r=0.96$). Correlations were generally weaker for the other two methods, $T_{lac-vis}$ and $T_{lac-log}$. The $D_{max}$ method showed good agreement between trials for power output and HR. For instance, limits of agreement for power output at $D_{max}$ between trials 1 and 2 ranged from $-15.9$ W to $+7.2$ W, lower than the actual mean increment used in the protocol of 18.4±1.2 W. Standard error of differences was 2.0 W and the confidence interval for bias was

−9.2 to +0.4 W between these two trials. Limits of agreement for the other three methods were much wider. For instance, limits of agreement for power output at $T_{lac-log}$ between trials 1 and 3 ranged from −84.1 W to +65.4 W. Generally limits of agreement were better between trials 1 and 2 than between trials 2 and 3, and agreement between trials 2 and 3 was better than between trials 1 and 3. Limits of agreement for HR at $D_{max}$ ranged from −14 beats.min$^{-1}$ to +3 beats.min$^{-1}$ between trials 1 and 2, −23 beats.min$^{-1}$ to +23 beats.min$^{-1}$ between trials 1 and 3, and from −16 beats.min$^{-1}$ to +27 beats.min$^{-1}$ between trials 2 and 3. Again, agreement for HR using the other methods was not as good. For instance limits of agreement for HR at $T_{lac}$-4 mM ranged from −62 beats.min$^{-1}$ to +49 beats.min$^{-1}$. The widest limits of agreement for $\dot{V}O_2$ were when using the $T_{lac-log}$ method between trials 1 and 3 (−1.90 to +1.57 l.min$^{-1}$), and the narrowest were for $T_{lac}$-4 mM between trials 1 and 2 (−0.69 to +0.82 l.min$^{-1}$).

**Table 1.** Mean (±SD) of variables at $D_{max}$, $T_{lac-vis}$, $T_{lac}$-4 mM, $T_{lac-log}$ and $T_{vent}$ for each of the 3 trials.

| Power Output (W) | Trial 1 | Trial 2 | Trial 3 |
|---|---|---|---|
| $D_{max}$ | 184.3 (35.0) | 188.6 (31.8) | 184.1 (25.7) |
| $T_{lac-vis}$ | 181.6 (32.3) | 186.7 (24.0) | 174.4 (31.4) |
| $T_{lac}$-4 mM | 198.7 (48.3) | 195.0 (54.7) | 202.6 (44.9) |
| $T_{lac-log}$ | 183.0 (34.8) | 191.4 (31.3) | 192.3 (31.9) |
| $T_{vent}$ | 177.6 (29.3) | 171.3 (26.0) | 183.9 (34.7) |
| **HR (beats.min$^{-1}$)** | | | |
| $D_{max}$ | 159 (18) | 165 (17) | 159 (7) |
| $T_{lac-vis}$ | 161 (14) | 162 (16) | 149 (15) |
| $T_{lac}$-4 mM | 157 (31) | 164 (16) | 163 (12) |
| $T_{lac-log}$ | 161 (17) | 165 (18) | 158 (10) |
| $T_{vent}$ | 159 (15) | 154 (18) | 154 (17) |
| **$\dot{V}O_2$ (l.min$^{-1}$)** | | | |
| $D_{max}$ | 3.27 (0.57) | 3.25 (0.66) | 3.26 (0.48) |
| $T_{lac-vis}$ | 3.13 (0.64) | 3.14 (0.54) | 2.95 (0.54) |
| $T_{lac}$-4 mM | 3.11 (1.30) | 3.27 (0.84) | 3.49 (0.68) |
| $T_{lac-log}$ | 3.17 (0.74) | 3.17 (0.72) | 3.33 (0.47) |
| $T_{vent}$ | 3.06 (0.67) | 2.89 (0.59) | 3.14 (0.68) |
| **RPE** | | | |
| $D_{max}$ | 14.5 (1.3) | 14.7 (1.3) | 14.1 (1.8) |
| $T_{lac-vis}$ | 12.5 (2.9) | 13.6 (2.4) | 12.1 (2.0) |
| $T_{lac}$-4 mM | 11.8 (5.7) | 13.9 (3.5) | 14.6 (3.1) |
| $T_{lac-log}$ | 13.2 (1.3) | 14.3 (2.6) | 13.5 (2.8) |
| $T_{vent}$ | 12.1 (3.1) | 12.0 (1.9) | 12.9 (1.8) |
| **Lactate (mmol.l$^{-1}$)** | | | |
| $D_{max}$ | 3.6 (0.7) | 3.9 (0.7) | 3.6 (0.7) |
| $T_{lac-vis}$ | 3.5 (0.8) | 3.8 (0.8) | 3.3 (0.5) |
| $T_{lac}$-4 mM | 4.04 (0.1) | 4.0 (0.0) | 4.0 (0.0) |
| $T_{lac-log}$ | N/A | N/A | N/A |
| $T_{vent}$ | 3.9 (1.7) | 3.6 (0.6) | 3.7 (0.9) |

The four methods used to determine $T_{lac}$ did not differ significantly ($p>0.05$) from one another, when power output, $\dot{V}O_2$, HR and RPE were used to describe the threshold (Table 2). The blood lactate concentrations at $D_{max}$ and $T_{lac-vis}$ were significantly lower than blood lactate concentration at $T_{lac}$-4 mM ($p=0.03$ and $p=0.005$ respectively). Mean power output for all three trials at $T_{vent}$ was significantly lower than mean power output at $T_{lac}$-4 mM and $T_{lac-log}$ ($p<0.05$), but was not significantly different from mean power output at $T_{lac-vis}$ ($p=0.49$), or $D_{max}$ ($p=0.31$). Mean HR at $T_{vent}$ was significantly lower ($p<0.05$) than that at $T_{lac-log}$ and mean RPE at $T_{vent}$ was significantly lower than mean RPE at $D_{max}$ and $T_{lac-log}$.

Table 2. Mean ($\pm$SD) of variables for all 3 trials for the 5 different methods used to attain a threshold.

| | Power Output (W) | $\dot{V}O_2$ (l.min$^{-1}$) | HR (beats.min$^{-1}$) | RPE | Lactate (mmol.l$^{-1}$) |
|---|---|---|---|---|---|
| $D_{max}$ | 185.7 ($\pm$29.8) | 3.26 ($\pm$0.55) | 161 ($\pm$14) | 14.4 ($\pm$1.4) | 3.7 ($\pm$0.7) |
| $T_{lac-vis}$ | 180.9 ($\pm$28.6) | 3.08 ($\pm$0.56) | 158 ($\pm$15) | 12.8 ($\pm$2.4) | 3.5 ($\pm$0.7) |
| $T_{lac}$-4 mM | 198.7 ($\pm$47.4) | 3.29 ($\pm$0.95) | 161 ($\pm$21) | 13.4 ($\pm$4.3) | 4.0 ($\pm$0.2) |
| $T_{lac-log}$ | 188.9 ($\pm$31.5) | 3.22 ($\pm$0.63) | 162 ($\pm$15) | 13.7 ($\pm$2.3) | N/A |
| $T_{vent}$ | 177.6 ($\pm$29.3) | 3.03 ($\pm$0.63) | 156 ($\pm$16) | 12.3 ($\pm$2.3) | 3.7 ($\pm$1.1) |

## 4. DISCUSSION

The purpose of the study was to determine reliability of the selected rowing protocol for detecting $T_{lac}$ using five different methods. From analysis of the data, it appears that using power output at $D_{max}$ to describe the threshold was the most reliable method for this protocol. There were no significant differences between trials, there were strong correlations ranging from $r=0.88$ to $r=0.99$, and limits of agreement, especially between the first two trials, were narrow. The most variable method when using power output to describe the threshold appeared to be the $T_{lac-log}$ method. These findings are not that surprising when considering that one of the aims of developing the $D_{max}$ method was to assess $T_{lac}$ in a reliable way (Cheng *et al.*, 1992). In the study of Cheng *et al.*, the test–retest correlation coefficient for blood lactate concentration at $D_{max}$ was $r=0.86$ and correlations were also strong for the other variables assessed ($\dot{V}E$, breathing frequency and $\dot{V}CO_2$). In the present study, correlations for HR and power output at $D_{max}$ were similar, ranging from $r=0.88$ to $r=0.99$, although correlations for $\dot{V}O_2$ and blood lactate concentration at $D_{max}$ were weaker. When devising and analysing the $T_{lac-log}$ method, focus has been on the accuracy of the best fit of the model (Beaver *et al.*, 1985; Hughson *et al.*, 1987; Myers *et al.*, 1994). The reliability of the $T_{lac-log}$ method on repeat tests has not been a primary concern. Hughson *et al.* (1987) commented that reproducibility of using the $T_{lac-log}$ method was 'far from perfect'. Hence, although the $T_{lac-log}$ method might be more accurate for describing or fitting the data, the use of the $D_{max}$ method appears more reliable when trials are repeated.

Generally power output was the most reliable variable to describe $T_{lac}$ using any of the five methods. In contrast, the least reliable was RPE due to greater variability in responses by subjects between trials. In studies where the reliability of RPE under identical conditions has been assessed, values of around $r=0.70$ have been found (Skinner *et al.*, 1973; Wenos *et al.*, 1996) with limits of agreement reported as being wide (Lamb *et al.*, 1999). As expected, when using RPE as a variable to describe $T_{lac}$, values were unreliable.

In comparing the four methods of $T_{lac}$ detection ($T_{lac-log}$, $D_{max}$, $T_{lac-vis}$, $T_{lac}$-4 mM), mean power output and $\dot{V}O_2$ were higher using the $T_{lac}$-4 mM method than the other three methods, and were lowest using the $T_{lac-vis}$ method (Table 1.2). This is consistent with findings of Bishop *et al.* (1998) in a comparison of the four methods. Similarly, Jones and Doust (1998) found velocity and HR at $T_{lac}$-4 mM to be significantly higher than those at $T_{lac-vis}$, and Yoshida *et al.* (1987) reported $\dot{V}O_2$ at $T_{lac}$-4 mM to be significantly higher than $\dot{V}O_2$ at $T_{lac-vis}$. The four methods, therefore, produce different values for $T_{lac}$, and may indicate different phenomena, or may represent different durations of endurance performance. This study did not attempt to relate the four methods to performance, although this is one of the reasons for determining $T_{lac}$. For this purpose, $T_{lac-vis}$ is the method often used. For instance, in a study by Jones and Doust (1998), strong correlations ($r=0.93$) were found between treadmill velocity at $T_{lac-vis}$ and 8-km running performance. Yoshida *et al.* (1987) found $T_{lac-vis}$ to correlate strongly with 12-min running performance. Similarly, $T_{lac}$-4 mM has been found to correlate with performance. Farrell *et al.* (1979) reported that a running velocity corresponding to $T_{lac}$-4 mM correlated more highly ($r=0.91$) with running performance (between 3.2 km and 42.2 km) than did $\dot{V}O_{2\,max}$ ($r=0.83$). However, the use of $T_{lac}$-4 mM to assess performance has been criticised. In work by Stegmann and Kindermann (1982), 5 of the 19 subjects tested could not complete 50 min of continuous cycling at an intensity equivalent to $T_{lac}$-4 mM, stopping after only 14 to 16 min. Similarly, other studies have shown that $T_{lac}$-4 mM cannot be used to establish steady state intensity or to predict time to exhaustion (Bourgois and Vrijens, 1998). The $T_{lac-log}$ and $D_{max}$ methods have been designed to improve the detection of $T_{lac}$. Although the $T_{lac-log}$ method is commonly used to determine a threshold (Jones and Doust, 1998; Moquin and Mazzeo, 2000), how the threshold relates to performance has not been specifically investigated. In a comparison of the various methods, Bishop *et al.* (1998) found the $D_{max}$ method was more highly correlated with endurance cycling lasting 60 min than were the $T_{lac}$-4 mM, $T_{lac-log}$ and $T_{lac-vis}$ methods. More research is required to determine whether the $D_{max}$ method, which appears reliable for repeat tests, is the most appropriate method for assessing a range of endurance performances.

There are practical limitations associated with the four methods. The $T_{lac-vis}$ is assessed subjectively via observers and with some of the plots a threshold, defined as the point where a curvilinear increase in blood lactate concentration occurs, was difficult to detect. This was either because no such increase occurred, or there appeared to be more than one point. In this study, a third investigator was used for 12 of the 24 plots when determining $T_{lac-vis}$, due to lack of agreement between the first two. The $T_{lac-log}$ method also requires the use of an observer to determine the division point subjectively, and as such, is no more sophisticated than the $T_{lac-vis}$ method. Lundberg *et al.* (1986) devised a computerised approach to determine the division point for $T_{lac-log}$, whereby the overall residual sum of squares is minimised. However, mean results of $T_{lac-log}$ assessed subjectively and objectively were very similar and did not differ significantly. Visual assessment of the log–log plots may, therefore, not improve the accuracy or reliability of $T_{lac}$ detection. For two of the trials $T_{lac}$-4 mM could not be determined correctly. For one subject on one of the trials, blood lactate concentration throughout the test was elevated, and on the first stage of the test exceeded 4 mmol.l$^{-1}$. For another subject in one of the trials, final stage blood lactate concentration was only 3.8 mmol.l$^{-1}$. The fixed value of 4 mmol.l$^{-1}$ is therefore unsuitable for all subjects, and may not be useful for rowing performance, since net lactate concentration differs due to changes in lactate dynamics as a consequence of adding the arms. For instance, Weltman *et al.* (1994) reported that $T_{lac\text{-}vis}$ occurred at a lower exercise intensity during rowing than during running. The $D_{max}$ method, in contrast to the other three methods, avoids the need for an observer and does not require a fixed value that must be met for all subjects.

The intention of the study is not to question why the $T_{lac}$ occurs or if a threshold, in the true sense of the word, occurs at all. Morton *et al.* (1994) claimed that using models to fit data in order to detect a threshold should be regarded with caution, since the models are phenomenological; they model the data, rather than considering why the data are produced. The word threshold is used here to be consistent with other research, and does not necessarily imply that there is a definite breakpoint in the data marking a transition from predominantly aerobic to anaerobic processes. Nor does it suggest that there is a change in lactate production and elimination.

The ventilatory threshold has often been used as a practical and non-invasive method of indicating $T_{lac}$ (Wasserman *et al.*, 1973; Caiozzo *et al.*, 1982). Ventilatory threshold usually occurs before the point associated with an increase in blood lactate concentration (Yeh *et al.*, 1983). In this study, $T_{vent}$ was also found to occur at a significantly lower exercise intensity than that at $T_{lac}$ assessed using $T_{lac}$-4 mM and $T_{lac\text{-}log}$ methods (Table 2). Glycogen depletion (through diet or training) results in a shift of $T_{lac}$ but not $T_{vent}$ (Hughes *et al.*, 1982). It has, therefore, been suggested that changes in ventilatory variables and blood lactate concentration are due to different underlying mechanisms (Walsh and Bannister, 1988). Despite this, correlations between power output at $T_{vent}$ and $T_{lac}$ (using the four methods) were strong and significant, and as Jones and Doust (1998) suggested, $T_{vent}$ can be used as a practical method to support $T_{lac}$ determination.

Based on the results of this study, power output at $D_{max}$ is the most reproducible method of attaining $T_{lac}$ when using a 3-min incremental rowing protocol. The $D_{max}$ method of assessing $T_{lac}$, as well as being reliable, has been found to correlate more highly with 60-min endurance performance than when using the $T_{lac}$-4 mM, $T_{lac\text{-}log}$ and $T_{lac\text{-}vis}$ methods (Bishop *et al.*, 1998). A further advantage of the $D_{max}$ method is that, unlike the $T_{lac\text{-}vis}$ and $T_{lac\text{-}log}$ methods, it does not require a subjective assessment of $T_{lac}$.

## REFERENCES

Beaver, W.L., Wasserman, K. and Whipp, B.J., 1985, Improved detection of lactate threshold during exercise using a log–log transformation. *Journal of Applied Physiology*, **59**, 1936–1940.

Bishop, D., Jenkins, D.G. and MacKinnon, L.T., 1998, The relationship between plasma lactate parameters, Wpeak and 1-h cycling performance in women. *Medicine and Science in Sports and Exercise*, **30**, 1270–1275.

Bland, J.M. and Altman, D.G., 1986, Statistical methods for assessing agreement between two methods of clinical measurement. *Lancet*, **i**, 307–310.

Borg, G., 1970, Perceived exertion as an indicator of somatic stress. *Scandinavian Journal of Rehabilitation and Medicine*, **2-3**, 92–98.

Bosquet, L., Mercier, D. and Léger, L., 1998, Validité de l'analyseur de lactate portatif Accusport™. *Science and Sports,* **13**, 138–141.

Bourgois, J. and Vrijens, J., 1998, Metabolic and cardiorespiratory responses in young oarsmen during prolonged exercise tests on a rowing ergometer at power outputs corresponding to two concepts of anaerobic threshold. *European Journal of Applied Physiology*, **77**, 164–169.

Caiozzo, V.J., Davis, J.A., Ellis, J.F., Azus, J.L., Vandagriff, R., Prietto, C.A. and McMaster, W.C., 1982, A comparison of gas exchange indices used to detect the anaerobic threshold. *Journal of Applied Physiology*, **53**, 1184–1189.

Calentano, F., Cortili, B.G., Di Prampero, P.E. and Cerretelli, P., 1974, Mechanical aspects of rowing. *Journal of Applied Physiology*, **36**, 642–647.

Cheng, B., Kuipers, H., Snyder, A.C., Keizer, H.A., Jeukendrup, A. and Hesselink, M., 1992, A new approach for the determination of ventilatory and lactate thresholds. *International Journal of Sports Medicine*, **13**, 518–522.

Farrell, P.A., Wilmore, J., Coyle, E., Billing, J. and Costill, D., 1979, Plasma lactate accumulation and distance running performance. *Medicine and Science in Sports and Exercise*, **11**, 338–344.

Forsyth, J.J. and Farrally, M.F., 2000, A comparison of lactate concentration in plasma collected from the toe, ear and fingertip after a simulated rowing exercise. *British Journal of Sports Medicine*, **34**, 35–38.

Green, H.J., Hughson, R.L, Orr, G.W. and Ranney, D.A., 1983, Anaerobic threshold, blood lactate and muscle metabolites in progressive exercise. *Journal of Applied Physiology*, **54**, 1032–1038.

Hahn, A., Bourdon, P. and Tanner, R., 2000, Protocols for the physiological assessment of rowers. In *Physiological Tests for Elite Athletes*, edited by Gore, C.J. (Champaign, IL: Human Kinetics), pp. 311–326.

Heck, J., Mader, A., Hess, G., Mücke, S., Müller, R. and Hollman, W., 1985, Justification of the 4–mmol/l lactate threshold. *International Journal of Sports Medicine*, **6**, 117–130.

Hughes, E.F., Turner, S.C. and Brooks, G.A., 1982, Effects of glycogen depletion and pedaling speed on anaerobic threshold. *Journal of Applied Physiology*, **52**, 1598–1607.

Hughson, R.L., Weisiger, K.H. and Swanson, G.D., 1987, Blood lactate concentration increases as a continuous function in progressive exercise. *Journal of Applied Physiology*, **62**, 1975–1981.

Jones, A.M. and Doust, J.H, 1998, The validity of the lactate minimum test for determination of the maximal lactate steady state. *Medicine and Science in Sports and Exercise*, **30**, 1304–1313.

Lamb, K.L., Eston, R.G. and Corns, D., 1999, Reliability of ratings of perceived exertion during progressive treadmill exercise. *British Journal of Sports Medicine*, **33**, 336-339.

Londeree, B.R., 1997, Effect of training on lactate/ventilatory thresholds: a meta-analysis. *Medicine and Science in Sports and Exercise*, **29**, 837–843.

Lundberg, M.A., Hughson, R.L., Weisiger, K.H. Jones, R.H. and Swanson, G.D., 1986, Computerized estimation of lactate threshold. *Computers and Biomedical Research*, **19**, 481–486.

Mader, A., Liesen, H., Heck, H., Philippi, H., Rost, R., Schürch, P. and Hollman, W., 1976, Zur Beurteilung der Sportartspezifischen Ausdauerleistungsfähigheit im Labor. Sportarzt Sportmedizin, 27, 108-112.

McLellan, T.M. and Cheung, K.S.Y., 1992, A comparative evaluation of the IAT and the critical power. *Medicine and Science in Sports and Exercise*, **24**, 543–550.

Morton, R.H., Fukuba, Y., Banister, E.W., Walsh, M.L., Kenny, C.T.C. and Cameron, B.J., 1994, Statistical evidence consistent with two lactate turnpoints during ramp exercise. *European Journal of Applied Physiology*, **69**, 445–449.

Moquin, A. and Mazzeo, R.S., 2000, Effect of mild dehydration on the lactate threshold in women. *Medicine and Science in Sports and Exercise*, **32**, 396–402.

Myers, J., Walsh, D., Buchanan, N., McAuley, P., Bowes, E. and Froelicher, V., 1994, Increase in blood lactate during ramp exercise: comparison of continuous and threshold models. *Medicine and Science in Sports and Exercise*, **26**, 1413–1419.

Sjödin, B. and Jacobs, I., 1981, Onset of blood lactate accumulation and marathon running performance. *International Journal of Sports Medicine*, **2**, 23–26.

Skinner, J.S., Hutsler, R., Bergsteinova, V. and Buskirk, E.R., 1973, Validity and reliability of a rating scale of perceived exertion. *Medicine and Science in Sports*, **5**, 94–96.

Smith, E.W., Skelton, M.S., Kremer, D.E., Pascoe, D.D. and Gladden, L.B., 1997, Lactate distribution in the blood during progressive exercise. *Medicine and Science in Sports and Exercise,* **29**, 654–660.

Stegmann, H. and Kindermann, W., 1982, Comparison of prolonged exercise tests at the individual anaerobic threshold and the fixed anaerobic threshold of 4 mmol.l$^{-1}$ lactate. *International Journal of Sports Medicine*, **3**, 105.

Stegmann, H., Kindermann, W. and Schnabel, A., 1981, Lactate kinetics and individual anaerobic threshold. *International Journal of Sports Medicine*, **2**, 160–165.

Walsh, M.L. and Banister, E.W., 1988, Possible mechanisms of the anaerobic threshold: a review. *Sports Medicine*, **5**, 269–302.

Wasserman, K., Whipp, B.J., Koyal, S.N. and Beaver, W.L., 1973, Anaerobic threshold and respiratory gas exchange during exercise. *Journal of Applied Physiology*, **35**, 236–243.

Weltman, A., Snead, D., Stein, P., Seip, R., Schurrer, R., Rutt, R. and Weltman J., 1990, Reliability and validity of a continuous incremental treadmill protocol for the determination of lactate threshold, fixed blood lactate concentrations and $VO_2$max. *International Journal of Sports Medicine*, **11**, 26–32.

Weltman, A., Wood, C.M., Womack, C.J., Davis, S.E., Blumer, J.L., Alvarez, J., Sauer, K. and Gaesser, G.A., 1994, Catecholamine and blood lactate responses to incremental rowing and running exercise. *Journal of Applied Physiology*, **76**, 1144–1149.

Wenos, D.L., Wallace, J.P., Surburg, P.R. and Morris, H.H., 1996, Reliability and comparison of RPE during variable and constant exercise protocols performed by older women. *International Journal of Sports Medicine*, **17**, 193-198.

Womack, C.J., Davis, S.E., Wood, C.M., Alvarez, K., Sauer, A., Weltman, A. and Gaesser, G.A., 1989, The blood lactate response during rowing ergometry as a predictor of rowing performance. *Medicine and Science in Sports and Exercise,* **21**, S122.

Yeh, M.P. Gardner, R.M., Adams, T.D., Yanowitz, F.G. and Crapo, R.O., 1983, 'Anaerobic threshold'; problems of determination and validation. *Journal of Applied Physiology*, **55**, 1178–1186.

Yoshida, T., 1984, Effect of exercise duration during incremental exercise on the determination of anaerobic threshold and the onset of blood lactate accumulation. *European Journal of Applied Physiology*, **53**, 196–199.

Yoshida, T., Chida, M., Ichioka, M. and Suda, A., 1987, Blood lactate parameters related to aerobic capacity and endurance performance. *European Journal of Applied Physiology*, **56**, 7–11.

# Part II
# PAEDIATRIC SCIENCE

# 7 Identifying Maturational Levels During Adolescence: A Methodological Problem

Isabel Fragoso[1], Marcos Fortes[2], Filomena Vieira[1]
and Luísa Canto e Castro[3]
[1]Faculty of Human Kinetics, Technical University of Lisbon,
Portugal
[2]Federal Centre of Technological Education Celso Suckow da
Fonseca, Rio de Janeiro-Brazil
[3]Faculty of Sciences, University of Lisbon, Portugal

## 1. INTRODUCTION

In theory, only those athletes with an ideal body shape will be able to be successful competitively. Although this seems theoretically simple, for adolescent performers, especially for elite young athletes, the confirmation is obviously difficult. Their physical characteristics are dependent on growth and maturation and one of the most important motor features, strength, is also dependent on LBM (lean body mass) which depends also on the maturation level. Motor skill levels and physical fitness tend to be optimised during adolescence but the onset and termination of this period may vary so much between boys and between girls as to hide their real physical capacity. The description of morphological events during adolescence, was systematized by Tanner (1962). However, it was only at the end of the 1960s that the complex hormonal physiology of pubertal events began to be better understood, above all because of the possibility of measuring hormonal concentrations with new techniques. There are today many ways to measure biological age but a methodology that can precisely divide adolescence in categories others than prepubescent, pubescent and after puberty is missing.

Knowing that the effects of different physical exercise programmes during growth depend on each body/organism, namely on its morphological characteristics and growth stage, the aim of our study was to evaluate different methods of maturation assessment in order to find one that can identify biological age, and that can also guarantee a fine differentiation among individuals, especially during adolescence.

## 2. METHODS

Altogether, 51 individuals aged between 8 and 18 years, who were members of the Marina Club Swimming Schools of Rio de Janeiro, Brazil were assessed in this study. Anthropometric measures were obtained according to Fragoso and Vieira (2000) and included weight, height, BMI, skeletal index, sitting height, arm span, arm length, leg length, biacromial and biiliocristal breadth, biepicondylar humerus and femur and stylion ulnar breadth, biceps, triceps, subscapular, iliac crest, abdominal, thoracic, axillary, thigh and medial calf skinfolds, arm, forearm, wrist, waist, gluteal (hip), thigh and mid-thigh, calf and ankle girths. Somatotype was calculated following the Heath-Carter method (1967) and body fat (%) was estimated by means of the equations of Slaughter *et al.* (1988). Lean body mass was calculated by subtracting fat body mass from the total body mass. The hand and wrist radiographs of 51 children were analysed by one experienced paediatric radiologist blinded to the chronological age of the subjects. Maturational measures consisted of bone maturation, assessed according to Greulich and Pyle (1959), and of sexual characteristics observed according to the classification of self-evaluation of Tanner (1962). The pubic hair was observed for both sexes (P1-P5), and genital (G1-G5) and breast development (M1-M5) just for boys and girls respectively. We used three sex maturational groups: (1) when the sum of the level of genitalia and pubic hair development is between 3 and 6; (2) when the sum of the level of genitalia and pubic hair development is equal to "7 and 8"; (3) when the sum of the genitalia and pubic hair is equal or superior to "9". We can observe in Table 1 that, according the stipulated sex maturational groups, almost all the boys' sample was classified within two very distant and distinct sex maturational groups (the first and the third). Therefore we can only use these ways of classification to differentiate girls' sex maturation.

**Table 1.** Total number of boys and girls in each level of genitalia and pubic hair development.

| Girls | | Breast Development | | | | |
|-------|-------|---|---|---|---|---|
| Public Hair | Level | 1 | 2 | 3 | 4 | 5 |
| | 1 | 4 | | | | |
| | 2 | 1 | 3 | | | |
| | 3 | | | 2 | | |
| | 4 | | | 4 | 3 | 3 |
| | 5 | | | | 1 | 1 |

| Boys | | Penis Development | | | | |
|------|-------|---|---|---|---|---|
| Pubic Hair | Level | 1 | 2 | 3 | 4 | 5 |
| | 1 | 3 | 5 | | | |
| | 2 | | 3 | | | |
| | 3 | 1 | 1 | | | |
| | 4 | | | 1 | 9 | 2 |
| | 5 | | | | 1 | 1 |

Another way to assess maturation level is through the hormone levels of IGF-I, IGFPB-3 and leptin. Blood was collected in the morning after at least a 6-hour fast. All the analyses were accomplished at the Laboratório Sérgio Franco. Serum

IGF-I, IGFBP-3, and plasma leptin concentrations were determined by immuno-radiometric assay.

For statistics, we used the SPSS program, version 11.0 for Windows. Descriptive statistics (mean values, standard deviation) were performed for all the sample and for each variable. The main goal was to determine a discriminant function that clearly separated the individuals according to their sex maturation category. Among all variables, X-ray bone age revealed the strongest discriminating power and so we thought it important to obtain a good prediction model to use in cases where this variable is not known. To achieve this objective we developed linear models for X-ray bone age and for the difference between X-ray bone age and chronological age. With a sample size of only 22 and 28 elements and such a long list of covariates, overfitting and co-linearity must be carefully analyzed. We calculated the intercorrelation for each group of variables (hormones, linearity, robustness, and fat related variables) and the correlation of each one with "age difference" and "bone age". We expected to reduce the dimensionality and find good representation for each group of variables, not losing those most related to "age difference" and "bone age". Statistical methodologies of classification and discrimination, proposed by Breiman *et al.* (1984) and by McLachlan (1992), were used and the best were obtained in order to limit any error of misclassification as low as possible. With this in mind, we divided the female sample into three sex maturation (sexmat) categories as indicated above. As already noted, this analysis could not be applied to the boys' sample because the number of subjects in each category was not well distributed.

## 3. RESULTS AND DISCUSSION

After determining the difference between X-ray bone age and chronological age, some preliminary analyses were performed. The results obtained strongly suggest a separate study for each sex. In Figure 1 it can be seen that 50% of the female sample presents less than one year of difference between bone and chronological age (quite symmetrically on both directions of the mean) while the central 50% of the boys' sample exceeded a negative difference of one year and a half and showed a mean variance of about 6 months. We can also observe that the female sample had a much smaller overall variability.

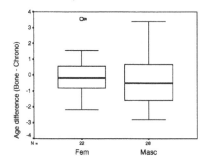

**Figure 1**. Box-Plots for age difference in both sexes.

In Tables 2 and 3 the observed mean and standard deviation values are revealed. The sample has a mean age around 12 years, the girls being one year older. However, boys were taller, had longer legs and longer arms. The girls weighed more and were fatter. The mean leptin hormone values were very similar to others reported by Bideci *et al.* (2002) and Andrade *et al.* (1995).

**Table 2.** Means and Standard Deviations of Age and Maturation Indicators.

| | Male (N=28) | | Female (N=22) | |
| --- | --- | --- | --- | --- |
| | Mean | SD | Mean | SD |
| Maturation Indicators | | | | |
| IGF1, ng.ml$^{-1}$ | 373.714 | 213.601 | 398.636 | 151.232 |
| IGFBP3, ng.ml$^{-1}$ | 4.573 | 1.034 | 4.750 | 0.974 |
| Leptin, ng.ml$^{-1}$ | 3.371 | 2.714 | 7.018 | 4.604 |
| Age | | | | |
| X-Ray (Bone age) | 11.839 | 3.577 | 13.091 | 3.127 |
| Chronological Age | 11.714 | 2.692 | 12.727 | 2.694 |

First, we looked for highly correlated variables hoping to reduce the dimensionality. The correlation matrix and the corresponding proximity tree showed that hormone concentration in male and female groups were only moderately correlated and therefore all the variables were retained in the hormone group. For the linearity group, there were larger intercorrelations so we chose one or two as representatives. The first one was "sitting height" in the female group and "height" in the male group as they had the highest correlation with "age diff" and "bone age", and as a second choice we had "leg or arm length" because they were less correlated with the first ones.

Finally, for the fat-related variables, we cut through the second level of the proximity tree, and selected as representative variables of this group "triceps", "thigh", "abdominal", "calf" and "biceps" for girls, and "axillary", "thoracic", "biceps", "calf and subscapular" for boys, reducing from nine to five variables the number of skinfolds for each sex group. According to the correlation matrix and dendrogram we selected "calf", wrist", "ankle", "waist" and "mid-thigh" girths were selected for the female group and "calf", "wrist", "waist", "mid-thigh", "ankle", "stylion-ulnar" and "biiliocristal" breadth for the male group.

A stepwise method was used to adjust a linear regression model for "age difference". The variables chosen for each group of variables (hormones, linearity, robusteness, and fat related variables) were obtained assuming that all the covariates could enter in the full model (Table 4).

With only four covariates – mid-thigh, ankle girths, triceps and calf skinfolds – almost 70% of the variability of the observed "age difference" in the female group was explained. If the model is well adjusted, predicted values would have a standard error of around 8 months.

**Table 3.** Means and standard deviations of anthropometric, body composition and somatotype measures.

| | Male (N=28) | | Female (N=22) | |
| --- | --- | --- | --- | --- |
| | Mean | SD | Mean | SD |
| Mass, kg | 48.882 | 14.322 | 48.291 | 9.719 |
| Height, m | 1.586 | 0.180 | 1.554 | 0.117 |
| BMI (kg / m$^2$) | 18.970 | 1.960 | 19.784 | 1.996 |
| Skelic Index | 94.323 | 11.576 | 91.980 | 6.226 |
| Sitting height | 0.817 | 0.093 | 0.811 | 0.069 |
| Arm span | 1.636 | 0.203 | 1.585 | 0.123 |
| Arm length | 0.713 | 0.090 | 0.691 | 0.052 |
| Leg length | 0.769 | 0.106 | 0.744 | 0.058 |
| Skinfolds, mm | | | | |
| Biceps | 6.732 | 3.632 | 9.091 | 3.692 |
| Triceps | 12.321 | 5.006 | 15.909 | 4.532 |
| Thigh | 15.518 | 5.379 | 19.886 | 4.892 |
| Calf | 12.450 | 4.174 | 16.205 | 5.342 |
| Subscapular | 8.357 | 3.082 | 10.545 | 4.251 |
| Axilar | 7.929 | 4.386 | 9.591 | 4.978 |
| Thoracic | 8.143 | 4.849 | 6.477 | 3.145 |
| Iliac crest | 8.975 | 4.630 | 12.341 | 4.917 |
| Abdominal | 12.536 | 6.288 | 16.477 | 5.086 |
| Girths, cm | | | | |
| Arm | 24.239 | 2.985 | 24.436 | 2.793 |
| Forearm | 22.743 | 2.924 | 21.977 | 1.416 |
| Wrist | 15.186 | 1.529 | 14.427 | 0.732 |
| Waist | 66.893 | 5.346 | 65.514 | 4.695 |
| Gluteal (hip) | 81.882 | 8.573 | 84.914 | 8.256 |
| Thigh | 48.604 | 4.538 | 50.309 | 4.754 |
| Mid-thigh | 45.332 | 4.170 | 45.668 | 4.296 |
| Calf | 31.486 | 3.767 | 30.918 | 2.709 |
| Ankle | 20.907 | 1.957 | 20.300 | 1.373 |
| Breadths, cm | | | | |
| Biacromial | 35.804 | 4.665 | 34.500 | 2.982 |
| Biiliocristal | 25.157 | 2.884 | 25.155 | 2.184 |
| Biepicondylar humerus | 6.607 | 0.808 | 6.345 | 0.350 |
| Stylion ulnar | 5.400 | 0.496 | 5.155 | 0.698 |
| Biepicondylar femur | 9.443 | 0.577 | 9.009 | 0.540 |
| Body Composition & Somatotype | | | | |
| Fat % | 15.178 | 5.518 | 20.530 | 5.257 |
| Endomorphy | 3.663 | 1.469 | 4.809 | 1.232 |
| Mesomorphy | 5.035 | 1.115 | 4.797 | 0.990 |
| Ectomorphy | 3.439 | 1.182 | 2.818 | 1.064 |

As reported by Veldre *et al.* (2001), these variables like skinfolds and extremity girths are exactly those that most correlate with breast and pubic development which according to Eveleth and Tanner (1990) and Beunen (1993) are highly correlated with bone age. The sample size was too small for arguing about its good adjustment, but the significance of the estimates and the analysis of residuals, that we can observe below (Figure 2), strongly suggest that this subject deserves further discussion. We have just presented the analysis of residuals for one of the regression models (Model 2). In a general way, it shows the residuals analysis of the regression model from which the predicted values to be used on the discriminant functions later on are obtained.

**Table 4.** Two adjusted linear regression models for "age difference" for Girls group. The coefficients the R squared, the adjusted R squared and the SEE (standard error of estimate) for each model.

| Girls | Model 1 Coef. | Model 2 Coef. |
|---|---|---|
| (Constant) | 11.221 | -1.432 |
| Mid-thigh girth | 0.476 | 0.264 |
| Waist girth | -0.261 | - |
| Wrist girth | -1.163 | - |
| Ankle girth | - | -0.546 |
| Triceps skinfold | - | 0.152 |
| Subscapular skinfold | 0.237 | - |
| Calf skinfold | -0.102 | -0.126 |
| $R^2$ | 0.714 | 0.682 |
| Adjusted $R^2$ | 0.625 | 0.607 |
| SEE | 0.752 | 0.770 |
| PIN and POUT | .05-.10 | .05-.10 |

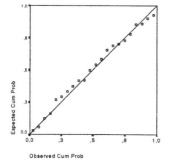 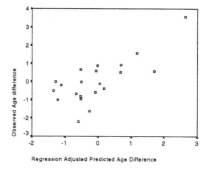

**Figure 2.** Normal P-P plot for residuals (Model 2, Girls sample) and predicted vs observed for age difference.

The same method was used to adjust three linear regression models for "bone age". The chosen variables are presented in Table 5.

Table 5. Three adjusted linear regression models for "bone age" (coefficients, R squared, adjusted R squared and SEE for each model).

| Girls | Model 3 Coef. | Model 4 Coef. | Model 5 Coef. |
|---|---|---|---|
| (Constant) | -12.574 | -13.608 | |
| Height | 18.829 | 18.630 | 9.387 |
| Subscapular skinfold | 0.177 | - | - |
| Thigh girth | 0.445 | 0.394 | - |
| Ankle girth | -1.229 | -1.087 | - |
| Calf skinfold | -0.178 | - | -0.130 |
| Leptin | - | - | 0.208 |
| Gluteal (hip) girth | - | - | 0.288 |
| Ankle girth | - | - | -0.976 |
| $R^2$ | 0.953 | 0.917 | 0.965 |
| Adjusted $R^2$ | 0.938 | 0.903 | 0.954 |
| SEE | 0.780 | 0.970 | 0.670 |
| PIN and POUT | .07-.10 | .05-.10 | .05-.10 |

With only three covariates, height, thigh and ankle girths, 92% of bone age variability can be explained and, if the model is well-adjusted, predicted values have a standard error around 11 months. Five anthropometric covariates explained 95% of bone age variability with an estimation error around 8 months. Finally, if we use the hormone group variables as covariates, the error of estimation decreases slightly (7 months). These results suggest that "age difference" is not associated with hormone variables (just slightly with leptin). Therefore, to have an estimation of "bone age" we do not need to know the serum concentrations of the hormones studied. According to Chicurel (2000), the fundamental purpose of leptin is to keep the brain informed of the "status" of energy storage in the organism. The amount of leptin segregated by the fat cells depends on their size. So it would be expected to find important associations, especially in pubescent girls, between this hormone and bone age maturation, but it seems sufficient to work with anthropometric variables.

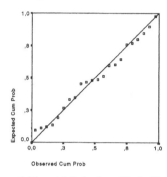
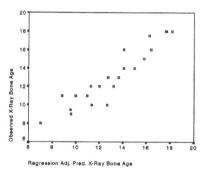

**Figure 3**. Normal P-P plot for residuals (Model 3, Girls sample) and predicted vs observed for X-ray bone age.

The sample size was small but the significance of the estimates and the analysis of residuals, shown in Figure 3 (we use the analysis of residuals of the regression Model 3), suggest that during adolescence bone age can be estimated with a small set of anthropometric variables.

The same strategy was used with the male sample. However, as boys' maturation varies much more and, as one of the 28 boys measured was 9 years old and had a bone age of 13 years, the prediction of bone age becomes more difficult and the error of estimation larger than that observed in the girls' sample. The regression models adjusted to the 28 boys to estimate their "age difference" showed an $R^2$ between 34% and 74% and a standard error between 8 and 13 months. These regression models are the result of the balance between 5 variables respectively hip girth, weight, calf skinfolds, body mass index, ankle girth, and IGF1, as shown in Table 6.

First, all the anthropometric covariates entered in the full model used an entering probability of 0.05. In this case, only the gluteal girth was chosen as an explanatory variable. Then we changed the entering probability to 0.18 and three anthropometric variables were chosen to explain age difference variability (gluteal girth, calf and sub-scapular skinfolds). This model explained 64% of the age difference variability. Finally, we took out one special case from the sample and tried to introduce hormone variables as covariates and the $R^2$ value increased to 74% (Model 4). These results differ from those already described for girls although the skinfolds and the extremity girths remained important explanatory variables. Boys had greater maturation variability and usually the difference between early and late maturers was greater than the differences between sexes. Besides, boys during puberty are particularly subject to variability in height, and height velocity and bone age velocity are poorly correlated (Benso *et al.*, 1997). Moreover, when we forced the decrease of inter-individual variability (Model 4), IGF1 was chosen as an explanatory variable which is a height-related variable (Andrade *et al.*, 1995, Gelander *et al.*, 1999, Bideci *et al.*, 2002).

**Table 6**. Four adjusted linear regression models for "age difference" – Boys sample – (coefficients, R squared, adjusted R squared and SEE for each model).

| Boys | Model 1 Coef. | Model 2 Coef. | Model 3 B | Model 4 B |
|---|---|---|---|---|
| (Constant) | -19.001 | -9.996 | -8.999 | -6.929 |
| Gluteal (hip) girth | 0.310 | 0.118 | 0.105 | 0.19 |
| Calf skinfold | - | -0.0848 | - | - |
| Subscapular skinfold | -0.192 | - | - | - |
| Weight | -0.108 | - | - | - |
| BMI | - | - | - | -0.308 |
| Ankle girth | - | - | - | -0.191 |
| IGF1 | - | - | - | 0.0016 |
| $R^2$ | 0.647 | 0.419 | 0.340 | 0.74 |
| Adjusted $R^2$ | 0.603 | 0.37 | 0.314 | 0.69 |
| SEE | 0.863 | 1.251 | 1.281 | 0.7856 |
| PIN and POUT | .10-.15 | .18-.20 | .05-.10 | .18-.20 |

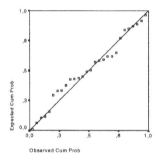 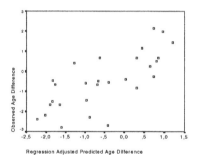

**Figure 4**. Normal P-P plot for residuals (Model 1, Boys' sample) and predicted vs observed for age difference.

Once again the sample size is small although larger than the female sample. The adjustment of Model 1 and the analysis of residuals are presented in Figure 4 and suggest a greater maturation variability as can be observed on the scatterplot of predicted values.

Finally, we adjusted five linear regression models to the boys' "bone age". Once again, we assumed all the covariates to enter in the full model except lean body mass (LBM) (Model 5), then we introduced also LBM (Model 6-9). The results show that we can estimate bone age with an error of 13, 14 months which is quite large. The best $R^2$ observed is related to Model 5 (91%), therefore, to estimate these variabilities needs five anthropometric variables namely, axillar skinfold, mid-thigh girth, height, calf skinfold and biiliocristal breadth. When using LBMl as covariate, although the $R^2$ was smaller (88%), the number of explanatory variables decreased (Model 7 and 8). Comparing the results of Model 8 and Model 9, we can say that hormone variables do not help much in the estimation of bone age variability.

**Table 7**. Five adjusted linear regression models for "bone age" – Boys sample – (coefficients, R squared, adjusted R squared and SEE for each model).

| Boys | Model 5 Coef. | Model 6 Coef. | Model 7 Coef. | Model 8 Coef. | Model 9 Coef. |
|---|---|---|---|---|---|
| (Constant) | -17.128 | 4.357 | 3.682 | -3.442 | 2.895 |
| Lean Body Mass | - | 0.219 | 0.214 | 0.163 | 0.185 |
| Axilar skinfold | -0.182 | 0.262 | 0.120 | - | - |
| Subscapular Skinfold | - | -0.237 | - | - | - |
| Mid-thigh girth | 0.25 | - | - | 0.215 | - |
| Height | 6.399 | - | - | - | - |
| Calf skinfold | -0.34 | - | - | - | - |
| Biiliocristal Breadth | 0.408 | - | - | - | - |
| IGFBP3 | | - | - | - | 0.595 |
| $R^2$ | 0.914 | 0.901 | 0.888 | 0.885 | 0.887 |
| Adjusted $R^2$ | 0.895 | 0.888 | 0.879 | 0.876 | 0.878 |
| SEE | 1.16 | 1.196 | 1.246 | 1.26 | 1.25 |
| PIN and POUT | .10-.15 | .10-.15 | .05-.10 | .10-.15 | .05-.10 |

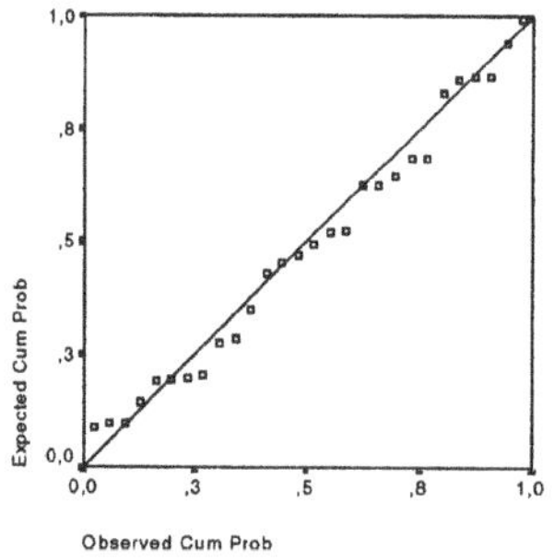

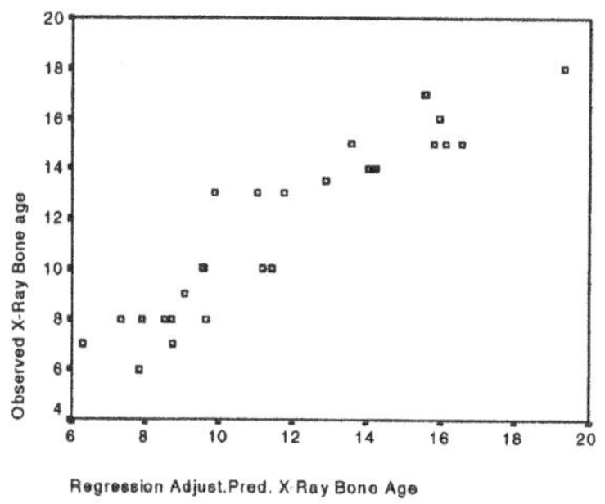

**Figure 5**. Normal P-P plot for residuals (Model 6, Boys sample) and predicted vs observed for X-ray bone age.

With the purpose of doing a discriminant analysis, the female sample was divided into three "sex maturation categories" as indicated in the methodology. We tried to discriminate the three female groups assuming all variables as covariates. This procedure was completed three times, but each time we used a different biological age. In the first discriminate model, we used the real bone age; in the second a predicted bone age which was obtained through the adjusted values of Model 1 plus decimal age; and finally we used the adjusted value from Model 5.

**Table 8.** Canonical Discriminant Function Coefficients for female sex maturation (group 1 and group 2). A - with observed bone age; B and C - with predicted values for bone age.

|  | A SEXMAT 1-2 | B SEXMAT 1-2 | C SEXMAT 1-2 |
|---|---|---|---|
| X-Ray (Bone age/Adjust bone age) | 0.589 | 0.570 | -1.523 |
| Leg length | - | - | 36.208 |
| Thigh skinfold | - | - | 0.498 |
| Mid-thigh girth | - | - | -0.344 |
| (Constant) | -7.611 | -7.430 | -2.210 |

Table 8 shows how to discriminate the two sex maturation groups. The discriminant function obtained by stepwise method in case A. for example, was $D = -7.611 + 0.589$ BA. An individual was classified in the more mature group if $D > 0$ and in the less mature group if $D < 0$.

**Table 9.** Classification results for maturation groups 1 and 2: observed group vs predicted group.

|  | A SEXMAT1 | A SEXMAT2 | B SEXMAT1 | B SEXMAT2 | C SEXMAT1 | C SEXMAT2 |
|---|---|---|---|---|---|---|
| SEXMAT1 | 6 (100%) | 0 (0%) | 6 (100%) | 0 (0%) | 6 (100%) | 0 (0%) |
| SEXMAT2 | 1 (14%) | 6 (86%) | 1 (14%) | 6 (86%) | 0 (0%) | 7 (100%) |
| correctly classified | 92% | | 92% | | 100% | |
| Cross validation | | | | | | |
| SEXMAT1 | 6 (100%) | 0 (0%) | 6 (100%) | 0 (0%) | 6 (100%) | 0 (0%) |
| SEXMAT2 | 1 (14%) | 6 (86%) | 2 (29%) | 5 (71%) | 0 (0%) | 7 (100%) |
| correctly classified | 92% | | 85% | | 100% | |

The anthropometric variables, leg length, thigh skinfold, mid-thigh girth and bone age seem to be the most important for discriminating the first two levels of maturation. The three canonical discriminant functions can discriminate between the two groups since all of them classified correctly more than 92% of all cases (Table 9). As far as girls are concerned, a discriminant function based on four anthropometric explanatory variables could classify correctly 100% of the female cases. It is particularly important that in this case we were working with adjusted bone age (Girls-Model 5). Another important conclusion is that bone age predicted by age difference can discriminate between sex maturation groups, as well as the real bone age.

**Table 10.** Canonical Discriminant Function Coefficients for female sex maturation (group 2 and 3).

|  | SEXMAT 2-3 |
|---|---|
| Sub-scapular skinfold | -1.291 |
| Thoracic skinfold | 0.894 |
| Mesomorphism | 3.387 |
| (Constant) | -7.027 |

To discriminate between categories 2 and 3 we do not need bone age but instead we need the subscapular skinfold, thoracic skinfold and to calculate girls' mesomorphy (Table 10). It is impressive how these anthropometric measures can correctly classify 100% of the female sample (Table 11). These results are in accordance with Veldre *et al.* (2001) who showed that increased mesomorphy is related to advanced stages of pubic hair development and with advanced maturation. The same author concluded that differences between skinfolds from stage M1 to M5 were twice greater than differences between age groups of 12 and 15 years old.

**Table 11.** Classification results for maturation groups 2 and 3: observed group vs predicted group.

|  | *SEXMAT2* | *SEXMAT3* |
|---|---|---|
| SEXMAT2 | 7 (100%) | 0 (0%) |
| SEXMAT3 | 0 (0%) | 5 (100%) |
| original grouped cases correctly classified | 100% | |
| SEXMAT2 | 7 (100%) | 0 (0%) |
| SEXMAT3 | 0 (0%) | 5 (100%) |
| cross-validated grouped cases correctly classified | 100% | |

Although the results are very satisfactory, it is important to confirm these findings with larger samples as well as with other predefined levels of maturation given by other categories of "sex maturation" and by other maturation indicators. This first study produced a good framework (1) to find a regression model that can offer a good evaluation and estimation of the difference between biological (bone age) and chronological age ("agedif" variable) during adolescence; (2) to discover the discriminant rules that can also guarantee a fine differentiation among individuals, especially during adolescence.

# REFERENCES

Andrade Olivie, M.A., Garcia-Mayor, R.V., Gonzalez Leston, D., Rodriguez Sousa, T., Segura Dominguez, A., Alvarez-Novoa, R. and Antelo Cortizas, J., 1995, Serum insulin-like growth factor (IGF) binding protein-3 and IGF-I levels during childhood and adolescence. A cross-sectional study. *Pediatric Research,* **38**, 149-155.

Benso, L., Vannelli, S., Pastorin, L., Benso, A., and Milani, S., 1997, Variation of bone age progression in healthy children. *Acta Paediatrica*, Suppl., **423**, 109-112.

Beunen, G., 1993, Biological maturation and physical performance, In *Kinanthropometry IV*, edited by Duquet, W. and Day, J.A.P. (London: E. & F. N. Spon), pp. 215-235.

Bideci, A., Cinaz, P., Hasanoglu, A. and Tumer, L., 2002, Leptin, insulin-like growth factor (IGF)-I and IGF binding protein-3 levels in children with constitutional delay of growth. *Journal of Pediatric Endocrinology and Metabolism,* **15**, 41-46.

Breiman, L., Friedman, J.H., Olshen, R.A. and Stone, C.J., 1984, *Classification and Regression Trees*. (California: Wadsworth, Belmont).

Chicurrel, M., 2000, Whatever happened to leptin? *Nature*, **40**, 538-540.

Eveleth, P.B. and Tanner, J.M., 1990, *Worldwide Variation in Human Growth.* (Cambridge: Cambridge University Press).

Fragoso, I. and Vieira, F., 2000, *Morfologia e Crescimento. Curso Prático.* (Cruz Quebrada: Edições FMH).

Gelander, L., Blum, W.F., Larsson, L., Rosberg, S. and Albertsson-Wikland, K., 1999, Monthly measurements of insulin-like growth factor I (IGF-I) and IGF-binding protein-3 in healthy prepubertal children: characterization and relationship with growth: the 1-year growth study. *Pediatric Research,* **45**, 377-383.

Greulich, W.W. and Pyle, S.I., 1959, *Radiographic Atlas of Skeletal Development of Hand and Wrist*. (Stanford: Standford University Press).

Heath, B.H. and Carter, J.E.L., 1967, A modified somatotype method. *American Journal of Physical Anthropology*, **27**, 57-74.

McLachlan, G. J., 1992, *Discriminant Analysis and Statistical Pattern Recognition*. (New York, Wiley).

Slaughter, M.H., Lohman, T.G., Boileau, R.A., Horswill, C.A., Stillma, R.J., Van Loan, M.D. and Bembem, D.A., 1988, Skinfold equations for estimation of body fatness in children and youth. *Human Biology*, **60**, 709-723.

Tanner, J. M., 1962, *Growth at Adolescence*, (Oxford: Blackwell Scientific Publications).

Veldre, G., Jurimae, T. and Kaarma, H., 2001, Relationships between Anthropometric Parameters and Sexual Maturation in 12- to 15-year-old Estonian Girls. In *Body Composition Assessment in Children and Adolescents*. Medicine and Sport Science, Vol. 44, edited by Jurimae, T. and Hills, A.P. (Basel: Karger), pp. 71-84.

# 8 Effects of Maximal and Sub-maximal Exercise on Growth Hormone Response in Athletic and Non-athletic Young Students

Abbas Ali Gaeini
Faculty of Physical Education and Sport Sciences,
University of Tehran, Iran

## 1. INTRODUCTION

Growth hormone (GH), as its name indicates, is responsible for stimulating growth of long bone of hands and feet. Consequently, it is the main factor regulating final height. In addition, this hormone controls the growth of lean tissues such as muscles and tendons (Sonksen, 1994; Peyreigne *et al.*, 1997), altering body composition in favour of increased lean body mass. Growth hormone also influences metabolism of carbohydrates, fats, and proteins. It increases the amount of fat consumption and mobilizes fatty acids from adipose tissue; it inhibits the entry of glucose into the muscle fibre and decreases its peripheral uptake. By increasing gluconeogensis in the liver, it influences carbohydrate metabolism (Sutton *et al.*, 1990). The most important metabolic activity of GH is stimulating the protein synthesis process. This hormone increases the level of protein synthesis in target cells (over time) (Sonksen, 1994; Borer, 1995).

Although there are no studies comparing directly anabolic steroids and GH, the effect of GH on protein synthesis process is several times greater than the effect of anabolic steroids (Sonksen, 1994).

Sleep and exercise are two of the major physiological stimulants for GH secretion (Vanhelder *et al.*, 1984; Macintyre, 1987). A few studies on the changes in GH due to exercise have been conducted (Roth *et al.*, 1963; Hunter and Greenwood, 1965; Shephard and Sidney, 1975; Sidney and Shephard, 1977; Sutton *et al.*, 1978; Kindermann *et al.*, 1982; Galbo, 1983; Bunt *et al.*, 1986; Kraemer *et al.*, 1994; Marin *et al.*, 1994; Bouix *et al.*, 1994; Borer, 1995; Eliakim *et al.*, 1998; De Vries *et al.*, 2000; Boisseau and Delamarche, 2000). It seems that this increase depends on various factors related to exercise (e.g. duration, intensity, anaerobiosis, blood lactate, hyperthermia).

Extensive research by Shephard and Sidney during the 1980s showed that exercise and physical activities were strong stimuli for GH secretion. It was concluded that the level of GH during exercise increased and this increase started earlier in high intensity activities (Shepherd and Sidney, 1975; Sidney and

Shephard, 1977). Sutton and Lazarus (1974) showed that 20 min of exercise at 75% to 90% of $\dot{V}O_{2\,max}$ resulted in GH response at a level comparable to that produced by hypoglycaemia due to insulin secretion (Macintyre, 1987).

Intensity, duration and type of exercise are the most important factors affecting GH secretion during exercise (Tanaka *et al.*, 1986). In one study, two groups of subjects with high and low work capacity exercised to exhaustion. Analysis revealed that the concentration of GH increased the same in both groups. The increase in subjects with low work capacity continued several hours after exercise (Sutton, 1978). In another study, subjects exercised under absolute and constant work (such activities are more difficult for the untrained); the increase in GH occurred only in untrained individuals (Bloom *et al.*, 1976; Sutton *et al.*, 1990). When the GH response was studied during a standard anaerobic run compared to an endurance aerobic run, it was found that GH response was significantly higher during anaerobic running (Kindermann *et al.*, 1982). It was claimed that the GH response to interval-based exercise is higher than in continuous exercise (Kozlwski *et al.*, 1983). In a subsequent study, it was shown that even if the total amounts of work performed by both type of exercise were equal, the GH response to interval exercises was greater (Vanhelder *et al.*, 1984).

Maturation-related differences in GH changes were studied in two groups of male and female subjects. The results showed that GH secretion increased with maturation. No significant difference in GH secretion was observed between the two sexes at various stage of maturation (Marin *et al.*, 1994). In another study, GH response and other hormones were studied in 56 pre-pubertal (40) and pubertal (16) subjects. The exercise-induced GH increase in pubertal children was significantly higher than in the pre-pubertal subjects. This group of children was selected from a population of children who showed growth delay (Bouix *et al.*, 1994).

Kauhanen (1990) studied GH secretion in two groups of athlete and non-athlete youths. The increase in GH secretion was significantly related to biological age rather than chronological age. Although the results of most studies show that physical exercise increases pulsatile release of GH at rest and during exercise (Peyreigne, 1997), several previous studies indicated that the level of GH during rest is not affected by exercise (McArdle *et al.*, 1991; Peyreigne *et al.*, 1997).

In general, it appears that GH response is related to personal attributes such as age, gender, physical composition and level of fitness in addition to type of exercise and environmental factors (Peyreigne, 1997; Sutton *et al.*, 1990). Although the crucial factor that causes stimulation and secretion of GH is not still known, it is evident that during exercise, probably lactic acid or change in acid-base level is a cause of GH secretion (Sutton and Lazarus, 1974).

Hansen (1971) claimed that probably two mechanisms are involved in GH secretion during exercise: 1) hormonal factors may be released locally in the muscle tissues during exercise and these factors in the blood stream will eventually affect GH control centres in the hypothalamus, 2) neural reflexes occur with blood circulation and respiration.

In explaining the low response of GH to exercise in trained individuals, it has been claimed that it is possible that during exercise alpha – adrenergic receptors are controlled. Therefore no pronounced change in GH response to exercise occurs, but by controlling the activities of beta-adrenergic receptors, GH secretion increases.

This view is accepted as the mechanism of central control of GH by some researchers (Sutton and Lazarus, 1974; Sutton *et al.*, 1976). Serotonergic neurotransmitters mediate the secretion of GH during exercise and researchers have claimed that a factor called cyproheptadine that counteracts serotonin action minimizes the secretion of GH (Smythe and Lazarus, 1974).

The aim of this research was to investigate the GH response of two groups of 15 and 17-year-old healthy athletic and non-athletic subjects expected to be at the peak level of GH- to two types of sub-maximal and maximal exercise protocols in order to examine GH response to exercise during the post-maturation period.

## 2. METHODOLOGY

### 2.1 Subjects

The subjects for this research included 91 adolescents between the age of 15 and 17 years. They were selected from two groups of athletic and non-athletic individuals.

From the total of 1076 volunteer non-athletic subjects qualified to participate in this research, 200 were randomly selected. Following careful inspection of their records collected by questionnaire for health and activity habits, 45 sedentary healthy subjects were selected as the non-athlete group (Table 1). For the athlete group, 100 adolescents athlete who were at least active for the last two years were identified through completion of a questionnaire administered to school and sport clubs.

At the second stage, a comprehensive questionnaire including education history, health status, sport and medical history was completed. Finally, 46 individuals who were active for the two previous years and exercised at least 3 time a week were selected as the athlete group (Table 1).

**Table 1**. Age of subjects in the athlete and non-athlete groups.

| Age (year) Groups | 15 | 16 | 17 | Total |
|---|---|---|---|---|
| Non-athlete | 14 | 16 | 15 | 45 |
| Athlete | 11 | 17 | 18 | 46 |
| Total | 25 | 33 | 33 | 91 |

### 2.2 Sub-maximal and maximal exercise protocols

The Bruce treadmill protocol was employed to determine the effect of physical activities on GH response. Even though this protocol has been criticized by some experts for its high increment in treadmill gradient every 3 min it was used because this protocol provides desirable maximal data (Niman, 1993). The subjects performed walking/running exercise for maximal effort. At any stage of the protocol when the subject demonstrated any sign of work intolerance (exercise fatigue, tumbling, inability to keep on with the work, paleness), the activity was terminated. In sub-maximal exercise, the modified version of this protocol was used (Hayward, 1991). The activity proceeded in a way that permitted the subjects to start the exercise protocol and if at any stage the subject's heart rate reached 150 beat.min$^{-1}$, the activity was kept constant until the subject showed signs of work intolerance. The two protocols were administered at a one-week interval; that is, in the first week sub- maximal activity and in the second week maximal activity was performed between 16:00 to 21:00 hours at a room temperature of 22°C with the humidity level 62%. For determining the GH response to the activities, 10 ml of venous blood was collected before and immediately following the termination of exercise. The blood sample was analysed immediately at a biochemistry laboratory by separating the serum and measuring the level of GH by radioimmunoassay.

## 3. RESULTS

Various statistical procedures including t-test and ANOVA were used to analyze the data. The results are as follow:

No significant difference was found between the body mass and height of athlete and non-athlete groups. There was a significant difference between the exercise responses of these two groups (Table 2).

Table 2. Means and SD of body mass, height, and exercise scores of the two groups.

| Characteristics | Athlete<br>M ±SD | Non-athlete<br>M ±SD | p-Value |
|---|---|---|---|
| Mass (kg) | 59.72 ± 8.9 | 57.9 ± 11.3 | 0.420 |
| Height (m) | 1.708 ± 0.932 | 1.6837 ± 0.07 | 0.311 |
| Exercise Score | 19.26 ± 1.33 | 17.05 ± 2.26 | 0.000 |

In the Bruce sub-maximal protocol, there were significant differences between all indices of athlete and non-athlete groups. The exception was the heart rate at the third stage (Table 3).

Table 3. Physiological indices of heart rate (beats min$^{-1}$), duration and the distance of activity in Bruce sub-maximal protocol in two groups of subjects.

| Groups<br>Indices | Athlete<br>M ±SD | Non-athlete<br>M ±SD | p-Value |
|---|---|---|---|
| Resting HR | 89±11 | 98±15 | 0.001 |
| HR end of 1$^{st}$ stage | 116±12 | 132±14 | 0.000 |
| HR end of 2$^{nd}$ stage | 130±12 | 143±10 | 0.000 |
| HR end of 3$^{rd}$ stage | 148±6 | 151±2 | 0.625 |
| HR end of 4$^{th}$ stage | 150±2 | - | - |
| Recovery HR | 103±12 | 110±12 | 0.001 |
| Duration of activity (min: s$^{-1}$) | 7:23±1:55 | 5:15±2:7 | 0.000 |
| Distance (m) | 529±174 | 356±152 | 0.000 |

In Bruce's maximal protocol, there were significant differences between the various indices of both groups in all stages (Table 4).

Maximal exercise resulted in 86.7% and 84.8% increase in GH secretion in athlete and non-athlete groups, respectively. The changes for sub-maximal exercise were 75.6% and 69.7% in athlete and non-athlete groups, respectively (Table 5), an indication of a marked effect of intensive exercise on GH secretion.

**Table 4.** Physiological indices of heart rate (beats min$^{-1}$), duration and the distance of activity in Bruce maximal protocol in two groups of subjects.

| Groups<br>Indices | Athlete<br>M ±SD | Non-athlete<br>M ±SD | P-Value |
|---|---|---|---|
| Resting HR | 86±11 | 99±12 | 0.000 |
| HR end of 1st stage | 107±11 | 129±12 | 0.000 |
| HR end of 2nd stage | 125±11 | 145±15 | 0.000 |
| HR end of 3rd stage | 148±12 | 169±15 | 0.000 |
| HR end of 4th stage | 168±12 | 187±12 | 0.000 |
| HR end of 5th stage | 184±12 | 192±9 | 0.001 |
| HR end of 6th stage | 191±9 | - | - |
| Recovery HR | 127±12 | 139±11 | 0.000 |
| Duration of activity (min: s$^{-1}$) | 14:27±1:47 | 11:40±1:56 | 0.000 |
| Distance (m) | 1300±239 | 942±334 | 0.000 |

**Table 5.** GH alteration percent (%) after maximal & sub-maximal exercises in two groups.

| Groups | Alterations<br>Exercise protocol | Increase | Decrease | No-change | Total |
|---|---|---|---|---|---|
| Non-athlete | Sub-maximal | %75.6 | %22.2 | %2.2 | %100 |
| | Maximal | %86.7 | %13.3 | - | %100 |
| Athlete | Sub-maximal | %69.3 | %28.5 | %2.2 | %100 |
| | Maximal | %84.8 | %13 | %2.2 | %100 |

Sub-maximal and maximal exercise caused significant increases in GH secretion (p<0.001, Table 6).

In addition, when the GH response due to sub-maximal and maximal exercise (M=5.35 vs. M=1.856 ng.ml$^{-1}$) was compared to the athlete group, there was a significant difference (p<0.001) between the GH responses.

The GH response to sub-maximal and maximal exercise in the non-athlete group (M=4.786 vs. M=6.342 ng.ml$^{-1}$) was significantly different (p<0.004). There was no significant difference between the GH secretion of athletes and non-athletes in response to sub-maximal and maximal exercise.

The statistical analysis performed using one and two-way analysis of variance to examine the joint effects of both groups and the type of exercise on the amount of secretion showed no significant difference between the two groups prior to exercise. The difference between the two groups after exercise was not significant. As far as the type of exercise was concerned, a significant difference (p=0.022) was found.

**Table 6**. Growth hormone (ng.ml$^{-1}$) response to maximal and sub-maximal exercise in two groups.

| Groups | Protocols | Before M±SD | After M±SD | p-Value |
|--------|-----------|-------------|------------|---------|
| Non-Athletic | Sub-maximal | 2.63±0.43 | 4.97±1.01 | 0.000 |
| | Maximal | 1.78±0.39 | 6.57±1.29 | 0.000 |
| Athletes | Sub-maximal | 2.58±0.58 | 4.44±0.98 | 0.000 |
| | Maximal | 2.45±0.32 | 7.19±1.33 | 0.000 |

## 4. DISCUSSION

The result of this study of the change in GH due to physical activities is in agreement with earlier reports showing the GH secretion increases in responses to sport activities and the more intensive the activity becomes, the greater the GH response. Therefore, it seems that sport activities regardless of being sub-maximal or maximal have a positive effect on GH secretion level. This effect is greater for maximal exercise, which means that such type of activity is a more powerful stimulus for GH secretion.

In addition, GH secretion due to maximal activity in adolescent athletes compared to non-athletes was greater while this level of secretion in sub-maximal activity in non-athletic adolescents compared to adolescent athletes was considerable. This indicates that sub-maximal activity in trained subjects is not considered a powerful stimulus for increasing GH secretion. On the other hand, since non-athlete adolescents probably are less physically fit compared to the athletic adolescents, the GH response following sub-maximal exercise was greater for them.

Meanwhile, the adolescent athletes probably could tolerate maximal exercise because of their better physical fitness. Therefore, the greater GH response in this group can be attributed to the increased duration of activity and increased work intensity. Thus, it can be concluded that:
i)   Physical activity and exercise have a positive effect on GH response.
ii)  There is a direct relation between the exercise intensity and GH response, especially in athletic adolescents.
iii) The GH response is greater in adolescent athletes during maximal exercise.

The first result of this study supports the findings of Marin *et al.* (1994) whose subjects had similar conditions and they concluded that the peak of GH secretion increases due to exercise. The main differences between the two studies were maturation classification criteria and the inclusion of sex as a variable in their research.

The second result of this study agrees with the findings of Shephard and Sydney (1975) who reported that GH levels increase during exercise, and the more intensive the exercise, the earlier this increase begins. Nauyen *et al.* (1984) also showed that GH levels following maximal exercise are greater than that of sub-maximal exercise. On the contrary, some authors observed no significant difference between GH response to exercise at various intensities (Sutton, 1978; Vanheledr *et al.*, 1984).

The third result of this study was that maximal exercise caused greater GH response in athletic adolescents while sub-maximal exercise caused greater GH response in non-athletic adolescents. This supports the results of Bunt *et al.* (1986) who found that male runners had higher levels of GH compared with a control group. Findings of two other earlier studies also support this result (Walsh *et al.*, 1984; Cheng *et al.*, 1986). On the other hand, Bloom *et al.* (1976) found greater GH response only in untrained subjects after maximal exercise. The same findings were also reported earlier by Shephard and Sydney(1975). Sutton *et al.* (1976) also found similar results in GH response between two trained and untrained groups following exhaustive exercise.

Despite extensive research conducted on the effect of sport activities on GH secretion, no significant findings have been obtained about the level of changes in GH secretion. Due to the diversity of results obtained and probable interference of other factors, generalization should be avoided. It seems that future research should aim at determining the effects of sport activities on GH secretion both in healthy individuals and patients. Also, the mechanisms associated with developing adaptability of the hypothalamic-pituitary system in GH secretion through the medium of exercise should be described.

## REFERENCES

Bloom, S.R., Johnson, R.H. Park, D.M., Rennie, M.J. and Sulaiman, W.R., 1976, Differences in the metabolic and hormonal response to exercise between racing cyclists and untrained individuals. *Journal of Physiology* (London), **258**, 1-18.

Boisseau, N. and Delamarche, P., 2000, Metabolic and hormonal responses to exercise in children and adolescents. *Sports Medicine*, **30**, 405-422.

Borer, K.T., 1995, The effects of exercise on growth. *Sports Medicine*, **20**, 375-397.

Bouix, O., Brun, J.F., Fedou, C., Raynaud, E., Kerdelhue, B., Lenoir, V. and Orsetti, A., 1994, Plasma beta-endorphin, corticotrophin and growth hormone responses to exercise in pubertal and prepubertal children. *Horm. Metab. Res.*, **26** (4), 195-119.

Bunt, J.C., Boileau, R.A., Bahr, J.M. and Nelson, R.A., 1986, Sex and training differences in human growth hormone levels during prolonged exercise, *Journal of Applied Physiology* (Bethesda), **61**, 1796-1801.

Cheng, F.E., Dodds, W.G., Sullivan, M., Kim, M.H and Malarkey, W.B., 1986, The acute effects of exercise on prolactin and growth hormone secretion: Comparison between sedentary women and women and women runners with normal and abnormal menstrual cycles. *Journal of Clinical Endocrinology and Metabolism*, **62**, 551-556.

De Vries, W.R., Bernards, N.T., de Rooij, M.H. and Koppeschaar, H.P., 2000, Dynamic exercise discloses different time related responses. *Psychosomatic Medicine*, 62, 866-72.

Eliakim, A., Brasel, J.A., Mohan, S., Wong, W.L. and Cooper, D.M., 1998, Increased physical activity and the growth hormone-IGF-I axis in adolescent males. *American Journal of Physiology*, 275, R 308-14.

Galbo, H., 1983, *Hormonal and Metabolic Adaptation to Exercise*, (NewYork: Georg Thieme Verlag).

Hansen, A.P., 1971, The effect of adrenergic receptor blockade on the exercise-induced serum growth hormone rise in normals and juvenile diabetics. *Journal of Clinical Endocrinology*, 33, 807-812.

Hayward, V.H., 1991, *Advanced Fitness Assessment & Exercise Prescription* (2nd ed). (Champaign, II: Human Kinetics).

Hunter, W.M. and Greenwood, F.C., 1965, Studies on the secretion of human pituitary growth hormone. *British Medical Journal*, 1, 804-806.

Kauhanen, H.L., 1990, Physiological performance capacity in different prepubescent athletic groups. *Sports Medicine*, 30, 57-66.

Kindermann, M.A., Schnabel, W.M., Schmitt, G., Biro, J., Cassens, A. and Weber, F., 1982, Catecholamines, growth hormone, cotisol, insulin, and sex hormones in anaerobic and aerobic exercise. *European Journal of Applied Physiology and Occupational Physiology*, 49, 389-399.

Kozlwski, S., Chwalbinskd-Moneta, J., Vigas, M., Kaciuba-Uscilko, H. and Nazar, K., 1983, Greater serum GH response to arm than to leg exercise performed at equivalent oxygen uptake. *European Journal of Applied Physiology*, 52, 131-135.

Kraemer, W.J, Gordon, S.E., Fleck, S.J., Marchitelli, L.J., Mello, R., Dziados, J.E., Friedl, K., Harman, E., Maresh, C. and Fry, A.C., 1991, Endogenous anabolic hormonal and growth factor responses to heavy resistance exercise in male and females. *International Journal of Sports Medicine*, 12, 228-235.

Macintyre, J.G., 1987, Growth hormone and athletes. *Sports Medicine*, 4, 129-142.

Marin, G.H.M., Domene, K.M., Barnes, B.J., Blackwell, F.G., Gassorla, M. and Culter, G.B., 1994, The effects of estrogen primary and puberty on the growth hormone response to standardized treadmill exercise and arginine insulin in normal girls and boys. *Journal of Clinical Endocrinology and Metabolism*, 79, 537-541.

McArdle, W.D., Katch, F.I. and Katch, V.L., 1991, *Exercise Physiology* (3rd Ed.) (Philadelphia: Lea & Febiger).

Nauyen, N.U., Wolf, J.P., Siomon, M.L., Henriet, M.T., Dumoulin, G. and Berthelay, S., 1984, Variations in circulating levels of prolactin and growth hormone during physical exercise in man: influence of the intensity of the workout. *Journal: Comptes rendus des séances de la societe de biologie et de ses filiales* (Paris), 178 (4), 450-457.

Nieman, D.C., 1993, Fitness and Your Health. (California: Bull Publishing Company).

Peyreigne, C., Brun, J.F., Monnier, J.F., Abecassis, M., Fedou, C., Raynaud, E. and Orsetti, A., 1997, Growth hormone somatomedins and muscular activity. *Science and Sports*, **12**(1), 4-18.

Roth, J., Glick, S.M., Yalow, R.S. and Berson, S.A., 1963, Secretion of human growth hormone: physiological and experimental modification. *Metabolism*, **12**, 557-559.

Shephard, R.J. and Sidney, K.H., 1975, Effects of physical exercise on plasma growth hormone and cortisol levels in human subjects. *Exercise and Sport Science Reviews*, **3**, 1-30.

Sidney, K.H. and Shephard, R.J., 1977, Growth hormone and cortisol age differences, effects of exercise and training. *Canadian Journal of Applied Sports Science*, **2**, 189-193.

Smythe, G.A., and Lazarus, L., 1974, Suppression of human growth hormone secretion by melatonin and cyproheptadine. *Journal of Clinical Investigation*, **54**, 116-121.

Sonksen, P., 1994, Growth hormone and sport. **Olympic Message 4**.

Sutton, J. and Lazarus, L., 1974, Effect of adrenergic blocking agents on growth hormone responses to physical exercise. *Horm. Metab. Res.*, **6**, 428-429.

Sutton, J.R., 1978, Hormonal and metabolic responses to exercise in subjects of high and low work capacities. *Medicine and Science in Sports*, **10**, 1-6.

Sutton, J.R., Farrell, P.A. and Harber, V.J., 1990, Hormonal adaptation to physical activity. In *Exercise, Fitness, and Health*, edited by Bouchard, C., Shephard, R.J., Stephens, T., Sutton, J.R. and McPherson, B.D. (Champaign, Illinois: Human Kinetics Books), pp. 217-259.

Sutton, J.R., Jones, N.L. and Toews, C.J., 1976, Growth hormone secretion in acid-base alterations at rest and during exercise. *Clinical Science and Molecular Medicine*, **50**, 241-247.

Tanaka, H., Shindo, M., Gutkowska, J., Kinoshita, A., Urata, H., Ikeda, M. and Arakawa, K., 1986 Effect of acute exercise on plasma immunoreactive-atrial natriuretic factor. *Life Science*, **39**, 1685-1693.

Vanhelder, W.P., Goode, R.C. and Radomski, M.W., 1984, Effects of anaerobic and aerobic exercise of equal duration and work expenditure on plasma growth hormone levels. *European Journal of Applied Physiology*, **52**, 255-257.

Walsh, B.T., Puig-Antich, J., Coetz, R., Cladis, M., Novacenko, H. and Classman, A.H., 1984, Sleep and growth hormone secretion in women athletes. *Electromyopathy and Clinical Neurophysiology (Louvain)*, **57** (6), 528-531.

# 9 Morphology and Sports Performance in Children Aged 10-13 Years: Identification of Different Levels of Motor Skills

Filomena Vieira[1], Isabel Fragoso[1], Luís Silva[1] and
Luísa Canto e Castro[2]
[1]Faculty of Human Kinetics, Technical University of Lisbon,
Portugal
[2]Faculty of Science, University of Lisbon, Portugal

## 1. INTRODUCTION

The association between morphological characteristics and motor performance has been, throughout time, the object of countless research studies. There is some correspondence between the level of participation in activities involving either body abilities or some morphological features like stature, arm span, the height of the centre of gravity, linearity, musculo-skeletal robustness and body composition (Slaughter *et al.*, 1982; Carter, 1988; Malina and Bouchard, 1991). However, there are few studies about which morphological variables better characterize successful and unsuccessful performances in different motor tests.

The aim of our work was to verify if the association between morphological characteristics and motor performance variables is identical for any level of motor performance. Therefore, we aimed to identify the contribution of each variable in the discrimination of successful and unsuccessful performances in different motor tests accomplished by children aged between 10 and 13 years.

## 2. METHODS

The sample consisted of 125 children aged between 10 and 13 years. The group studied was formed of children resident in Lisbon and attending Casa Pia of Lisbon.

Two major groups of variables were considered: anthropometric measures and motor performance tests. The former were obtained according to Lohman *et al.* (1988), which included, besides height and weight, 4 lengths (upper extremity, forearm, lower extremity and calf), 4 breadths (biacromial, biiliocristal, biepicondylar humerus, biepicondylar femur), 5 girths (thoracic (xiphoidal), arm relaxed, arm flexed and tensed, mid-thigh and calf), and 6 skinfolds (subscapular, abdominal, iliac crest, triceps, front thigh and medial calf). The sum of skinfolds (SUM SK) was used as the indicator of total fat and somatotype was assessed according to Heath-Carter's method (Heath and Carter, 1967).

Motor performance was assessed with the motor tests reported by Neto (1987). In other words, distance throw (DT), speed (SPD), precision throw (PT), strength (STG), flexibility (FLEX) and balance (BAL) were employed.

Motor variables were transformed in order to render the data symmetrical, through a Box-Cox modification from the equation (1.1):

$$y = \frac{x^P - 1}{p} \tag{1.1}$$

Due to bias of some of these variables in the estimation of the exponent of the transformation power, we opted for a robust methodology as described in Hoaglin, Mosteller and Tukey (1983). Starting from the transformed data for each motor variable, children were divided into two groups according to their level of motor performance – successful and unsuccessful. The criterion used to define these groups was mean $\pm$ SD. In other words, motor performance was classified as successful whenever the values obtained were greater than or equal to the mean + SD and classified as unsuccessful if it was less than or equal to the mean – SD.

Considering that motor variables are usually good predictors of performance in other motor tests, we created a new variable that represented the mean of general success in motor tests, which we called global performance. To do so, we normalized the results of the different tests, working with the transformed variables and not considering their absolute values but their correspondent percentile within the group analysed. In this way, the child's global performance is given by the arithmetic mean of the percentile of each motor test, being classified in the successful group when that mean was greater than or equal to percentile 75 and in the unsuccessful group when the mean of the percentiles was less than or equal to percentile 25.

Statistically, we used ANOVA and Scheffe techniques of comparison to assess the existence of significant differences among the several motor tests for each age group. Discriminant analysis (McKay and Campbell, 1982) was used to classify the individuals into successful and unsuccessful groups and to identify the variables that most condition motor performance in each motor test and for each group of motor performance.

The data were analysed in four different ways (anthropometric variables, motor variables, anthropometric and motor variables together, and somatotype variables) avoiding in the same analysis level-correlated variables. However, concerning the variables balance, speed, strength and global performance, we did not obtain results for the four levels of analysis. In some cases, none of the independent variables revealed a significant contribution according to the entrance criterion used in the stepwise method. Therefore, the tables of presentation of results for these variables just include the analysis levels that showed at least one variable with a significant discriminant contribution. The probabilities of F for entrance and exit of the stepwise were 0.05 and 0.10 for all the variables except for speed of the 12-13 year-old group where, due to the low dimension of the sample we considered as a probability of entrance 0.10, and as probability of exit 0.20.

In the statistical analysis of the data, we used the SPSS 11.0 software for Windows.

## 3. RESULTS AND DISCUSSION

The comparison of motor performance in the different tests and for the different ages revealed significant differences between the 10-11 and the 12-13 year-old groups only for speed and strength tests (Table 1). Age was not taken into account as far as flexibility, balance, distance throw and precision throw were concerned, and the results of the motor tests were globally analysed independently of age. Speed and strength tests were studied separately for both 10-11 and 12-13 years-old groups.

Research on distance throw tests showed that the variables that better explained motor performance were, independently of sex, the biepicondylar humerus and biepicondylar femur breadths (BCH and BCF), the quotient between the shoulder and hip breadths and the sum of triceps, subscapular, iliac crest and medial calf skinfolds (Nelson *et al.*, 1986), biacromial breadth and calf girth (Lopes, 1992). It seems, however, that throw task performances are strongly influenced by sexual dimorphism (Nelson *et al.*, 1986; Nelson and Thomas, 1991).

**Table 1**. Performance comparison of each motor test for each age group (levels of probability obtained according to ANOVA and Scheffe test).

| | ANOVA | SCHEFFE | |
|---|---|---|---|
| **Task** | **p value** | **Ages** | **p value** |
| **PT** | 0.506 | | |
| **DT** | 0.279 | | |
| **BAL** | 0.433 | | |
| **FLEX** | 0.392 | | |
| **SPD** | **0.004**[*] | **13 years-10 years** | **0. 028**[*] |
| | | **11 years** | **0. 007**[*] |
| | | 12 years | 0.141 |
| **STG** | **0.001**[*] | **13 years -10 years** | **0. 007**[*] |
| | | **11 years** | **0. 025**[*] |
| | | 12 years | 0.589 |

*p$\leq$ 0.05

In this research, we verified that precision throw, biepicondylar femur breadth, the sum of skinfolds and endomorphy are the variables that better classify the individuals in the successful and unsuccessful group for distance throw (Table 2). In fact, taking the discriminant analysis as an example and adopting as independent variables anthropometric and motor variables, the discriminant function according to stepwise method was:

D=-9.4+0.41PT+0.897BCF-0.019SUM SK                    (1.2)

being an individual classified in the successful group if D>0 and in the unsuccessful group if D<0.

Table 2. Canonical Discriminant Function Coefficients – Distance Throw (DT).

|  | ANT + MOT | ANT | MOT | SOM |
|---|---|---|---|---|
| PT | 0.410 | - | 0.448 | - |
| ENDO | - | - | - | -0.946 |
| BCF | 0.897 | - | - | - |
| SUM SK | -0.019 | -0.038 | - | - |
| (Constant) | -9.400 | 2.392 | -3.484 | 2.364 |

Results showed that success on distance throwing, seemed to be associated with better performances on precision throw, with low quantities of body fat and with smaller biepicondylar femur breadths.

Table 3. Classification results – Distance Throw (DT).

|  | ANT + MOT | | ANT | | MOT | | SOM | |
|---|---|---|---|---|---|---|---|---|
|  | unsuc. | suc. | unsuc. | suc. | unsuc. | suc. | unsuc. | suc. |
| Unsuccessful | 21 *91%* | 2 *9%* | 15 *65%* | 8 *35%* | 19 *83%* | 4 *17%* | 13 *57%* | 10 *44%* |
| Successful | 3 *12%* | 23 *89%* | 5 *19%* | 21 *81%* | 5 *19%* | 21 *81%* | 1 *4%* | 25 *96%* |
| Cases correctly classified | 90% | | 74% | | 82% | | 78% | |

The percentage of correct classifications in the successful and unsuccessful groups varied according to the considered group of variables, varying between 74% and 90% (Table 3). As Nelson *et al.* (1986) reported, we confirmed that the sum of skinfolds and endomorphy discriminated better the successful individuals. Lack of success on distance throw may possibly be discriminated through precision throw results.

Table 4. Canonical Discriminant Function Coefficients – Precision Throw (PT).

|  | ANT + MOT | ANT | MOT | SOM |
|---|---|---|---|---|
| BAL | 0.020 | - | 0.018 | - |
| DT | 0.199 | - | 0.230 | - |
| ENDO | - | - | - | -0.857 |
| SUM SK | -0.013 | -0.035 | - | - |
| (Constant) | -5.188 | 2.158 | -6.754 | 2.143 |

Table 5. Classification results – Precision Throw (PT).

| | ANT + MOT | | ANT | | MOT | | SOM | |
|---|---|---|---|---|---|---|---|---|
| | unsuc. | suc. | unsuc. | Suc. | unsuc. | suc. | unsuc. | suc. |
| **Unsuccessful** | 25 *86%* | 4 *14%* | 15 *52%* | 14 *48%* | 24 *83%* | 5 *17%* | 15 *52%* | 14 *48%* |
| **Successful** | 2 *7%* | 29 *94%* | 4 *13%* | 27 *87%* | 3 *10%* | 28 *90%* | 3 *10%* | 28 *90%* |
| **Cases correctly classified** | 90% | | 70% | | 87% | | 71% | |

Although we have not found studies relating to precision test performances that allow us to compare the results of this work, they seem to indicate that children with smaller amounts of fat and better performances on balance and distance throw tests (Table 4) are the ones who are successful on a precision throw. These variables discriminate correctly 70% to 90% of the individuals in the respective successful or unsuccessful group, the percentage of classifications in the successful group being greater for all the groups analysed (Table 5).

Our results indicate that precision throw and the sum of skinfolds discriminated 88% of the cases in the respective successful and unsuccessful groups in the balance test, representing 91% of the individuals correctly classified in the unsuccessful group and 86% in the successful group (Table 7). This result confirmed the conclusions of Lopes (1992) and Pissanos *et al.* (1983) who claimed that balance performance tests were positively related to age and the sum of triceps, subscapular, iliac crest, abdominal and medial calf skinfolds.

representing

Table 6. Canonical Discriminant Function Coefficients – Balance (BAL).

representing

| | ANT + MOT | MOT |
|---|---|---|
| **PT** | 0.518 | 0.465 |
| **SUM SK** | 0.019 | - |
| **(Constant)** | -5.374 | -3.756 |

Table 7. Classification results – Balance (BAL).

| | ANT + MOT | | MOT | |
|---|---|---|---|---|
| | unsuc. | suc. | unsuc. | suc. |
| **Unsuccessful** | 20 *91%* | 2 *9%* | 20 *91%* | 2 *9%* |
| **Successful** | 3 *14%* | 18 *86%* | 3 *14%* | 18 *86%* |
| **Cases correctly classified** | 88% | | 88% | |

Again, it seems that the best precision throw tests results are the ones that better discriminate successful individuals on balance tests. The sum of skinfolds was selected for the analysis only when anthropometric and motor variables were considered together. When we analysed anthropometric variables and somatotype variables separately, none of them was considered relevant to discriminate between both groups (Table 6).

Researchers have shown that flexibility is specific of each articulation and decreases with age in males, being relatively constant in females (Docherty and Bell, 1985) and is related to anthropometric measures, height being the one most frequently referred to as a decisive factor on this kind of test (Docherty and Bell, 1985; Gabbard and Tandy, 1988; Bénéfice, 1992). According to Docherty and Bell (1985) there are high correlations between balance and linearity measures which include, besides height, upper-arm, forearm, upper extremity, thigh, calf, lower extremity lengths, and cervical height.

The results obtained contradict these conclusions. They seem to denote that the more flexible children are those with less linearity, explained by the lowest values of ectomorphy, with greater calf girths and less precision on throwing (Table 8).

Table 8. Canonical Discriminant Function Coefficients – Flexibility (FLEX).

|  | ANT + MOT | ANT | MOT | SOM |
|---|---|---|---|---|
| **PT** | -0.218 | - | -0.394 | - |
| **ECTO** | - | - | - | -1.041 |
| **CALF GIRTH** | 0.428 | 0.486 | - | - |
| **(Constant)** | -11.167 | -14.375 | 2.730 | 2.621 |

Table 9. Classification results – Flexibility (FLEX).

|  | ANT + MOT | | ANT | | MOT | | SOM | |
|---|---|---|---|---|---|---|---|---|
|  | unsuc. | suc. | unsuc. | suc. | unsuc. | suc. | unsuc. | suc. |
| **Unsuccessful** | 16 *84%* | 3 *16%* | 16 *84%* | 3 *16%* | 13 *68%* | 6 *32%* | 14 *74%* | 5 *26%* |
| **Successful** | 4 *15%* | 22 *85%* | 4 *15%* | 22 *85%* | 6 *23%* | 20 *73%* | 8 *31%* | 18 *69%* |
| **Cases correctly classified** | 84% | | 84% | | 73% | | 71% | |

Considering that the percentage of cases correctly identified as successful or unsuccessful group members is equal either when we analysed the anthropometric and motor variables together, or when we only considered the anthropometric variables (Table 9), we can infer that, if only using calf girth, we can correctly identify 84% of the cases, classifying slightly better the successful group members.

The significant differences in motor performance for speed and strength tests of the 10-11 and 12-13 year-old groups seem to confirm the views of several authors including Slaughter *et al.* (1982), Pissanos *et al.* (1983), Bénéfice (1992) and Lopes (1992). They found age a significant factor in performance prediction on speed tests.

They

Table 10. Canonical Discriminant Function Coefficients – Speed (SPD).

|  | 10-11y ANT + MOT | 10-11y ANT | 10-11y SOM | 12-13y ANT + MOT | 12-13y SOM |
|---|---|---|---|---|---|
| **STRENGTH** | 0.766 | - | - | 0.492 | - |
| **TIB. MED. - SPHY. TIB.** | - | -0.389 | - | - | - |
| **BCF** | - | 3.140 | - | - | - |
| **ECTO** | - | - | 1.101 | - | - |
| **MESO** | - | - | - | - | 1.009 |
| **(Constant)** | -2.149 | -11.087 | -2.856 | -2.366 | -4.061 |

Table 11. Classification results – Speed (SPD).

|  | 10-11y ANT + MOT | | 10-11y ANT | | 10-11y SOM | | 12-13y ANT + MOT | | 12-13y SOM | |
|---|---|---|---|---|---|---|---|---|---|---|
|  | unsuc. | suc. | unsuc. | suc. | unsuc. | suc. | unsuc. | suc. | unsuc. | suc. |
| **Unsucessful** | 8 *89%* | 1 *11%* | 7 *78%* | 2 *22%* | 8 *89%* | 1 *11%* | 6 *67%* | 3 *33%* | 6 *67%* | 3 *33%* |
| **Sucessful** | 1 *10%* | 9 *90%* | 1 *10%* | 9 *90%* | 1 *10%* | 9 *90%* | 2 *33%* | 4 *67%* | 2 *33%* | 4 *67%* |
| **Cases correctly classified** | 90% | | 84% | | 90% | | 67% | | 67% | |

Bénéfice (1992) considered that age, height and arm muscle area explained 43% of the variance observed on speed tests and Lopes (1992) noted a negative association between calf girth and speed test results, possibly due to the fact that calf girth measures included the amount of fat mass negatively associated with motor performance. We confirmed in our study that among the variables that better discriminated between successful and unsuccessful groups on speed tests we could identify for the 10-11 year-old group strength, ectomorphy, tibiale mediale-sphyrion tibiale length and biepicondylar femur breadth. Through these variables, we could correctly classify 84% to 90% of children respectively in the successful and unsuccessful groups, the best classifications being for the successful group (Tables 10 and 11). It seems that stronger children with higher ectomorphy are the most successful ones as far as speed tests are concerned for younger groups. Regarding the 12-13 year-old group, the percentage of correct classifications in successful and unsuccessful groups was much lower (67%), success being related to higher mesomorphy and muscular strength.

These results can easily be explained if we note that successful motor performance on short-duration speed tests, which involve a maximum whole body engagement, necessitates anaerobic tolerance, muscular strength and coordination to ensure a high frequency of limb movement. It seems, however, that at lower ages, while coordination problems are not yet solved, low weight is more important with physical robustness becoming critical in the 12-13 year-old group. According to Komi (1992) and Sale (1988), strength training in youngsters gives rise to neuromuscular changes due, at first, to improvement in the neural system and has repercussions both on inter and intra-muscular coordination and on the reduction of antagonist muscle intervention.

Table 12. Canonical Discriminant Function Coefficients – Strength (STG).

|  | 10-11y | 12-13y | 12-13y |
|  | ANT + MOT | ANT + MOT | ANT |
|---|---|---|---|
| TIB. MED. - SPHY. TIB. | - | - | 0.45 |
| BCF | 1.890 | - | - |
| SPEED | -3.415 | -6.095 | - |
| (Constant) | -0.271 | 24.28 | -16.62 |

As expected, for any age group, stronger children are also the ones who have better results on speed tests (Table 12). Success on strength tests also seems to be related to larger bone breadths in the 10-11 year-old group, and bigger tibiale mediale-sphyrion tibiale lengths in the 12-13 year-old group. In older children, we managed to get a greater percentage of correct classifications in the successful and unsuccessful groups (92%) (Table 13).

These results may be influenced by the children's maturational level, where boys with advanced maturation had better results on strength tests (Beunen *et al.*, 1981; Freitas, 2001). Jones *et al.* (2000) found correlations of 0.73 between handgrip strength and sexual maturation in United Kingdom children and adolescents of both sexes.

Table 13. Classification results – Strength (STG).

|  | 10-11y | | 12-13y | | 12-13y | |
|  | ANT + MOT | | ANT + MOT | | ANT | |
|  | unsuc. | suc. | unsuc. | suc. | unsuc. | suc. |
|---|---|---|---|---|---|---|
| Unsuccessful | 9 75% | 3 25% | 6 86% | 1 14% | 6 86% | 1 14% |
| Successful | 1 14% | 6 86% | 0 0% | 5 100% | 1 20% | 4 80% |
| Correctly cases classified | 79% | | 92% | | 83% | |

Lastly, our data seem to show that age is the fundamental factor to differentiate successful and unsuccessful global performances (Table 14) in children. This variable enabled us to discriminate correctly 80% of children for both performance groups (Table 15).

Table 14. Canonical Discriminant Function Coefficients – Global Performance.

|  | ANT |
| --- | --- |
| AGE | 0.921 |
| (Constant) | -10.620 |

Table 15. Classification results – Global Performance.

|  | ANT | |
| --- | --- | --- |
|  | unsuc. | suc. |
| Unsucessful | 7 *78%* | 2 *22%* |
| Sucessful | 1 *17%* | 5 *83%* |
| Correctly classified cases | 80% | |

In summary, it seems that, in general, it becomes easier to discern successful children than unsuccessful ones according to the different tests. Motor and anthropometric aspects that were more often chosen as discriminant factors for both groups included precision throw, summed skinfolds, BCF, ENDO and ECTO. Our results corroborate those of Silva (2000) who claimed that the number of anthropometric and motor performance variables that contribute to the interpretation of success on certain motor tests, is smaller than the number of variables needed to explain lack of success.

Although we have found general classifications of 80-90%, it is important to confirm these results in other studies using larger samples and where children are grouped according to their motor performance and maturational level.

# REFERENCES

Bénéfice, E., 1992, Growth and motor performance of healthy Senegalese preschool children. *American Journal of Human Biology*, **4**, 717-728.

Beunen, G., Ostyn, M., Simons, J., Renson, R. and Van Gerven, D., 1981, Chronological and biological age as related to physical fitness in boys 12 to 19 years. *Annals of Human Biology*, **8**, 321-331.

Carter, L., 1988, Somatotypes of children in sports. In *Young Athletes. Biological, Psycological and Educational Perspectives*, edited by Malina, R., (Champaign, IL: Human Kinetics).

Docherty, D. and Bell, R.D., 1985, The relationship between flexibility and linearity measures in boys and girls 6-15 years of age. *Journal of Human Movements Studies*, **11**, 279-288.

Freitas, D.L., 2001, *Crescimento somático, maturação biológica, aptidão física, actividade física e estatuto sócio-económico de crianças e adolescentes madeirenses.* Phd Thesis, (Porto: FCDEF-UP).

Gabbard, C. and Tandy, R., 1988, Body composition and flexibility among prepubescent males and females. *Journal of Human Movement Studies*, **14**, 153-159.

Heath, B.H. and Carter, J.E.L., 1967, A modified somatotype method. *American Journal of Physical Anthropology*, **27**, 57-74.

Hoaglin, D., Mosteller, F. and Tukey, J., 1983, *Understanding Robust and Explanatory Data Analysis*, (Chichester: John Wiley & Sons, Inc.).

Jones, M., Hitchen, P. and Stratton, G., 2000, The importance of considering biological maturity when assessing physical fitness measures in girls and boys aged 10 to 16 years. *Annals of Human Biology*, **27**, 57-65.

Komi, P.V., 1992, *Strength and Power in Sport*, (Oxford: Blackwell Scientific).

Lohman, T.G., Roche, A.F. and Martorell, R., 1988, *Anthropometric Standardisation Reference Manual*, (Champaign, IL: Human Kinetics).

Lopes, V.P., 1992, *Desenvolvimento motor – Indicadores bioculturais e somáticos do rendimento motor em crianças de 5/6 anos.* Master Thesis, (Lisboa: FMH-UTL).

Malina, R. and Bouchard, C., 1991, *Growth Maturation and Physical Activity*, (Champaign, IL: Human Kinetics).

McKay, R.J. and Campbell, N.A., 1982, Variable selection techniques in discriminant analysis. *British Journal of Mathematical and Statistical Psychology*, **35**, 1-41.

Nelson, J.K. and Thomas, J.R., 1991, Longitudinal change in throwing performance: gender differences. *Research Quarterly for Exercise and Sport*, **62**, 105-108.

Nelson, J.K., Thomas, J.R., Nelson, K.R. and Abraham, P.C., 1986, Gender differences in children's throwing performance: biology and environment. *Research Quarterly for Exercise and Sport*, **57**, 280-287.

Neto, C., 1987, *Motricidade e Desenvolvimento. Estudo do comportamento de crianças de 5-6 anos relativo à influência de diferentes estímulos pedagógicos de habilidades fundamentais de manipulação.* PhD Thesis (Lisboa: ISEF-UTL).

Pissanos, B.W., Moore, J.B. and Reeve, T.G., 1983, Age, sex, and body composition as predictors of children's performance on basic motor abilities and health-related fitness items. *Perceptual and Motor Skills*, **56**, 71-77.

Sale, D.G., 1988, Neural adaptationto resistance training. *Medicine and Science in Sports and Exercise*, **20**, S135-145.

Silva, L., 2000, Morfologia e prestação motora em crianças dos 10 aos 13 anos de idade. Masters Thesis, (Lisboa: FMH,UTL).

Slaughter, M.H., Lohman, T.G. and Boileau, R.A., 1982, Relationship of anthropometric dimensions to physical performance in children. *Journal of Sports Medicine and Physical Fitness*, **22**, 377-385.

# 10   The Slow-component Response of $\dot{V}O_2$ to Heavy Intensity Exercise in Children

Samantha G. Fawkner and Neil Armstrong
Children's Health and Exercise Research Centre, University of
Exeter, St. Lukes, Havertree Road, Exeter, EX1 2LU, UK

## 1. INTRODUCTION

With adults, following the onset of an exercise intensity set above an individual's ventilatory threshold (Tvent), oxygen uptake ($\dot{V}O_2$) rises rapidly during a short cardiodynamic phase 1, which is followed by an exponential process that projects towards a theoretical steady state. This steady state in $\dot{V}O_2$ may not be achieved due to an additional slow component in $\dot{V}O_2$. The amplitude and nature of this slow component are dependent upon the intensity domain in which subjects exercise (Gaesser and Poole, 1996). When exercise is above the Tvent but below critical power (CP) (i.e. in the heavy-intensity domain), a steady state in $\dot{V}O_2$ will eventually be achieved (Poole et al., 1988).

The slow component response to heavy-intensity exercise in children has traditionally been investigated by setting exercise intensities with respect to $\dot{V}O_{2peak}$ and Tvent usually as a percentage of the difference between Tvent and $\dot{V}O_{2peak}$ ($\Delta$) (Armon et al., 1991; Hebestreit et al., 1998; Williams et al., 2001) but without reference to CP. Although it has been assumed that, by using these indicators, children are exercising at the same relative exercise intensity and within the same intensity domain, this has yet to be confirmed. There are currently no data that suggest that CP is sex or age independent and the slow component has not previously been investigated in children with respect to CP, the upper boundary of the heavy intensity domain. The purpose of this study was therefore to investigate the magnitude of the slow component with respect to Tvent, $\dot{V}O_{2peak}$ and CP in prepubertal children.

## 2. METHODS

### 2.1 Subjects

Eighteen pre-pubertal healthy 11-12 year old children (9 boys, 9 girls) volunteered to take part in the study. Written informed consent was obtained from subjects and their parents.    Ethical approval was granted by the local Research Ethics Committee. Subjects were not currently undertaking any regular exercise training.

## 2.2 Resting measures

Subjects visited the laboratory on at least six occasions.  Age was calculated at the date of the first exercise test. Stature was measured using a Holtain stadiometer (Holtain, Crymych, Dyfed, UK) and body mass was determined using Avery beam balance scales (Avery, Birmingham, UK) during a habituation session, in which the children were familiarised with the equipment, protocols, and experimenters. Sexual maturity was assessed visually using the indices of pubic hair described by Tanner (1962).  All observations were made by the same nurse. Exercise was carried out on the same electronically-braked cycle ergometer (Lode Excalibur Sport, Groningen, the Netherlands) with the seat height, handlebar height and crank length adapted to each child and subsequently maintained throughout the testing period.

## 2.3 Measurement of $\dot{V}O_{2peak}$ and Tvent

Both $\dot{V}O_{2peak}$ and Tvent were determined using a ramp test to voluntary exhaustion. During exercise, gas exchange variables were measured and displayed on-line using an EX670 mass spectrometer and analysis suite (Morgan Medical Ltd, Kent, UK) which was calibrated according to the manufacturers' instructions using a single calibration gas mixture (BOC, Guildford, UK), and room air.  Expired volume was measured using a turbine flow meter (Interface Associates, California, USA) with a dead space volume of 90 ml.  Volume calibration was achieved using a hand held calibration syringe (Hans Rudolph, Kansas City, USA) over a range of flow speeds. The sum of the gas transport and analyser response delay terms was determined and appropriate adjustments made in the software.  All calibration procedures were repeated prior to each experimental test.    Breath-by-breath responses were subsequently interpolated to 1-s intervals.

Following a 3-min warm-up of unloaded pedalling, the resistance increased continuously at either 10 or 15 W·min[-1] in order to attain a test approximately 8-10 min in duration.  Subjects pedalled at a cadence of $70 \pm 5$ rev·min[-1], and the children were actively encouraged to continue until voluntary exhaustion. Maximal effort was considered to have been given if, in addition to subjective indications of intense effort (e.g. excessive hyperpnea, facial flushing, sweating, discomfort), RER reached a value $> 1.00$.  All subjects satisfied these criteria.  Peak $\dot{V}O_2$ was taken as the highest recorded 10-s stationary average value during the maximal exercise test. The Tvent was determined non-invasively using the V-slope method (Tv-slope) (Beaver *et al.*, 1986; Fawkner *et al.*, 2002).

## 2.4 Constant work rate exercise tests

On subsequent visits, subjects completed a step change exercise test that consisted of 6 min of unloaded pedalling, followed instantaneously by a transitional (Tr) work rate designed to elicit 40% of the difference between the $\dot{V}O_2$ at Tv-slope and $\dot{V}O_{2\,peak}$ (40%Δ) for 10 min. A pedal cadence of 70 ± 5 rev·min$^{-1}$ was maintained throughout. Fingertip blood samples were taken immediately following the end of exercise and assayed for lactate concentration using a whole-blood automated and self-calibrating analyser (YSI 2300 Stat Plus, Yellow Springs Instruments, Ohio, USA). Heart rate (HR) was monitored using an electrocardiograph (LifePulse, HME, UK).

A single transition was completed on each visit, and at least three, but in most cases four transitions were completed in total. The responses for each individual to each rest-to-exercise transition were time aligned to the start of exercise and averaged together to form a single data set for analysis. The final 60 s of data were excluded since during this period the children's responses can be affected by pre-empting the end of the exercise test.

The duration of phase 1 was estimated from the averaged response profile, according to the methods outlined by Whipp *et al.* (1982). The following model (equation 1) was applied to the averaged response file, and parameters estimated using least squares non-linear regression analysis (Sigma Plot, Jandal Scientific, San Rafael, CA).

$$\Delta \dot{V}O_{2(t)} = A_1 \bullet \left(1 - e^{-(t-\delta_1)/\tau_1}\right) + A_2 \bullet \left(1 - e^{-(t-\delta_2)/\tau_2}\right) \ (t > \text{phase 1}) \qquad (1)$$

where: $\Delta \dot{V}O_2$ (t) is the increase in $\dot{V}O_2$ at time t above the prior control level which was calculated as the mean $\dot{V}O_2$ from the last minute of baseline pedalling; $A_1$ and $A_2$, $\tau_1$ and $\tau_2$ and $\delta_1$ and $\delta_2$ are the amplitudes, time constants and independent time delays of each exponential respectively.

The amplitude of the secondary process (A2') was assessed as the change in $\dot{V}O_2$ between $A_1$ and the $\Delta \dot{V}O_2$ tot, where $\Delta \dot{V}O_2$ tot is the total change in $\dot{V}O_2$ after 9 min (taken as the mean $\Delta \dot{V}O_2$ for the last 30s). A2' was expressed as a percentage of the $\Delta \dot{V}O_2$ tot (A2'/$\Delta \dot{V}O_2$ %) and represents the slow component.

## 2.5 Measurement of critical power (CP)

Gas exchange was not measured during CP tests. The children completed three constant load exercise tests to voluntary exhaustion in one day with at least 3 hours passive rest between tests. The prescribed power outputs were chosen in order for the length of the three tests to range between 2 and 15 min (Fawkner and Armstrong, 2002). Exercise tests were preceded by a warm up of unloaded pedalling for 2 min. The work rate was imposed instantaneously and the subject was encouraged throughout the exercise test to maintain the cadence at 70 ± 5 rev·min$^{-1}$. The test was ended when the child was no longer capable of maintaining a minimum cadence of 50 rev·min$^{-1}$ despite strong verbal encouragement. Use of the electronically braked cycle ergometer ensured that power output remained constant independent of pedal cadence throughout the exercise test. The time to exhaustion was recorded to the nearest second, and the subject continued for a further 3 min of unloaded pedalling for recovery. The same investigator carried out all tests. For each subject, CP was estimated by least squares linear regression analysis using the power-time$^{-1}$ model (Sigma Plot, Jandal Scientific, San Rafael, CA). The $\dot{V}O_2$ at CP (CP-$\dot{V}O_2$) was derived from the ramp test response profile.

## 2.6 Statistical analysis

Peak $\dot{V}O_2$ was expressed relative to body mass as a ratio (ml·kg$^{-1}$·min$^{-1}$) and as a power function ratio (PFR) (ml·kg$^{-b}$·min$^{-1}$). The 'b' exponent represents the gradient of the $\log_e$ peak $\dot{V}O_2$ (l·min$^{-1}$) – $\log_e$ body mass (kg) relationship, and was derived using log-linear analysis of covariance (ANCOVA).

The difference between the exercise intensity at 40%Δ and CP was assessed in absolute terms (watts and predicted $\dot{V}O_2$), and relative to $\dot{V}O_{2peak}$. Sex differences in the response parameters were investigated using ANOVA, and relationships amongst the response variables assessed using correlation coefficients. Significance was set at the p < 0.05 level.

## 3. RESULTS

Table 1. Physical characteristics and peak exercise responses.

|  | Boys (n=9) | Girls (n=9) |
|---|---|---|
| Age (years) | 10.8 ± 0.2 | 10.8 ± 0.3 |
| Body Mass (kg) | 35.8 ± 7.6 | 35.1 ± 4.9 |
| Stature (m) | 1.42 ± 0.09 | 1.44 ± 0.05 |
| RER at $\dot{V}O_{2peak}$ | 1.26 ± 0.06 | 1.25 ± 0.07 |
| Peak $\dot{V}O_2$ (l·min$^{-1}$) | 1.67 ± 0.29* | 1.39 ± 0.20 |
| Peak $\dot{V}O_2$ (ml·kg$^{-1}$·min$^{-1}$) | 47.0 ± 4.8* | 40.1 ± 7.9 |
| Peak $\dot{V}O_2$ (ml·kg$^{-0.54}$·min$^{-1}$) | 241.4 ± 22.8* | 197.1 ± 32.9 |
| Peak Lactate (mmol·l$^{-1}$) | 7.2 ± 1.7 | 6.5 ± 2.0 |
| Peak HR (beats·min$^{-1}$) | 201 ± 6 | 205 ± 6 |

n, number of subjects; RER, respiratory exchange ratio; $\dot{V}O_{2peak}$ oxygen uptake.
Significant sex differences * (p < 0.05)

Table 1 presents the subjects' physical characteristics and peak responses to the ramp test. The children were all stage 1 for pubic hair. The ANCOVA for $\dot{V}O_2$

peak identified a common 'b' exponent for the whole group (0.54, SE 0.10). The boys had a significantly higher $\dot{V}O_{2peak}$ expressed in absolute terms ($l \cdot min^{-1}$) relative to body mass ($ml \cdot kg^{-1} \cdot min^{-1}$) and as a PFR ($ml \cdot kg^{-0.54} \cdot min^{-1}$).

Table 2 presents the Tv-slope, CP and transitional (Tr) exercise intensity. There were no significant differences in Tv-slope as a percentage of $\dot{V}O_{2peak}$, or Tr-VO2 as a percentage of $\dot{V}O_{2peak}$. Critical power was higher in the boys than the girls, in both absolute terms, and as a percentage of $\dot{V}O_{2peak}$. Critical power was higher than the transitional exercise intensity (Tr-W) in all the boys and seven of the girls. The difference between Tr-$\dot{V}O_2$ and CP-$\dot{V}O_2$ was significantly greater in the boys than the girls.

**Table 2.** Parameters of Tv-slope, CP and the transitional (Tr) exercise intensity.

|  | Boys (n=9) | Girls (n=9) |
| --- | --- | --- |
| Tv-slope-$\dot{V}O_2$ % | 52.8 ± 6.0 | 54.5 ± 4.8 |
| Tr-$\dot{V}O_2$ % | 71.7 ± 3.6 | 72.9 ± 2.8 |
| Tr -W (W) | 74 ± 16 | 61 ± 13 |
| CP (W) | 99 ± 17* | 76 ± 12 |
| CP-$\dot{V}O_2$ ($l \cdot min^{-1}$) | 1.36 ± 0.23* | 1.06 ± 0.17 |
| CP-$\dot{V}O_2$ % | 81.8 ± 3.7* | 76.1 ± 5.1 |
| CP-Tr (W) | 15 ± 7* | 5 ± 8 |
| CP-Tr ($l \cdot min^{-1}$) | 0.17 ± 0.08* | 0.04 ± 0.10 |
| CP-Tr% | 10.1 ± 5.1* | 3.2 ± 7.2 |

Tv-slope- $\dot{V}O_2$ %, percentage of $\dot{V}O_{2peak}$ at which Tv-slope occurred; Tr-VO2%, projected transitional $\dot{V}O_2$ as a percentage of $\dot{V}O_{2peak}$; Tr-W, change in exercise intensity in watts; CP, critical power; CP-$\dot{V}O_2$, $\dot{V}O_2$ at CP; CP-$\dot{V}O_2$ %, percentage of $\dot{V}O_{2peak}$ at which CP occurred; CP-Tr, difference between the transitional power output and CP; CP-Tr%, difference between Tr-$\dot{V}O_2$ % and CP-$\dot{V}O_2$ %. Significant sex differences * ($p < 0.05$)

Table 3 presents the subjects' responses to the step change tests. The slow component was significantly greater in the girls than the boys and the HR at the end of exercise was also significantly higher in the girls.

**Table 3.** Subjects' responses to step change tests.

|  | Boys (n=9) | Girls (n=9) |
|---|---|---|
| A2'/Δ $\dot{V}O_2$ % (slow component) | 9.2 ± 2.9* | 13.1 ± 4.1 |
| Δ $\dot{V}O_2$ tot% | 78.7 ± 5.7 | 81.0 ± 3.3 |
| EEHR (beats·min⁻¹) | 179 ± 9* | 188 ± 6 |
| EELactate (mmol·l⁻¹) | 3.4 ± 0.9 | 3.8 ± 1.6 |

Δ $\dot{V}O_2$ tot%, Δ $\dot{V}O_2$ tot as a percentage of $\dot{V}O_{2peak}$; EEHR, end exercise heart rate; EELactate, end exercise blood lactate (10 min).
Significant sex differences * (p < 0.05)

Table 4 presents the linear correlation coefficients between exercise variables, and the slow component. In the boys only, a significant negative relationship between the slow component and the difference between CP- $\dot{V}O_2$ and Tr- $\dot{V}O_2$ as a percentage of $\dot{V}O_{2peak}$ was found.

**Table 4.** Linear correlation coefficients.

|  | Boys (n=9) | Girls(n=9) |
|---|---|---|
|  | $A_2$'/ΔVO$_2$% (slow component) | $A_2$'/ΔVO$_2$% (slow component) |
| CP- $\dot{V}O_2$ % | -0.470 | 0.083 |
| CP-Tr% | -0.826** | -0.182 |
| EELactate (mmol·l⁻¹) | 0.185 | 0.153 |

Significant relationship ** (p < 0.01)

accurately

## 4. DISCUSSION

Studies with adults have clearly shown that the slow component is dependent upon the relative exercise intensity at which subjects exercise (Poole *et al.*, 1988). Studies with children to date have, however, been hindered due to an inability to discern intensity domains accurately. We have therefore recently identified methods suitable for identifying the upper boundaries of both moderate and heavy intensity exercise with children, Tv-slope and CP (Fawkner *et al.*, 2002; Fawkner and Armstrong, 2002), in order to be able to investigate children's responses to exercise within well-defined domains.

In all but two of the girls, the exercise intensity corresponding to 40%Δ was below that corresponding to CP. There were no sex differences in the $\dot{V}O_2$ at Tv-slope or the transitional $\dot{V}O_2$. Therefore, as designed, with respect to $\dot{V}O_{2peak}$ and Tv-slope, the boys and girls were exercising at the same relative exercise intensity and the majority of the subjects were indeed exercising within the heavy intensity domain.

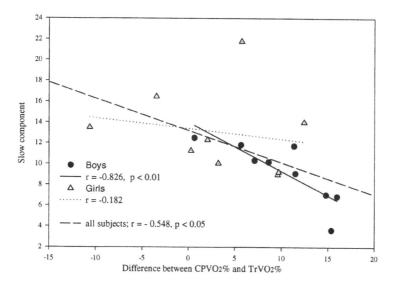

**Figure 1**. The relationship between the difference between CP- $\dot{V}O_2$ % and Tr- $\dot{V}O_2$ % and the slow component.

There were significant sex differences in CP, both in absolute terms and relative to $\dot{V}O_{2peak}$, as well as significant differences in the deviation of Tr- $\dot{V}O_2$ from CP-VO$_2$. This implies that on average, at 40%Δ the girls were exercising closer to their CP than the boys. The girls also displayed a larger slow component than the boys, and there was a strong relationship between the slow component and the difference between Tr- $\dot{V}O_2$ and CP- $\dot{V}O_2$ in the boys, although not in the girls (Figure 1). This suggests that sex differences in the slow component may be associated with the fact that the boys were exercising at a lower exercise intensity relative to CP.

Although the mechanisms controlling the slow component remain essentially elusive, current consensus suggests a predominant role of fibre type recruitment patterns and the availability of oxygen to the active muscle fibres (Gaesser and Poole, 1996; Burnley *et al.*, 2000). Equally the factors limiting CP are obscure but it is considered that they lie with the ability to utilise and deliver $O_2$ to the working muscle (Moritani *et al.*, 1981; Poole *et al.*, 1990). It does not appear that there are any studies that have considered the relationship between CP and fibre type profiles, although a reduction in $O_2$ availability by breathing hypoxic gas has been shown to reduce CP significantly with adults (Moritani *et al.*, 1981). These results may therefore be indicative of sex differences in the delivery of $O_2$ during heavy intensity exercise, but this clearly requires further examination.

We have previously demonstrated the limits of agreement within which both Tvent and CP may be estimated with children of this age (Fawkner *et al.*, 2002; Fawkner and Armstrong, 2002). The results of this study should be interpreted within the context of these limitations.

## 5. CONCLUSIONS

Assessment of CP with children has shown that at 40%Δ, children are generally exercising within the heavy intensity domain. Critical power occurs at a higher percentage of $\dot{V}O_{2peak}$ in boys than in girls and this may explain why at 40%Δ girls have a larger slow component than boys.

### Acknowledgements

We gratefully acknowledge the technical support of David Childs.
The work was supported by the National Lottery Charities Board for Health and Social Research and the Darlington Trust.

## REFERENCES

Armon, Y., Cooper, D.M., Flores, R., Zanconato, S. and Barstow, T.J., 1991, Oxygen uptake dynamics during high-intensity exercise in children and adults. *Journal of Applied Physiology*, **70**, 841-848.

Beaver, W.L., Wasserman, K. and Whipp, B.J., 1986, A new method for detecting anaerobic threshold by gas exchange. *Journal of Applied Physiology*, **60**, 2020-2027.

Burnley, M., Jones, A.M., Carter, H. and Doust, J.H., 2000, Effects of prior heavy exercise on phase II pulmonary oxygen uptake kinetics during heavy exercise. *Journal of Applied Physiology*, **89**, 1387-1396.

Fawkner, S.G. and Armstrong, N., 2002, Assessment of critical power in children. *Pediatric Exercise Science*, **14**, 259-268.

Fawkner, S.G., Armstrong, N., Childs, D.J. and Welsman, J.R., 2002, Reliability of the visually identified ventilatory threshold and V-slope in children. *Pediatric Exercise Science*, **14**, 181-192.

Gaesser, G.A. and Poole, D.C., 1996, The slow component of oxygen uptake kinetics in humans. In *Exercise and Sports Science Reviews*, edited by Holloszy, J.O., (USA: Williams and Wilkins), pp. 35-70.

Hebestreit, H., Kreimler, S., Hughson, R.L. and Bar-Or, O., 1998, Kinetics of oxygen uptake at the onset of exercise in boys and men. *Journal of Applied Physiology*, **85**, 1833-1841.

Moritani, T., Nagata, A., DeVries, H.A. and Muro, M., 1981, Critical power as a measure of physical work capacity and anaerobic threshold. *Ergonomics*, **24**, 339-350.

Poole, D.C., Ward, S.A., Gardner, G.W. and Whipp, B.J., 1988, Metabolic and respiratory profile of the upper limit for prolonged exercise in man. *Ergonomics*, 31, 1265-1279.

Poole, D.C., Ward, S.A. and Whipp, B.J., 1990, The effects of training on the metabolic and respiratory profile of high-intensity cycle ergometer exercise. *European Journal of Applied Physiology*, **59**, 421-429.

Tanner, J.M., 1962, *Growth at Adolescence*. (Oxford: Blackwell), pp. 28-39.

Whipp, B.J., Ward, S.A., Lamarra, N., Davis, J.A. and Wasserman, K., 1982, Parameters of ventilatory and gas exchange dynamics during exercise. *Journal of Applied Physiology*, **52**, 1506-1513.

Williams, C.A., Carter, H., Jones, A.M. and Doust, J.H., 2001, Oxygen uptake kinetics during treadmill running in boys and men. *Journal of Applied Physiology*, **90**, 1700-1706.

# Part III

# ANTHROPOMETRY IN SPORTS

# 11 Anthropometry of Team Sports

J.E. Lindsay Carter
Department of Exercise and Nutritional Sciences
San Diego State University
San Diego, CA, 92182-7251, USA

## 1. INTRODUCTION

Anthropometry is the measurement of shape and form in humans, while kinanthropometry is defined as the quantitative study of size, shape, proportion, composition and maturation in relation to gross motor function (Ross and Marfell-Jones, 1990). Team sports include such well-known sports as rugby and basketball, but exclude sports in which individual scores may be totaled for a "team" score, e.g. gymnastics. Physique and performance in team sports are both affected by age and maturation, selection process, competitive level, playing position, tactics, and gender (Carter, 1985).

Many factors are involved in the development of the elite athlete including biochemistry, physiology, psychology, genetics, sociology and economics. Thus the physique (i.e. anthropometry) of the elite athlete reflects the "end product" of complex processes which may begin many years beforehand. Human athletic performance is usually a combination of (but is not limited to) such characteristics as speed, stamina, strength, suppleness, skill, psychology and tactics. These characteristics are of different importance in various sports, at various stages of development of the athlete and at different times within the competitive season. Although cellular processes are important in the function of tissues, it is wise to study the physique as a whole in relation to a sport. The athlete takes his/her whole body to the contest, not just selected systems or sub-systems. On the other hand, while some athletes succeed because they have the "right" physique, others may succeed because they have an unusual physique that may confer a specific biomechanical or physiological advantage.

Early studies describing the range and specificity in physiques of Olympic athletes from 1928 to 1976 in a variety of sports were summarized Borms and Hebbelinck (1984), and other sports by Carter and Heath (1990). Theoretical models of physique and performance have been provided by Tittel and Wutscherk (1972), Tittel (1978), Hay and Reid (1988). Carter (1985) noted that "Absolute and relative size, somatotype, composition, and maturation are morphological factors that may limit human performance. It is inferred that athletes who have, or acquire, the optimal physique for an event are more likely to succeed than those who lack these characteristics. Quantification of physique through kinanthropometry can provide a better basis for understanding the limits related to the biomechanics and physiology of performance." (p. 115.)

Norton *et al.* (1996) described a process called "morphological optimization" and "selection pressures", along with "anthropometric profiling", that provides a framework for evaluating the elite athlete. They also cautioned that differences in profiles are influenced by the level of competition and early versus later data for many sports (p. 289). The concept of morphological optimisation "...is the process whereby the physical demands of a sport lead to selection of body types (structure and composition) best suited to that sport. This is most obvious at the professional level of sport. The anatomical features are not fixed with the athletic population. Rather, they are continually undergoing refinement within each generation as a response to training and along generations as humans evolve, rules and technologies are altered, and the status of sports changes. All of these characteristics impact upon the sport to modify the potential population from which athletes are selected." (p. 352).

The purpose of this report is to review findings from recent studies on the anthropometry of athletes in selected team sports. Morphological prototypes, in terms of absolute and relative size, somatotype and composition are described and compared with respect to playing position, the level of competition, order of finish, and sexual dimorphism.

The teams sports examined in this review consist of 13 samples from seven sports, 1,114 males, and 456 females, for a total of 1,570 athletes. These are chosen for review because they are from recent studies and have used essentially the same anthropometric methods which facilitates comparisons. In addition, the author was associated with each of the studies. Seven team sports were examined: Basketball (females, N = 168), World Championships, 1994; Rugby (males), primary (N = 237) and secondary (N = 369) South African schoolboys, USA University (N = 42) and National (N = 64) teams, 1990s; Soccer (males, N = 110), Copa America 1995; Synchronized swimming (females, N = 118), World Championships, 1991; Underwater hockey (males, N = 90, females, N = 59), World Championships 1992; Volleyball (males, N = 11, females, N = 15), USA National teams, 1988; Water polo (males, N = 190, females, N = 96), World Championships, 1991.

## 2. METHODS

Essentially the same anthropometric variables and methods were used in these studies, thereby facilitating within and among sport comparisons. The anthropometry and proportionality analysis followed the methods of Ross and Marfell-Jones (1990), and of the International Society for the Advancement of Kinanthropometry (ISAK, 2001). Somatotypes were calculated according to Carter and Heath (1990). The main descriptive statistics within sports by gender are summarized in Tables 1-2, and Figures 1-2. Basketball and synchronized swimming for women are presented first, followed by the two football sports for men, rugby and soccer, then by underwater hockey, volleyball, and water polo, which have both men's and women's teams.

## 3. RESULTS

### 3.1 Basketball

Absolute size and proportionality characteristics of female basketball players at the World Championships in Australia 1994 were examined by Ackland *et al.* (1996, 1997).

Table 1. Descriptive statistics (M ± SD) for female team sports players.

| Sample | N | Age (yr) | Stature (m) | Mass (kg) | ∑6skf* (mm) | Somatotype | SAM ** |
|---|---|---|---|---|---|---|---|
| BASKETBALL[1] | 168 | 25.0 | 1.801 | 73.2 | 88.6 | 3.0-3.5-3.0 | 1.4 |
|  |  | 3.5 | 0.095 | 9.3 | - | 0.9 1.0 1.0 | 0.7 |
| Guards | 64 | 25.4 | 1.719 | 66.1 | 84.9 | 2.9-3.9-2.6 | 1.4 |
|  |  | 3.3 | 0.061 | 6.2 | - | 0.9 1.0 0.9 | 0.7 |
| Forwards | 57 | 25.2 | 1.813 | 73.3 | 84.4 | 2.8-3.5-3.2 | 1.4 |
|  |  | 3.8 | 0.059 | 5.1 | - | 0.9 0.9 1.0 | 0.7 |
| Centres | 47 | 24.1 | 1.898 | 82.6 | 98.7 | 3.2-3.1-3.4 | 1.5 |
|  |  | 3.1 | 0.064 | 8.2 | - | 0.9 1.1 1.0 | 0.7 |
|  |  |  |  |  |  |  |  |
| SYNCHRONIZED SWIMMING[2] | 118 | 21.7 | 1.688 | 56.5 | 81.8 | 3.3-3.5-3.2 | 1.4 |
|  |  | 2.6 | 0.059 | 5.3 | 22.7 | 1.0 0.9 1.0 | 0.8 |
|  |  |  |  |  |  |  |  |
| UNDERWATER HOCKEY[3] | 59 | 27.3 | 1.685 | 62.2 | 93.5 | 3.8-4.3-2.6 | - |
|  |  | 5.2 | 0.051 | 6.7 | 26.7 | 1.1 0.9 1.0 |  |
|  |  |  |  |  |  |  |  |
| VOLLEYBALL[4] | 15 | 23.7 | 1.788 | 67.7 | 68.8 | 2.8-3.3-3.6 | 1.5 |
|  |  | 3.4 | 0.083 | 6.2 | 10.6 | 0.6 1.1 1.4 | 0.6 |
|  |  |  |  |  |  |  |  |
| WATER POLO[5] | 109 | 23.7 | 1.713 | 64.8 | 89.8 | 3.6-4.0-2.8 | 1.3 |
|  |  | 3.4 | 0.059 | 7.2 | 23.8 | 1.0 0.9 0.9 | 0.5 |

\* ∑6skf = triceps, subscapular, supraspinale, abdominal, front thigh, medial calf.
\** SAM = somatotype attitudinal mean.
[1] Ackland *et al.* (1996, 1997)
[2] Carter and Ackland (1994)
[3] Marfell-Jones and Carter (1993)
[4] Carter *et al.* (1994)
[5] Carter and Ackland (1994)

In total, 168 players from 14 national teams were measured using 38 variables, including breadths, girths, lengths and skinfolds. Analyses were conducted according to playing position, guards (n = 4), forwards (n = 57) and centres (n = 47), and team performance. There were differences in absolute size between the three positions, but the forwards and centres were similar on several variables, especially in relative size of upper body dimensions. Guards demonstrated a different proportionality profile from the forwards and centres. Guards in four top teams were longer in five absolute length variables than guards in four bottom teams. Forwards in four top teams were also longer in five absolute length variables than forwards in four bottom teams and were also larger in relative hip breadth and girth, and waist girth.

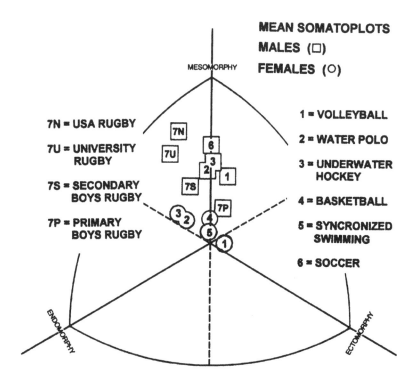

**Figure 1**. Mean somatoplots for the seven sports.

In terms of somatotypes (unpublished), there were no differences among positions in somatotype attitudinal means (SAMs), but there were differences among the mean somatotypes in that the guards differed from forwards and centres due to the guards being more mesomorphic and less ectomorphic than forwards and centres. In addition, both the guards and forwards on the four top teams were taller and more ectomorphic than their counterparts on the four low teams. The skinfold patterns of six skinfolds were similar for the three playing positions, but the centres were larger than the other two groups at all sites and in sum of six skinfolds.

## 3.2 Synchronized swimming

Synchronized swimmers (N = 118) competed in the team event at the World Championships in Perth, 1991, (Carter and Ackland, 1994). When the three best teams were compared to the other 10 teams, the best were older by 1.6 years and had greater neck, flexed arm and mid-thigh girths, smaller wrist and ankle girths, greater biacromial breadth, and shorter forearm length. The sum of six skinfolds was greater in teams from the Netherlands, Australia and China, than in teams from Japan and Spain, but there was no consistent difference by final placing. The proportions of the top teams were also compared with those of the lower placed teams. The former had relatively longer arm spans, smaller forearm and thigh lengths, longer foot lengths, and wider biacromial and biiliocristal breadths. They also had smaller wrist and ankle girths and were smaller in seven out of eight skinfolds – the exception being the iliac crest site.

A wide range of somatotypes was found for team synchronized swimmers; however, they clustered around a mean of 3½-3½-3 (Central), with the largest variation in somatoplots along the ectomorphic axis. Although there were no differences in mean somatotypes among teams, there were some differences in endomorphy and mesomorphy components taken separately, but these were not related to final team ranking.

## 3.3 Rugby Union football

Early studies on rugby focused primarily on British Commonwealth players (e.g. Bell, 1979). In general these studies had small numbers and usually divided players into forwards and backs who were compared in terms of body size, somatotype and adiposity. Most of the studies showed the size of the differences between forwards and backs in many variables.

De Ridder (1993) and De Ridder *et al.* (1995) studied 237 primary schoolboy players (age = 13.1 years) and 369 secondary schoolboy players (age = 18.1 years) in South Africa and showed many differences in 10 playing positions and the two levels of play. Compared to the primary players, the secondary players were taller and heavier, more mesomorphic and less ectomorphic in most positions. These changes were consistent by position and expected due to growth and maturation.

Although USA rugby is not yet at the top level internationally, two recent studies have looked at the national team and a club team to compare them by position and playing level. In the first study (Carlson *et al.*, 1994) anthropometric and performance data were collected on 65 national level USA rugby players (age = 26.3 years) in order to compare them by player position (forwards, backs) and performance level (national team, junior national, development). Discriminant function analyses (DFA) showed that forwards were taller, heavier and had more subcutaneous adiposity than backs, were more endo-mesomorphic and more variable in somatotype. In motor performance the variables that best discriminated between backs and forwards were repeated jumps, push-ups, and standing vertical jump. Classification into three playing levels was unsatisfactory using either anthropometric or motor performance variables. These results suggest that at the national level it is the rugby skills and experience (and probably coach's judgment) that separates the playing levels when the players are similar in physique and performance.

In a second study by Kieffer *et al.* (2000), anthropometric data were collected on 42 university level rugby players (age = 21.9 years) to make comparisons on these characteristics by playing position and by performance level and to compare university and national players. Prior studies divided rugby players into forwards and backs. This study further subdivided forwards into tight and loose forwards due to perceived differences in their role during play. Measures taken included stature, mass, skinfolds, girths, and breadths. Descriptive statistics, skinfold patterns, and somatotypes were calculated for the total two samples and playing position subgroups. Discriminant function analyses were employed to determine which combination of variables best discriminated among positions at each level, and between levels for each position. The tight forwards were taller, heavier, and had more subcutaneous adiposity than backs or loose forwards. Loose forwards tended to be similar to backs at the university level and to tight forwards at the national level. No significant differences were found in somatotype between loose forwards and backs, but tight forwards differed significantly from both other positions. The DFA differentiated the three positions reasonably well at both levels of play, post-hoc analyses correctly classifying 80% or more of all players at each level. Loose forwards were most often misclassified, usually as backs. The DFA differentiated players at all positions by playing level, with 90% or more of players correctly classified.

The results of this study indicate that there were some significant differences between loose forwards and tight forwards at both the national and university levels of play. Loose forwards appear at both levels to be more similar in aspects of body size, composition, and somatotype to backs than they are to tight forwards. Furthermore, when players remain separated in the three playing groups, there are significant differences between players at the university level and their counterparts at the national level in most aspects studied. Due to the significant differences in morphology displayed by loose forwards and tight forwards, it would seem that future studies of rugby players would be well advised to separate these two groups.

**Table 2**. Descriptive statistics (M ± SD) for male team sports players.

| Sample | N | Age (yr) | Stature (m) | Mass (kg) | ∑6skf* (mm) | Somatotype | SAM** |
|---|---|---|---|---|---|---|---|
| RUGBY | | | | | | | |
| Primary Schoolboys[1] | 237 | 13.1 0.3 | 1.639 0.086 | 55.0 10.2 | 62.6 27.2 | 2.6-4.2-3.2 1.2 0.9 1.1 | 1.3 0.8 |
| Backs | 110 | 13.1 0.3 | 1.600 0.079 | 49.0 7.8 | 51.4 14.1 | 2.2-4.0-3.5 0.7 0.8 0.9 | 1.2 0.6 |
| Forwards | 127 | 13.1 0.3 | 1.673 0.077 | 60.2 9.1 | 72.3 31.8 | 3.0-4.4-2.8 1.4 1.0 1.3 | 1.5 2.0 |
| | | | | | | | |
| Secondary Schoolboys[1] | 369 | 18.1 0.7 | 1.801 0.075 | 80.6 11.3 | 68.6 30.7 | 2.9-4.7-2.1 1.2 1.2 1.0 | 1.7 0.9 |
| Backs | 170 | 18.1 0.7 | 1.762 0.059 | 72.9 6.6 | 55.7 17.5 | 2.9-4.5-2.3 0.8 1.0 0.8 | 1.8 0.9 |
| Forwards | 199 | 18.1 0.7 | 1.833 0.073 | 87.3 10.3 | 79.5 35.1 | 3.3-5.0-1.9 1.4 1.2 1.0 | 1.7 0.9 |
| | | | | | | | |
| San Diego State Univ[2] | 42 | 21.9 1.9 | 1.792 0.060 | 84.1 6.1 | 85.1 25.7 | 3.5-5.9-1.6 1.1 1.0 0.8 | 2.0 1.0 |
| Backs | 23 | 21.6 2.1 | 1.775 0.059 | 77.5 6.3 | 66.9 20.3 | 2.8-5.4-2.0 0.9 1.0 0.9 | 1.6 1.0 |
| Loose Forwards | 7 | 21.9 1.1 | 1.789 0.049 | 81.8 4.0 | 66.5 18.4 | 2.9-5.8-1.7 0.9 1.1 0.5 | 1.3 0.9 |
| Tight Forwards | 12 | 22.4 1.9 | 1.825 0.071 | 98.0 6.9 | 130.7 38.2 | 5.3-6.8-0.9 1.5 1.0 0.9 | 3.0 1.2 |
| | | | | | | | |
| USA National[2] | 65 | 26.3 2.5 | 1.832 0.075 | 90.6 12.3 | 67.9 17.4 | 2.8-6.3-1.5 0.9 1.0 0.8 | 1.4 0.8 |
| Backs | 30 | 25.8 2.3 | 1.789 0.053 | 80.8 7.2 | 55.4 12.6 | 2.4-5.9-1.8 0.6 0.8 0.7 | 1.2 0.6 |
| Loose Forwards | 12 | 26.4 2.4 | 1.887 0.048 | 94.4 6.7 | 64.2 17.5 | 2.5-5.9-1.9 0.6 1.1 0.8 | 1.3 0.8 |
| Tight Forwards | 23 | 27.0 2.9 | 1.859 0.081 | 101.5 9.3 | 86.2 22.7 | 3.5-7.1-0.9 1.0 0.9 0.6 | 1.6 0.9 |
| SOCCER[3] | 110 | 26.1 4.1 | 1.777 0.057 | 76.4 7.0 | 46.5 - | 2.1-5.3-2.2 0.5 0.8 0.6 | 1.0 0.5 |
| Goalkeepers | 15 | 27.9 5.2 | 1.824 0.049 | 84.6 6.6 | 57.9 - | 2.6-5.5-1.9 0.7 0.6 0.5 | 0.9 0.5 |
| Other Positions | 95 | 25.8 3.7 | 1.770 0.055 | 75.0 6.3 | 44.7 - | 2.0-5.3-2.2 0.5 0.8 0.6 | 1.0 0.5 |
| | | | | | | | |
| UNDERWATER HOCKEY[4] | 90 | 28.5 5.5 | 1.810 0.060 | 77.5 7.8 | 63.6 21.9 | 2.6-5.5-2.6 0.9 0.9 0.9 | - |
| | | | | | | | |
| VOLLEYBALL[5] | 11 | 25.2 2.1 | 1.934 0.070 | 87.6 6.9 | 50.3 6.8 | 1.9-4.7-3.3 0.3 0.9 0.7 | 1.0 0.6 |
| | | | | | | | |
| WATER POLO[6] | 190 | 25.2 3.8 | 1.865 0.065 | 86.1 8.4 | 62.5 17.5 | 2.5-5.3-2.4 0.8 1.0 0.9 | 1.3 0.7 |

* ∑6skf = triceps, subscapular, supraspinale, abdominal, front thigh, medial calf.
** SAM = somatotype attitudinal mean.
[1] De Ridder (1993, 1995)
[2] Kieffer *et al.* (2000)
[3] Rienzi *et al.* (1998)
[4] Marfell-Jones and Carter (1993)
[5] Carter *et al.* (1994)
[6] Carter and Ackland (1994)

### 3.4 Association football (Soccer)

The Copa America tournament in Uruguay, 1995, was the basis for a study of the kinanthropometry and motion analysis of players from six national teams (N = 110) (Rienzi and Mazza, 1998). The teams were Argentina (n = 22), Bolivia (n = 20), Columbia (n = 14), Ecuador (n = 22), Paraguay (n = 10) and Uruguay (n = 22). Data were collected on 41 anthropometric variables and were analyzed in terms of absolute and relative body size, somatotype, and body composition. There were 60 Whites, 34 Mestizos and 16 Blacks, whose professional playing experience ranged from 1 to 21 years, with a median of 7.0 years.

Comparisons were made between goalkeepers (GK, n = 15) and other position players (OTH, n = 95); among teams without GK; and among the seven positions: GK, central (CD = 20) and lateral (LD = 17) defenders, defensive (DM = 20) and lateral (OM = 14) midfielders, central (CS = 9) and lateral (LS = 15) strikers. Goalkeepers averaged 27.9 (±5.2) years, 1.824 (±0.049) m and 84.6 (±6.6) kg. Other positions averaged 25.8 (±3.7), 1.770 (±0.055) m and 75.0 (±6.3) kg. There were no significant differences between any of the comparisons in terms of age which was 26.1 (±4.0) years (N = 110). The results of the ANOVAs showed that GK and CD were taller than OM, LD and LS (p<0.001). For body mass, GK CS and CD were heavier than OM, LD and LS, and CS were heavier than DM (p<0.001). There were no significant differences among teams in stature or body mass. The scatter of somatotypes about their respective means (SAMs) was not different for any comparison. When mean somatotypes (Š) were compared, there were no significant differences among teams, or by playing position, but GK (Š = 2.6-5.5-1.9) were more endomorphic (p<0.01) than OTH (Š = 2.0-5.3-2.2). When endomorphy was compared among positions, GK were more endomorphic than LS (Š = 1.8-5.4-2.1), CD (Š = 1.9-5.3-2.3) and LD (Š = 2.0-5.3-2.1). Based on DFA using age, stature, body mass and somatotype, the goalkeepers were slightly different from other players as a group, and some of the six other positions separately. The differences were attributed to greater body mass and endomorphy in the goalkeepers. Overall the biggest differences in physique were between GK and OTH players, with a tendency for the GK, CD and CS to be more alike, and also LD, OM and LS tended to be more like each other. It was concluded that although there is a wide range in age, professional playing experience, and body size, there is considerable similarity and limited distributions in somatotypes for the non-GK positions.

When compared to other players, GK had significantly larger skinfolds at all six sites, and for sum of six, but the skinfold patterns were similar. With respect to absolute of other variables and relative size, the most common differences were between goalkeepers, who were larger in several variables, and players in outfield positions. There was considerable variation in many variables among the outfield positions. Proportionally, GK were heavier, higher in muscle girths and skinfolds compared to other playing positions. For both absolute and relative size, there was evidence that GK, CD and CS were more like each other on several variables, especially body mass, biacromial breadth and arm span. Not all teams had "large" CS and coaches may have selected different "types" of strikers to suit their preferred tactics, or vice versa. Overall, the field positions had similar proportionality profiles, which tended to be smaller than those of the GK. When the six teams were compared, excluding GK, there were no important differences in any of the major areas of comparison. Discriminant analyses were unable to separate the teams on the basis of body size or somatotype.

### 3.5 Underwater hockey

A study of underwater hockey players was conducted at the World Underwater Hockey Championships in New Zealand in 1992 (Marfell-Jones and Carter, 1993). Anthropometry (42 variables) was taken on women's teams from five countries (N = 59), and men's teams from eight countries (N = 90). The women's teams differed in age, with the United States older than New Zealand and France, and South Africa older than New Zealand. There were no differences in mass, but South Africa was taller than Australia. The mean somatotype was 4-4½-2½ (Mesomorph-Endomorph). The Australian team had a greater somatotype attitudinal mean (SAM) than the United States or France, but there were no differences among somatotype means.

Among the men's teams there were differences in age with the USA older than France, New Zealand and Australia, but there were no differences in mass or stature. There were some differences in the sum of six skinfolds, with France being the lowest. The mean somatotype was 2½-5½-2½. The SAMs did not differ, and there were no differences among means.

### 3.6 Volleyball

Sexual dimorphism in physique and performance characteristics in the 1988 USA women's (N = 15) and USA men's (N = 11) National volleyball teams were examined by Carter *et al.* (1994). Age, 22 anthropometric variables, three jumping and three muscular strength measures were obtained. As the sample was small, no comparisons in anthropometry by position were made.

Males were heavier and taller than females, but similar in age (25.2 vs. 23.6 years). Males had larger arm girth, and wider bones in five of seven measures. Males and females had similar trunk skinfolds, but females had higher extremity sites and males were lower in sum of skinfolds and percent fat (9.5% vs. 16.0%). The females had smaller proportional values for arm girth, humerus and femur breadths, antero-posterior and transverse chest dimensions, as well as larger values for triceps, thigh and calf skinfolds. Mean somatotypes differed (males = 2-4½-3½, females = 3-3½-3½), but had similar dispersions (SAMs). Relative to their stature, the vertical jump for males was 45% and 40% for females. Relative to body mass, females bench-pressed 97%, and males 124%. It is concluded that volleyball players are typically tall, lean, muscular athletes with strong upper bodies and good jumping ability. Their sexual dimorphism is consistent with that found in other sports.

### 3.7 Water polo

Female water polo players from nine countries at the World Championships in Perth, 1991, were examined by Carter and Ackland (1994). Water polo players (WP) designated their primary playing position as centre forward (CF), centre back (CB), goalkeeper (GK), or offensive/defensive wing, denoted as other positions (OTH). Differences in morphology were examined among players in these positions, as well as among teams.

The mean somatotype for all female WP (N = 109) was 3½-4-3 (central). The analysis of players by position showed that OTH were significantly smaller and lighter than CF and CB. These differences were shown in many absolute and proportional size variables. Centre forwards in particular, had greater proportional weight which was accounted for by greater musculature (higher absolute and proportional breadths and girths) as well as greater adiposity (higher proportional skinfold thicknesses). Female GK were more ectomorphic than players in all other positions, with similar absolute girth and breadth values to OTH, but they had linear dimensions more similar to CF and CB. Goalkeepers also had lower proportional weight and lower proportional values for five breadths and six girths compared to OTH.

The male water polo players (N = 190) were from 15 countries at the World Championships in Perth, 1991 (Carter and Ackland, 1994). Their primary playing position were the same as for females (see above). Differences in morphology were examined between players in these positions. The mean somatotype was 2½-5½-2½ (balanced Mesomorph). The only difference between positions was in ectomorphy, where GK were significantly more ectomorphic than CF. Centre backs and OTH players were similar in somatotype to the CF players.

Although similar in somatotype to the CF and CB, the OTH players were significantly smaller and lighter. The OTH players were smaller in body mass, stature and four segment lengths, 13 girths and seven breadths. Centre forwards and, to a lesser extent, CB were therefore the largest and most robust of all players. CF had a significantly higher proportional weight compared to OTH and this is possibly due to higher proportional skinfold thicknesses and waist girth. Clearly however, CF possess higher levels of skinfolds in proportion to their size than OTH players. The advantage of greater size for CF enhances their ability to provide a large focal point for the team when attacking the opponent's goal, as well as a protection from constant physical contact by the CB.

Goalkeepers were similar to OTH on most girth and breadth dimensions but were more like CF and CB with respect to stature as well as individual segment lengths and higher relative skeletal mass compared to CF. Similarly, GK possessed significantly lower proportional weight compared to OTH. This result appears to be due to lower proportional girth measures particularly with respect to the upper body – an attribute which would indicate reduced upper limb inertia and thus would facilitate relative quickness of movement to protect the goal.

Male and female WP teams were also categorized in terms of their eventual placing and players comprising the teams which made the finals (best) were compared with those in the teams which finished in the lowest order (rest). Using these groupings, very few differences between best and rest were noted for either male or female WP in somatotype, absolute size or body composition variables. Due to the large variation in body size and shape for positional players within each team, the lack of differences is not unexpected. In future analyses, it may be more useful to partition the teams into respective player positions before running this analysis. However, with respect to proportionality, male WP players in the best teams had a smaller proportional weight than the rest. This is explained by lower proportional values for two lengths, two breadths, five girths and two skinfold thicknesses. A similar trend was shown for the females who have lower proportional values for hip and thigh girths as well as for two skinfolds. These results serve to reinforce the notion that even though WP players were among the largest of aquatic athletes and that a certain body size and structure is required for success in the sport, body morphology alone is not the key to success. Clearly, the players with the greatest size did not ensure the success of the team.

There were differences in physique between male and female water polo players. This sexual dimorphism was expressed in absolute and relative size, as well as body composition and somatotype. Differences were expected in absolute size, but there were also differences in relative size.

• 6sk(hc) (mm)

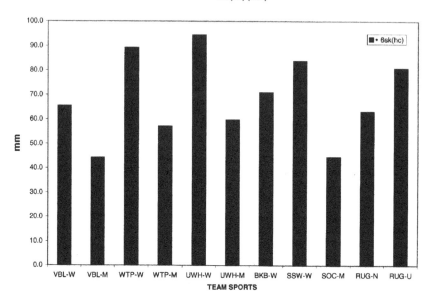

**Figure 2**. Height corrected sum of six skinfolds for team sports: VBL-W = volleyball women; VBL-M = volleyball men; WTP-W = water polo women; WTP-M = water polo men; UHW-W = underwater hockey women; UHW-M = underwater hockey men; BKB-W = basketball women; SSW-W = synchronized swimming women; SOC-M = soccer men; RUG-N = USA national men; RUG-U = university men.

## 4. SUMMARY

Playing position: Size and somatotype differences were evident in water polo (both genders), basketball and rugby (at all levels). Few differences were found in soccer, but goalkeepers were generally different in size, composition and somatotype from field players. The latter differed little from each other except that in some size variables centre backs and central strikers tended to be larger.

Level of competition: In rugby, as expected, the primary and secondary schoolboys differed from each other in most measures of body size and shape, and they differed from the University and National teams, which also differed slightly from each other.

Order of finish: Physique differences in several absolute and relative size variables were found between the top and lower placed teams in synchronised swimmers, between basketball forwards versus guards in segment lengths, and in a few variables in both male and female water polo players. In soccer, among teams (excluding goalkeepers) players did not differ from each other.

Sexual dimorphism: Differences in all areas of physique assessment were observed in underwater hockey, water polo, and volleyball.

Comparison among sports: For women, basketball players are clearly the tallest and heaviest. They have high absolute sum of skinfolds, but are lower than both water polo players, underwater hockey players and synchronized swimmers when adjusted for stature. Volleyball players have the lowest skinfolds, both in absolute and relative values. Mean somatotypes are distributed along the ectomorphic axis with volleyball players the most and underwater hockey and water polo players the least ectomorphic. For men, the soccer players are lighter than all other groups, while the heaviest are adult rugby tight forwards. Volleyball players are the tallest, and along with soccer players they have the lowest skinfolds, in absolute and relative values. For somatotype, the most endo-mesomorphic are the rugby players, especially the tight forwards, and the volleyball players the most ecto-mesomorphic. Soccer, water polo and underwater hockey players are clustered around balanced mesomorphy.

## 5. CONCLUSIONS

Although physique is only one of several aspects of successful physical performance, it is a very important foundation upon which success is built. Morphological prototypes needed for success at various levels both within and among these sports are well defined. There is more variability in some team sports than in others. These prototypes can be used in talent selection and the assessment of training status. This review of seven sports supports the concept of "morphological optimization" as a useful reflection of selection pressures, training status, and talent selection in both male and female athletes.

## REFERENCES

Ackland, T.R., Schreiner, A.B. and Kerr, D.A., 1996, Technical note: Anthropometric normative data for female international basketball players. *The Australian Journal of Science and Medicine in Sport*, **29**, 22-24.

Ackland, T.R., Schreiner, A.B. and Kerr, D.A., 1997, Absolute size and proportionality characteristics of World Championship female basketball players. *Journal of Sports Sciences*, **15**, 485-490.

Bell, W., 1979, Body composition of rugby union football players. *British Journal of Sports Medicine*, **13**, 19-23.

Borms, J. and Hebbelinck, M., 1984, Review of studies on Olympic athletes. In *Physical Structure of Olympic Athletes, Part II, Kinanthropometry of Olympic Athletes*, edited by Carter, J.E.L., (Basel: Karger), pp. 7-27.

Carlson, B.R., Carter, J.E.L., Patterson, P., Petti, K., Orfanos, S.M. and Noffal, G.J., 1994, Physique and motor performance characteristics of USA national rugby players. *Journal of Sports Sciences*, **1**, 403-412.

Carter, J.E.L., 1985, Morphological factors limiting human performance. In *The Limits of Human Performance, The American Academy of Physical Education Papers, No. 18.*, edited by Eckert, H.M., and Clarke, D.H. (Champaign, Il: Human Kinetics), pp. 106-117.

Carter, J.E.L. and Heath, B.H., 1990, *Somatotyping: Development and Applications*, (Cambridge: Cambridge University Press).

Carter, J.E.L. and Ackland, T.R., 1994, *Kinanthropometry in Aquatic Sports – A Study of World Class Athletes*, (Champaign, IL: Human Kinetics).

Carter, J.E.L., Powell-Santi, L.A. and Rodriguez Alonso, C., 1994, Physique and performance of USA volleyball players. In *Access to Active Living, Proceedings for the 10th Commonwealth & International Scientific Congress, 10-14 August, 1994*, edited by Bell, F.I. and Van Gyn, G.H. (Victoria, B.C., Canada), pp. 311-316.

De Ridder, J.H., 1993, '*N morphologiese profile van junior en senior Cravenweek rugbyspelers* (A morphological profile of junior and senior Cravenweek rugby players). Ph.D. Thesis, Potchestroom University for CHE, Potchestroom, South Africa.

De Ridder, J.H., Van der Walt, T.S.P. and Carter, J.E.L., 1995, Los somatotipos descolares Sudafricaonos jugadores de rugby de elite. In *Actas del CongresoCientifico Olimpico, 1992, Biomecanica y Cineanthropometria*, Vol. V, edited by C. Garcia Lopez, (Malaga: Instituto Andaluz del Deporte), pp. 292-301.

Hay, J.G. and Reid, J.G., 1988, *Anatomy, Mechanics and Human Motion*, 2nd ed, (Englewood Cliffs, NJ: Prentice Hall).

ISAK, 2001, *International Standards for Anthropometric Assessment*, (Underdale, SA: International Society for the Advancement of Kinanthropometry).

Kieffer, S., Carter, L., Held-Sturman, M., Patterson, P. and Carlson, R., 2000, Physique characteristics of USA national and university level rugby players. In *Kinanthropometry VI: Proceedings of the Sixth Conference of the International Society for the Advancement of Kinanthropometry*, edited by Norton, K., Olds, T. and Dollman, J. (Underdale, SA: International Society for the Advancement of Kinanthropometry), pp. 53-77.

Marfell-Jones, M.J. and Carter, J.E.L., 1993, *World underwater hockey anthropometric project, 1992*, (Trentham, New Zealand: Central Institute of Technology).

Norton, K., Olds, T., Olive, S. and Craig, N., 1996, *Anthropometry and sports performance*. In Anthropometrica, edited by Norton, K. and Olds. T., (Sydney: University of New South Wales Press), pp. 287-364.

Rienzi, E. and Mazza, J.C., 1998, *Futbolista Sudamericano de Elite: Morphologia, Analysis del Juego y Performance*, edited by Rienzi, E., Mazza, J.C., Carter, J.E.L. and Reilly, T., (Buenos Aires/Rosario: Biosystem Servicio Educativo).

Ross, W.D. and Marfell-Jones, M.J., 1990, Kinanthropometry. In *Physiological Testing of the High-Performance Athlete*, edited by MacDougall, J., Wenger, H.A. and Green, H.J., (Champaign, IL: Human Kinetics), pp. 223-308.

Tittel, K. 1978, Tasks and tendencies of sports anthropometry's development. In *Biomechanics of Sport and Kinanthropometry*, edited by Landry, F., and Orban, W.A.R., (Miami: Symposia Specialists), pp. 283-296.

Tittel, K., and Wutscherk, H., 1972, *Sportanthropometrie*, (Leipzig: J.A. Barth).

# 12   Anthropometric Characteristics of Rugby Sevens Players: An Evaluation During Two Consecutive International Events

E. Rienzi, M. Pérez, M. Stefani, C. Maiuri and G. Rodríguez
UNISPORT, Centro de Evaluación y Orientación Físico Deportiva,
Montevideo KIP Club

## 1. INTRODUCTION

Rugby Sevens is possibly one of the team sports that has developed greatly in the past decade. Since its creation, by Ned Haig (Melrose Rugby Football Club), in Scotland in 1883, Rugby Sevens has experienced great changes, and is now played by many fully professional players. A World Cup takes place every four years, and the IRB (International Rugby Board) has also created the World Sevens Series, now in its third season.

One of the most traditional events in Rugby Sevens takes place in Punta del Este, Uruguay, organized by The British Schools Old Boys Club from Montevideo, Uruguay. During the tournaments of 1996 and 1997 (this tournament being a qualifying round for the Hong Kong World Cup), we developed a kinanthropometric project (SEASIDE UKP: Seven-a-Side Uruguayan Kinanthropometric Project), in order to assess the anthropometric characteristics of players involved in this rugby speciality.

## 2. MATERIAL AND METHODS

Altogether, 246 players from 28 different countries, were measured, providing us with the widest sample obtained in Rugby Sevens up to that time. The countries represented in this study were: Western Samoa, Papua New Guinea, Cook Islands, New Zealand, Fiji, Tahiti, Australia, South Africa, Israel, Namibia, Wales, Spain, Germany, France, Russia, Italy, Portugal, Romania, Trinidad and Tobago, Bermuda, Bahamas, Canada, U.S.A., Argentina, Brazil, Chile, Paraguay, and Uruguay. National sides with very different playing standards were analysed, but in every case, players were internationals representing their countries.

In this research, 43 anthropometric measurements were performed on each player, following ISAK recommendations (nine lengths, eight skinfolds, thirteen girths, nine breadths, stature, sitting height, body mass and arm span). The equipment used consisted of four Centurion Kits (Rosscraft), four Harpenden skinfold calipers, and a weighing scale. The measurements were performed during two days prior to the start of each tournament. Playing position in Rugby Sevens was considered.

The first comparison established dividing the sample into backs (n=138) and forwards (n=108) and performing ANOVA for the 43 anthropometric measurements. Percentage body fat (Durnin and Womersley, 1974), absolute and relative muscle mass (Drinkwater and Mazza, 1994), absolute and relative bone mass (Drinkwater and Mazza, 1994), and somatotype (Carter, 1992) were calculated for the two groups.

Considering the different playing standards of the players taking part in these two tournaments, it was decided to analyse differences between best and worst performers in the abovementioned events. We considered best performers to be those players whose teams finished in the top four positions in each tournament (New Zealand, Fiji, France, Australia, Argentina, Western Samoa and Cook Islands), and as worst performers, those who finished in the final four positions (U.S.A., Bermuda, Brazil, Chile, Tahiti, Bahamas and Paraguay). We obtained a sample of n=61 best performers, and n=65 as worst performers. Analysis of variance was conducted for this comparison.

Finally, the groups of best and worst performers were divided in two, considering their role (position) in the game (backs n=35 and forwards n=26 for the best group; backs n=38 and forwards n=27 for the worst group). Statistic differences were explored by means of ANOVA.

## 3. RESULTS

Performing ANOVA on the whole sample, as seen in Tables 1 and 2, statistical differences were observed for the 43 measurements (p<0.001) between forwards and backs.

**Table 1.** Differences between forwards and backs for 43 anthropometric measurements according to ANOVA: lengths and skinfolds (means for all the sample).

|  | Forw. | Backs | p< |
|---|---|---|---|
| Lengths (cm) |  |  |  |
| Acromiale-radiale | 35.62 | 33.86 | 0.001 |
| Radiale-stylion | 27.69 | 26.54 | 0.001 |
| Stylion-dactylion | 21.10 | 20.20 | 0.001 |
| Iliospinale | 102.85 | 98.04 | 0.001 |
| Trochanterion | 96.14 | 92.08 | 0.001 |
| Trochanterion-tibiale | 46.80 | 44.84 | 0.001 |
| Tibiale laterale | 49.73 | 47.55 | 0.001 |
| Tibiale mediale | 41.76 | 39.63 | 0.001 |
| Foot length | 27.84 | 26.59 | 0.001 |
| Skinfolds (mm) |  |  |  |
| Triceps | 9.50 | 7.96 | 0.001 |
| Subscapular | 12.28 | 9.98 | 0.001 |
| Biceps | 4.36 | 3.74 | 0.001 |
| Iliac crest | 12.37 | 9.63 | 0.001 |
| Supraspinale | 9.01 | 7.44 | 0.001 |
| Abdominal | 17.49 | 12.91 | 0.001 |
| Front thigh | 11.92 | 9.85 | 0.001 |
| Medial calf | 7.69 | 6.19 | 0.001 |

**Table 2.** Differences between forwards and backs for 43 anthropometric measurements according to ANOVA: girths, breadths, stature, sitting height, arm span and mass (means for all the sample).

| Girths (cm) | | | |
|---|---|---|---|
| Head | 57.76 | 56.71 | 0.001 |
| Neck | 41.09 | 38.72 | 0.001 |
| Arm relaxed | 35.00 | 32.58 | 0.001 |
| Arm fully flexed and tensed | 37.18 | 34.80 | 0.001 |
| Forearm | 30.47 | 28.97 | 0.001 |
| Wrist | 18.17 | 17.23 | 0.001 |
| Thigh subgluteus | 63.33 | 60.18 | 0.001 |
| Thigh medium | 60.86 | 57.69 | 0.001 |
| Calf | 40.79 | 38.91 | 0.001 |
| Ankle | 24.25 | 22.93 | 0.001 |
| Chest | 105.67 | 99.75 | 0.001 |
| Waist minimum | 87.46 | 82.01 | 0.001 |
| Hip maximum | 102.55 | 97.27 | 0.001 |
| Breadths (cm) | | | |
| Biacromial | 43.58 | 41.86 | 0.001 |
| Biiliocristal | 30.86 | 29.27 | 0.001 |
| Chest depth | 22.03 | 20.63 | 0.001 |
| Transverse chest | 32.81 | 31.05 | 0.001 |
| Biepicondylar humerus | 7.46 | 7.13 | 0.001 |
| Wrist | 6.23 | 5.96 | 0.001 |
| Biepicondylar femur | 9.92 | 9.40 | 0.001 |
| Bimalleolare | 8.35 | 7.90 | 0.001 |
| Stature (m) | 1.832 | 1.764 | 0.001 |
| Sitting height (cm) | 95.99 | 93.40 | 0.001 |
| Arm span (cm) | 190.84 | 183.10 | 0.001 |
| Mass (kg) | 91.71 | 79.86 | 0.001 |

The ANOVA comparisons for body composition and somatotype variables yielded statistical differences (see Table 3): absolute muscle mass (forwards: 56.58 ± 5.77 kg, and backs 49.33 ± 6.87 kg; $p < 0.001$), relative muscle mass (NS), absolute bone mass (forwards: 11.39 ± 1.45 kg, and backs: 9.79 ± 0.86 kg, $p < 0.001$), relative bone mass (NS), percentage body fat (forwards: 13.86 ± 3.72%, and backs: 11.83 ± 3.20%; $p < 0.001$).

Observations for somatotype were: endomorphy (forwards: 3.04 ± 1.07; and backs: 2.51 ± 0.88; $p < 0.001$), and corrected endomorphy (forwards: 2.85 ± 1.00, and backs: 2.43 ± 0.86; $p < 0.001$); mesomorphy (forwards: 6.12 ± 1.05, and backs; 5.67 ± 0.94; $p < 0.001$) and ectomorphy (forwards: 1.29 ± 0.71, and backs: 1.54 ± 0.72; $p < 0.005$).

**Table 3**. Differences in body composition and somatotype means between forwards and backs according to ANOVA (all the sample).

|  | Forw. | Backs | p< |
|---|---|---|---|
| Body Composition |  |  |  |
| Absolute muscle mass (kg) | 56.58 | 49.33 | 0.001 |
| Relative muscle mass (%) | 61.39 | 62.05 | NS |
| Absolute bone mass (kg) | 11.39 | 9.79 | 0.001 |
| Relative bone mass (%) | 12.44 | 12.28 | NS |
| % body fat | 13.86 | 11.83 | 0.001 |
| Somatotype |  |  |  |
| Endomorphy | 3.04 | 2.51 | 0.001 |
| Endomorphy corrected | 2.85 | 2.43 | 0.001 |
| Mesomorphy | 6.12 | 5.67 | 0.001 |
| Ectomorphy | 1.29 | 1.54 | 0.005 |

When the sample was divided between best and worst performers, statistical differences were observed (ANOVA $p < 0.05$) in 30 of the 43 measurements (see Tables 4 and 5).

**Table 4**. Comparisons on 43 anthropometric measurements between best and worst performers using ANOVA: lengths and skinfolds (means).

|  | Best | Worst | p< |
|---|---|---|---|
| Lengths (cm) |  |  |  |
| Acromiale radiale | 35.01 | 34.39 | 0.02 |
| Radiale-stylion | 27.28 | 26.91 | NS |
| Stylion-dactylion | 21.08 | 20.26 | 0.001 |
| Iliospinale | 101.02 | 99.54 | 0.03 |
| Trochanterion | 94.59 | 93.30 | 0.04 |
| Trochanterion-tibiale | 45.69 | 45.42 | NS |
| Tibiale laterale | 49.00 | 48.23 | 0.04 |
| Tibiale mediale | 40.72 | 40.30 | NS |
| Foot | 27.56 | 26.74 | 0.001 |
| Skinfolds (mm) |  |  |  |
| Triceps | 8.01 | 9.27 | 0.005 |
| Subscapular | 10.77 | 11.98 | 0.05 |
| Biceps | 3.95 | 4.16 | NS |
| Iliac crest | 10.32 | 12.56 | 0.015 |
| Supraspinale | 7.40 | 9.54 | 0.001 |
| Abdominal | 14.47 | 16.96 | NS |
| Front thigh | 9.99 | 11.24 | 0.04 |
| Medial calf | 6.22 | 7.63 | 0.04 |

**Table 5.** Comparisons on 43 anthropometric measurements between best and worst performers using ANOVA: girths, breadths, stature, sitting height, arm span and mass (means).

|  | Best | Worst | p< |
|---|---|---|---|
| Girths (cm) |  |  |  |
| Head | 57.68 | 57.03 | 0.01 |
| Neck | 40.66 | 39.46 | 0.001 |
| Arm relaxed | 34.31 | 33.42 | 0.01 |
| Arm fully flexed and tensed | 36.71 | 35.37 | 0.001 |
| Forearm | 30.31 | 29.09 | 0.001 |
| Wrist | 18.04 | 17.38 | 0.001 |
| Thigh subgluteus | 62.27 | 60.95 | 0.02 |
| Thigh medium | 60.19 | 58.46 | 0.001 |
| Calf | 40.66 | 39.28 | 0.001 |
| Ankle | 24.02 | 23.24 | 0.001 |
| Chest | 103.34 | 101.80 | NS |
| Waist minimum | 84.49 | 84.26 | NS |
| Hip maximum | 100.00 | 98.77 | NS |
| Breadths (cm) |  |  |  |
| Biacromial | 43.00 | 42.40 | 0.050 |
| Biiliocristal | 30.12 | 29.75 | NS |
| Chest depth | 21.01 | 21.06 | NS |
| Transverse chest | 31.87 | 31.67 | NS |
| Biepicondylar humerus | 7.28 | 7.20 | NS |
| Wrist | 6.18 | 5.97 | 0.001 |
| Hand | 8.87 | 8.62 | 0.004 |
| Biepicondylar femur | 9.75 | 9.58 | 0.04 |
| Bimalleolare | 8.16 | 8.01 | 0.04 |
| Stature (m) | 1.806 | 1.780 | 0.01 |
| Sitting height (cm) | 95.38 | 93.71 | 0.002 |
| Arm span (cm) | 188.50 | 185.06 | 0.01 |
| Mass (kg) | 86.97 | 82.56 | 0.005 |

When body composition and somatotype variables were compared between best and worst performers, we found in almost all of them, statistical differences between groups (Table 6). In absolute muscle mass, the means and SD were: best: $53.00 \pm 6.98$ kg, and worst: $50.38 \pm 4.79$ kg ($p<0.001$), and in relative muscle mass, we also found statistical differences: best: $62.25 \pm 3.48\%$, and worst: $60.84 \pm 4.11\%$ ($p<0.001$). In absolute bone mass was found: best: $10.42 \pm 1.24$ kg, worst: $10.13 \pm 1.06$ kg ($p<0.004$), and NS differences in relative bone mass comparison. The % body fat was significantly less in the best performers ($12.01 \pm 3.06\%$), than in the worst ones ($13.98 \pm 4.20\%$) ($p<0.002$). In somatotype components, there were significant differences in endomorphy (best: $2.71 \pm 0.75$, worst: $3.01 \pm 1.19$; $p<0.001$), and in mesomorphy between groups (best: $5.95 \pm 1.02$, worst: $5.76 \pm 0.98$; $p<0.02$). No significant differences were found in ectomorphy.

When only best performers were considered, divided between forwards and backs, there were statistical differences in all the anthropometric measurements (p<0.05), except head girth and seven of the eight skinfolds analysed (see Tables 7 and 8).

Table 6. Means in body composition and somatotype variables between best and worst performers; ANOVA results.

|  | Best | Worst | p< |
|---|---|---|---|
| Body Composition |  |  |  |
| Absolute muscle mass (kg) | 53.00 | 50.38 | 0.001 |
| Relative muscle mass (%) | 62.25 | 60.84 | 0.001 |
| Absolute bone mass (kg) | 10.42 | 10.13 | 0.004 |
| Relative bone mass (%) | 11.34 | 11.02 | NS |
| % body fat | 12.01 | 13.98 | 0.002 |
| Somatotype |  |  |  |
| Endomorphy | 2.71 | 3.01 | 0.001 |
| Mesomorphy | 5.95 | 5.76 | 0.02 |
| Ectomorphy | 1.42 | 1.46 | NS |

Table 7. Means of 43 anthropometric measurements of best performers divided considering their role in the game : lengths and skinfolds (forwards and backs). Results of ANOVA.

|  | Forw. | Backs | p< |
|---|---|---|---|
| Lengths (cm) |  |  |  |
| Acromiale-radiale | 35.03 | 34.22 | 0.001 |
| Radiale-stylion | 28.00 | 26.74 | 0.001 |
| Stylion-dactylion | 21.69 | 20.65 | 0.001 |
| Iliospinale | 104.84 | 98.23 | 0.001 |
| Trochanterion | 96.99 | 94.50 | 0.001 |
| Trochanterion-tibiale | 46.62 | 45.15 | 0.02 |
| Tibiale laterale | 50.75 | 47.60 | 0.001 |
| Tibiale mediale | 42.24 | 39.60 | 0.001 |
| Foot | 28.53 | 26.90 | 0.001 |
| Skinfolds (mm) |  |  |  |
| Triceps | 8.30 | 7.76 | NS |
| Subscapular | 11.66 | 10.12 | 0.04 |
| Biceps | 4.02 | 3.92 | NS |
| Iliac crest | 10.36 | 10.24 | NS |
| Supraspinale | 7.43 | 7.31 | NS |
| Abdominal | 13.96 | 11.97 | NS |
| Front thigh | 10.55 | 9.59 | NS |
| Medial calf | 6.54 | 5.95 | NS |

**Table 8**. Means of 43 anthropometric measurements of best performers divided considering their role in the game : girths, breadths, stature, sitting height, arm span and mass (forwards and backs). Results of ANOVA.

| | Forw. | Backs | p< |
|---|---|---|---|
| Girths (cm) | | | |
| Head | 57.86 | 57.58 | NS |
| Neck | 42.00 | 39.64 | 0.001 |
| Arm relaxed | 35.40 | 33.52 | 0.001 |
| Arm fully flexed and tensed | 37.92 | 35.84 | 0.001 |
| Forearm | 31.18 | 29.70 | 0.001 |
| Wrist | 18.68 | 17.57 | 0.001 |
| Thigh subgluteus | 63.64 | 61.23 | 0.007 |
| Thigh medium | 61.48 | 59.25 | 0.005 |
| Calf | 41.75 | 39.82 | 0.002 |
| Ankle | 24.70 | 23.52 | 0.001 |
| Chest | 105.80 | 101.36 | 0.001 |
| Waist minimum | 86.54 | 82.91 | 0.001 |
| Hip maximum | 102.16 | 98.30 | 0.001 |
| Breadths (cm) | | | |
| Biacromial | 43.99 | 42.25 | 0.001 |
| Biiliocristal | 31.03 | 29.43 | 0.001 |
| Chest depth | 21.60 | 20.53 | 0.001 |
| Transverse chest | 32.88 | 31.05 | 0.001 |
| Biepicondylar humerus | 7.56 | 7.07 | 0.001 |
| Wrist | 6.37 | 6.04 | 0.001 |
| Hand | 9.14 | 8.67 | 0.001 |
| Biepicondylar femur | 10.11 | 9.48 | 0.001 |
| Bimalleolare | 8.47 | 7.93 | 0.001 |
| Stature (m) | 1.854 | 1.77 | 0.001 |
| Sitting height (cm) | 97.05 | 94.06 | 0.001 |
| Arm span (cm) | 193.92 | 184.53 | 0.001 |
| Mass (kg) | 92.70 | 82.65 | 0.001 |

No statistical differences ($p < 0.05$) were found on any of the three somatotype components between best performing forwards and backs. Differences also disappeared in percent body fat, and percent muscle mass. Absolute muscle mass, remained greater in forwards (forwards: $56.09 \pm 5.47$ kg, backs: $50.26 \pm 5.74$ kg; $p < 0.001$), and for the first time, relative bone mass appeared to be greater in forwards than in backs (forwards: $12.62 \pm 0.88$ %, backs: $12.03 \pm 0.83$ %; $p < 0.005$) (see Table 9).

When the worst performing group was divided into forwards and backs, statistical differences were found in 42 of the 43 anthropometric measurements done ($p < 0.05$) (see Tables 10 and 11).

Statistical differences were found too in almost all somatotype and body composition components between worst performing forwards and backs. Only in relative muscle mass were differences not significant (see Table 12).

**Table 9.** Comparisons for means in body composition and somatotype in best performers divided in forwards and backs (ANOVA results).

|  | Forw. | Backs | p< |
|---|---|---|---|
| Body Composition |  |  |  |
| Absolute muscle mass (kg) | 56.09 | 50.26 | 0.001 |
| Relative muscle mass (%) | 60.73 | 59.92 | NS |
| Absolute bone mass (kg) | 11.78 | 9.93 | 0.001 |
| Relative bone mass (%) | 12.62 | 12.03 | 0.005 |
| % body fat | 12.66 | 11.52 | NS |
| Somatotype |  |  |  |
| Endomorphy | 2.50 | 2.33 | NS |
| Mesomorphy | 6.34 | 6.00 | NS |
| Ectomorphy | 1.46 | 1.32 | NS |

**Table 10.** Comparisons on 43 anthropometric measurements of worst performers divided considering their role in the game: lengths and skinfolds (forwards and backs). Results of ANOVA are indicated.

|  | Forw. | Backs | p< |
|---|---|---|---|
| Lengths (cm) |  |  |  |
| Acromiale-radiale | 34.39 | 33.86 | 0.001 |
| Radiale-stylion | 26.91 | 26.65 | 0.04 |
| Stylion-dactylion | 20.58 | 20.26 | 0.02 |
| Iliospinale | 101.01 | 99.54 | 0.01 |
| Trochanterion | 95.91 | 93.30 | 0.006 |
| Trochanterion-tibiale | 49.76 | 45.42 | 0.01 |
| Tibiale laterale | 48.23 | 47.10 | 0.02 |
| Tibiale mediale | 40.30 | 39.88 | 0.05 |
| Foot | 27.10 | 26.49 | 0.02 |
| Skinfolds (mm) |  |  |  |
| Triceps | 10.44 | 9.27 | 0.005 |
| Subscapular | 16.17 | 11.98 | 0.001 |
| Biceps | 4.16 | 3.84 | 0.002 |
| Iliac crest | 13.30 | 11.90 | 0.004 |
| Supraspinale | 9.54 | 8.70 | 0.03 |
| Abdominal | 16.96 | 13.45 | 0.05 |
| Front thigh | 14.27 | 11.24 | 0.01 |
| Medial calf | 7.63 | 6.63 | 0.004 |

Table 11. Means of 43 anthropometric measurements of worst performers divided considering their role in the game: girths, breadths, stature, sitting height, arm span and mass (forwards and backs). Results of ANOVA are indicated.

|  | Forw. | Backs | p< |
|---|---|---|---|
| Girths (cm) |  |  |  |
| Head | 57.03 | 56.30 | 0.001 |
| Neck | 40.67 | 38.60 | 0.001 |
| Arm relaxed | 34.86 | 32.40 | 0.001 |
| Arm fully flexed and tensed | 36.58 | 34.52 | 0.001 |
| Forearm | 29.77 | 28.61 | 0.001 |
| Wrist | 17.80 | 17.08 | 0.001 |
| Thigh subgluteus | 62.95 | 59.54 | 0.001 |
| Thigh medium | 60.28 | 57.17 | 0.001 |
| Calf | 40.36 | 38.52 | 0.001 |
| Ankle | 23.90 | 22.78 | 0.001 |
| Chest | 104.91 | 99.60 | 0.001 |
| Waist minimum | 87.27 | 82.12 | 0.001 |
| Hip maximum | 101.78 | 96.64 | 0.001 |
| Breadths (cm) |  |  |  |
| Biacromial | 43.36 | 41.72 | 0.001 |
| Biiliocristal | 30.15 | 29.47 | 0.05 |
| Chest depth | 21.77 | 20.55 | 0.001 |
| Transverse chest | 32.18 | 31.31 | 0.04 |
| Biepicondylar humerus | 7.26 | 7.16 | NS |
| Wrist | 6.04 | 5.91 | 0.05 |
| Hand | 8.86 | 8.46 | 0.003 |
| Biepicondylar femur | 9.77 | 9.44 | 0.004 |
| Bimalleolare | 8.19 | 7.88 | 0.002 |
| Stature (m) | 1.803 | 1.764 | 0.003 |
| Sitting height (cm) | 94.82 | 92.93 | 0.02 |
| Arm span (cm) | 187.55 | 183.28 | 0.02 |
| Mass (kg) | 88.25 | 78.52 | 0.001 |

Table 12. Comparisons for means in body composition and somatotype in worst performers divided in forwards and backs (ANOVA results).

|  | Forw. | Backs | p< |
|---|---|---|---|
| Body Composition |  |  |  |
| Absolute muscle mass (kg) | 54.08 | 48.14 | 0.001 |
| Relative muscle mass (%) | 60.42 | 61.21 | NS |
| Absolute bone mass (kg) | 10.65 | 9.77 | 0.001 |
| Relative bone mass (%) | 11.99 | 12.41 | 0.04 |
| % body fat | 15.61 | 12.95 | 0.01 |
| Somatotype |  |  |  |
| Endomorphy | 3.57 | 2.85 | 0.02 |
| Mesomorphy | 6.05 | 5.55 | 0.03 |
| Ectomorphy | 1.38 | 1.41 | NS |

## 4. DISCUSSION .

The size of the whole sample (n=246), and the number of anthropometric measurements made, clearly suggest, in line with the results obtained, that there are at least two different morphological types in  Rugby Sevens, related to the playing position on the field (forwards and backs). The significant statistical differences found in the 43 anthropometric measurements are very consistent with this idea. Further analysis of body composition indicators showed statistical differences in absolute muscle and bone masses, in % body fat, and in the three components of somatotype.

Even though all the subjects were international players, it is known that the development of this sport is not the same all around the world. The comparison made on morphological type between best and worst performers reinforces this observation. There were statistical differences in 32 of the 43 anthropometric measurements made (6 of the 9 lengths, 6 of the 8 skinfolds, 10 of the 13 girths, 6 of the 9 breadths, stature, sitting height, arm span and body mass). There were also statistical differences in absolute and relative muscle mass, absolute bone mass, % body fat, and in two of the three components of somatotype (endomorphy and mesomorphy). Evidently, there are morphological differences associated with the playing standard in Rugby Sevens.

When the best players were divided into forwards and backs, there were statistical differences in 35 of the 43 anthropometric measurements made (the 9 lengths, only one of the 8 skinfolds, 12 of the 13 girths, the 9 breadths, stature, sitting height, arm span and body mass). When the worst players were divided into forwards and backs, there were statistical differences in 42 of the 43 anthropometric measurements. The above results are further confirmation that there are, at least from the morphological point of view, two types of players, in relation to their playing position on the field. The absence of differences in almost all the skinfolds measured, % body fat, relative muscle mass, and in the three components of the somatotype in the best group, is very suggestive. In the same way, the presence of statistical differences in almost all body composition and somatotype components in the worst group, probably reflects a poor training and nutritional condition in the less successful players.

At the high performance level, a low percentage of body fat was found, with no statistical differences between groups. In muscle mass, absolute values were still larger in forwards, but in relative terms, those differences disappeared. In bone mass, for the very first time in this study, statistical differences were found in absolute and relative values, clearly related to the different performance requirements of forwards and backs. In the somatotype components, no differences were found.

Considering the massive changes the game of rugby has experienced in the last decade (laws, coaching, fitness training, playing gear, etc.), extensive research is needed in all aspects of both the full game and the abbreviated code. Sports scientists (in all disciplines) must work hard to keep pace with the constant changes, in order to make the game safer for the players and more exciting for the spectators.

## 5. CONCLUSIONS

We can conclude that in Rugby Sevens, there are at least two different morphological types: forwards and backs. This difference must be taken into consideration for talent selection in this sport.

The high-level players were taller, heavier, bigger, more muscular and leaner than the low-level counterparts. Similar relative values in muscle mass and in % body fat (both forwards and backs), confirm the importance of training, and nutritional aspects in these athletes. The differences found in bone mass, in elite players, strongly suggest the importance of skeletal frame for success in this game.

Even when technical and tactical aspects of every team sport have great importance, anthropometry is a very valuable tool in the selection of talent in Rugby Sevens. It is useful also in monitoring responses of physique to the training process.

## REFERENCES

Carter, J.E.L., 1992, *The Heath-Carter Anthropometric Somatotype. Instruction Manual*, (San Diego: San Diego State University).

Drinkwater, D.T. and Mazza, J.C., 1994, Body composition. Chapter 6. pp. 102-137. *Kinanthropometry in Aquatic Sports*, edited by Carter, J.E.L. and Ackland, T.R. (Champaign, Il: HK Sport Science Monograph Series).

Durnin, J.V.G.A., and Womersley, J., 1974, Body fat assessed from total body density and its estimation from skinfold thicknesses: Measurements on 481 men and women aged 16 to 72 years. *British Journal of Nutrition*, **32**, 77-97.

# 13 Whole-body and Regional Bone Mineral Density and Bone Mineral Mass in Rugby Union Players: Comparison of Forwards, Backs and Controls

W. Bell[1], W.D. Evans[2], D.M. Cobner[1] and R. Eston[3]

[1]University of Wales Institute Cardiff, Cyncoed, Cardiff CF23 6XD
[2]University of Wales Hospital, Heath Park, Cardiff CF14 4XW
[3]University of Wales, Bangor, Gwyneddd LL57 2PX

## 1. INTRODUCTION

Rugby Union football is a physical contact game which places considerable emphasis on absolute size, strength, speed and power. Since the effects of exercise, training, and performance on bone mineral density (BMD) are thought to be site-specific, and not generalised throughout the skeleton, differences between athletes in different sports, or differences between athletes involved in the same sport, are likely to be observed only at specific anatomical locations (Beck and Marcus, 1999). The effects of physical activity on bone remodelling, therefore, will depend to some extent on the nature of the activity and the application of the principles and practice of training programmes.

It is fairly well established that physical activity of one kind or another confers beneficial effects on the modelling and remodelling of bone. This is true in both males and females, in children and adults, and at competitive and recreational levels of sports performance. In general, studies which have compared different athletic groups, or athletic groups with controls, have confirmed that athletes undertaking a training programme of skeletal loading, such as weight-training or weight-bearing activities, demonstrate enhanced bone remodelling. On the other hand, some authors have reported that extreme levels of physical activity or training are detrimental to bone remodelling (McDougall et al., 1992; Chilibeck et al., 1995; Beck and Marcus, 1999). Considering the extent of participation in Rugby Union football, there is a surprising lack of information regarding the skeletal characteristics of players. Apart from the constrasting playing requirements and training regimes of forwards and backs, a full-body contact game such as Rugby Union football increases the potential for injury, especially if bone health is compromised. Rates of injury vary according to playing position, there being a marked contrast between forwards and backs. Forwards sustain a greater proportion of injuries to the upper-body, whereas backs sustain a greater proportion to the lower limbs (Bird *et al.*, 1998). Bearing in mind the above considerations, the objective of the present study was to contrast the differences in whole-body and regional BMD and bone mineral mass (BMM) between forwards, backs and controls.

## 2. MATERIALS AND METHODS

### 2.1 Participants

Thirty competitive young adult rugby players aged 21.1 ± 2.1 years (M ± SD) and 21 controls (22.3 ± 5.1 years)  participated in the study. The criterion for inclusion was that players had played representative rugby at a junior level of the game. The majority had competed at regional level and twenty had attained international honours. Although players were not considered to be elite performers, a number will go on to play first-class rugby in the UK. At this stage of their career, individuals will have trained and played competitive rugby for about 9 years. Players were assigned to playing units on the basis of individual playing position as either forwards (n=15) or backs (n=15). The control group (n=21) consisted of recreationally active individuals. Informed consent was obtained from individuals and all procedures were approved by the appropriate ethics conmmittee.

### 2.2 Anthropometry and bone mineral mass

Stature was measured to the nearest 0.1 cm using a Harpenden stadiometer and body mass to the closest 0.1 kg on digital scales.

Measurements of BMM were made by dual-energy X-ray absorptiometry (DXA) using Hologic QDR/1000W and QDR/1500W scanners (Hologic, Waltham, MA, USA). A detailed account of procedures and calibration can be found in Bell *et al.* (1995). Briefly, each subject was aligned with the long axis of the couch and remained motionless during the scan. The technique is based on the differential attenuation of radiation at two energies as it passes through bone and soft tissue. The attenuation data are displayed as a digital image with each picture element (pixel) corresponding to individual measurement points through the subject. Pixels containing bone are identified by their value of differential attenuation and decomposed into bone mineral and soft-tissue masses. Pixels not containing bone are decomposed into lean and soft-tissue components using a soft-tissue phantom which is scanned simultaneously with the subject. When this process is complete, the total masses of bone mineral, fat and lean tissue compartments are obtained by summing the corresponding values for individual pixels. Recent discussions of the validity and reliability of DXA can be found in Lohman (1996) and Lohman *et al.* (2000).

The digital image of each subject was then partitioned into regional anatomical segments comprising the head, right and left arms, trunk, and right and left legs. Whole-body and regional analyses for BMD and BMM were carried out for mean arms, mean legs, pelvis, lumbar spine and thoracic spine.

## 2.3 Analytical procedures

Bone mineral mass was checked for normality using probability plots. Correlations between standard scores and raw scores ranged between 0.97-0.98. The cut-off point for normality was 0.96, consequently BMM was considered Gaussian. There were only minor differences in BMM between right and left arms and right and left legs, thus the mean was calculated and used in all analyses. Raw measurements were used for the pelvis, lumbar and thoracic spine.

Descriptive data are presented as means ± SDs. A simple analysis of variance (ANOVA) was employed to identify differences between groups. Where significance occurred post-hoc comparisons utilised Tukey's HSD method (Daniel, 1995). A probability level of $p=0.05$ was prescribed for all tests. Power was calculated for all variables. Apart from the pelvis, which had a value of 0.5, all variables had values upwards of 0.9.

All BMD values are reported as areal densities ($g.cm^2$). Since BMD does not adequately adjust for bone and body size, BMM was corrected (BMMc) using BMM as the dependent variable and bone area, body mass, and stature, as independent variables in multiple regression analysis (Prentice *et al.*, 1994).

## 3. RESULTS

Table 1 summarises the descriptive data for forwards, backs and controls. Forwards were significantly taller and heavier than both backs and controls ($p=0.004 - p=0.0001$), and although not significant the backs were taller and heavier than controls.

Results for BMD can be seen in Table 2. Whole-body and lower-limb BMD values were larger in forwards than either backs or controls ($p=0.0001$); there were no differences between backs and controls. In the upper limbs differences occurred between all three groups; forwards had greater values than backs and controls, and backs greater values than controls ($p=0.0001$). Differences between groups were not apparent in the pelvis. In the lumbar spine BMD for forwards and backs contrasted with that of controls (p=0.0001); in the thoracic spine forwards had greater values than backs and controls (p=0.001).

**Table 1**. Descriptive characteristics for forwards, backs and controls

|  | Forwards | Backs | Controls |
|---|---|---|---|
| Age (years) | 20.6 ± 1.4 | 20.7± 2.6 | 22.3 ± 5.5 |
| Stature (m) | 1.844 ± 0.056 ab | 1.788 ± 0.052 b | 1.775 ± 0.067 a |
| Body mass (kg) | 99.8 ± 10.3 ab | 80.3 ± 5.5 b | 74.3 ± 8.7 a |

Significance: a = fowards vs controls      b = forwards vs backs

**Table 2**. BMD (g.cm$^2$ ) for whole-body, arms, legs, pelvis, lumbar and thoracic spine

|  | Forwards | Backs | Controls |
|---|---|---|---|
| Whole-body | 1.383 ± 0.09 ab | 1.283 ± 0.07 b | 1.263 ± 0.07 a |
| Arms | 1.070 ± 0.07 ab | 0.983 ± 0.05 bc | 0.876 ± 0.05 ac |
| Legs | 1.624 ± 0.12 ab | 1.516 ± 0.10 b | 1.460 ± 0.11 a |
| Pelvis | 1.398 ± 0.09 | 1.309 ± 0.11 | 1.335 ± 0.14 |
| Lumbar spine | 1.343 ± 0.15 a | 1.271 ± 0.13 c | 1.160 ± 0.11 ac |
| Thoracic spine | 1.138 ± 0.15 ab | 0.978 ± 0.09 b | 1.023 ± 0.09 a |

Significance: a = fwds vs controls      b = fwds vs backs      c= backs vs controls

Data for BMM corrected for size are given in Table 3. Corrected BMM at the arms, legs, pelvis, lumbar and thoracic spine was significantly greater in forwards than controls, and in forwards than backs (p=0.001 – p=0.0001). Backs and controls differed at the arms, pelvis and thoracic spine (p=0.0001).

**Table 3.** BMMc (g) for whole-body, arms, legs, pelvis, lumbar and thoracic spine

|  | Forwards | Backs | Controls |
|---|---|---|---|
| Whole-body | 3885 ± 280 ab | 3304 ± 269 bc | 3010 ± 263 ac |
| Arms | 309 ± 31 ab | 242 ± 37 bc | 204 ± 29 ac |
| Legs | 769 ± 53 ab | 653 ± 42 b | 622 ± 55 a |
| Pelvis | 452 ± 21 ab | 410 ± 21 bc | 390 ± 20 ac |
| Lumbar spine | 90 ± 14 ab | 79 ± 6 b | 74 ± 13 a |
| Thoracic spine | 229 ± 21 ab | 188 ± 15 bc | 170 ± 19 ac |

Significance: a = fwds vs controls    b = fwds vs backs    c = backs vs controls

## 4. DISCUSSION

Forwards are a much more disparate group of players than backs, because their contribution to the game is different from that of backs. The variation in size, between these two playing units (Table 1), and the contrasting high-intensity impact activities during competition and training, are the potential determinants influencing bone adaptation in Rugby Union players.

Forwards were at the 90th centile for stature, and backs and controls the 70th centile. For body mass, forwards were at the 99th centile, backs the 90th centile, and controls the 75th centile (Freeman *et al.*, 1995). Overall, forwards had a greater body mass per unit stature than backs.

Individuals exercising at relatively high skeletal loads have shown a consistently greater whole-body BMD than those exercising at lower skeletal loads. Hamdy *et al.* (1994), for example, found that weight-lifters (1.324 g.cm$^2$) had a larger BMD (adjusted for body mass) than either cross-trained athletes (1.311g.cm$^2$), runners (1.259 g.cm$^2$), or those involved in recreational activities (1.256 g.cm$^2$). Likewise, Smith and Rutherford (1993) found rowers (1.272 g.cm$^2$) to have larger BMD values than either triathletes (1.211 g.cm$^2$) or sedentary individuals (1.197 g.cm$^2$). Moderate exercise may not provide sufficient stimulus to the skeleton to initiate an adaptive response.

In the present study, whole-body BMD (Table 2) was significantly greater in forwards than backs (1.383 vs 1.283 g.cm$^2$) and controls (1.383 vs 1.263 g.cm$^2$). A contributory reason for this is the larger body mass of forwards, which will tend to increase the gravitational load on the skeleton.

In general, most studies show a positive relationship between body mass and BMD. For example, Smith and Rutherford (1993) found a significant moderate correlation between BMD and body mass in male rowers and triathletes (r=0.42, p=0.014). Hamdy *et al.* (1994) recorded a value of 0.73 for their mixed group of athletes. These figures compare with the present groups of forwards (r=0.73, p=0.001), backs (r=0.92, p=0.01) and controls (r=0.46, p=0.1). The relationship between BMD and body mass in rugby players is clearly much higher than that of controls.

Due to the similarity of chronological age in the three groups, T scores (mean and population SD at peak bone mass) were used as the reference point for comparison. Values were well above normal (greater than −1.0) in both forwards and backs (2.368 vs 1.305 units, p=0.001), percentages being 119% and 110% respectively.

There is considerable evidence which suggests that the response of bone to mechanical loading is site-specific (Hamdy *et al.*, 1994; Chilibeck *et al.*, 1995). In forwards, particularly at the scrummage, there is vigorous use of the arms and legs. The arms are used to provide a compact and safe scrummaging unit, whilst the legs are used to propel the scrum forward, or alternatively, to maintain it in a static position, depending on the strategy being employed. Specific confrontational encounters of this kind are not carried out by backs, although they are expected to engage vigorously in rucks and mauls. It might be expected, therefore, that differences in BMD of the upper and lower limbs would exist between forwards and backs. Table 2 confirms that this is so. Furthermore, both groups of players had significantly greater values in the arms than the control group. There were significant differences between forwards, and backs  and controls in the legs, but not between backs and controls. Bone mineral density was uniformly greater in the legs than the arms in all three groups.

Because of the flexed position adopted by players at the scrum, there will be considerable horizontal loading to the spine. In fact, most spinal injuries occur at the scrum, where the combined force of the two opposing packs at engagement of the scrum is of the order of 14,995 N (Milburn, 1993). To a lesser extent, vertical loading will occur at the spine in those players involved in jumping and landing at the line-out. Differences were observed between forwards and backs in the thoracic spine (1.138 vs 0.978 g.cm$^2$) and although there were no differences between forwards and backs in the lumbar spine, both these groups demonstrated larger BMD values than controls (Table 2).

The training of Rugby Union players is usually individual and position-specific, involving regimes of aerobic, anaerobic, strength and power training. Both groups of players engage in systematic pre-season and in-season weight-training, but generally speaking, training will be more intensive and varied in forwards than backs, largely because of the extensive nature of the game they play.

Weight-training stimulates an increase in BMM and BMD. This occurs as a consequence of  the direct action of muscle pulling on bone, or when heavy weights are supported by the skeleton. Hamdy *et al.* (1994), for example, found higher BMD values of the lumbar vertebrae in weight-lifters (1.211 g.cm$^2$) compared with cross-trained (1.311 g.cm$^2$), running (1.259 g.cm$^2$) and recreational young adults (1.256 g.cm$^2$). In elite junior Olympic weight-lifters (Conroy *et al.*, 1993), BMD values at the spine (1.41 g.cm$^2$) and femoral neck (1.30 $g.cm^2$) were found to be greater than those of age-matched controls (1.06 and 1.05 $g.cm^2$ respectively). Rowers, who also engage in heavy weight-training programmes, have higher BMD values at the spine, arms, legs, pelvis and ribs, compared with triathletes and sedentary controls (Smith and Rutherford, 1993).

The use of BMD ($g.cm^2$), an expression derived by dividing BMM (g) by the scanned area of bone, is an important clinical tool in the assessment of fracture risk and the clinical management of patients with bone disease. Its weakness, however, is that it fails adequately to correct BMM for bone and body size. Prentice *et al.* (1994) advised that the simplest way to avoid size-related artifacts is to use BMM as the dependent variable, and to include bone area, body mass, and stature, as independent variables in multiple regression models. It is suggested that this procedure is applicable to all skeletal sites, irrespective of study group, instrumentation and scanning protocol.

When adjustments were made for size (Table 3) forwards had significantly larger corrected  BMM values than backs for whole-body, as well as all regional sites. It is reasonable to attribute these differences to the contrasting playing and training requirements of the two playing units, although it would require some direct experimental evidence to support this claim. The corrected BMM values between forwards and controls are more striking than those between backs and controls. This is not unexpected since both groups of players are involved in different playing and training practices, which will tend to load the skeleton differently.

It is concluded that there are substantional differences in whole-body and regional BMD and BMMc between forwards and backs, and that these are the likely result of contrasting playing and training requirements. Comparisons between forwards and controls were more diverse than those between backs and controls.

## REFERENCES

Beck, B. and Marcus, R., 1999, Skeletal effects of exercise in men. In *Osteoporosis in Men: the effects of gender on skeletal health*, edited by Orwell, E.S. (London: Academic Press), pp. 129-155.

Bell, W., Davies, J.S., Evans, W.D. and Scanlon, F.M., 1995, The validity of estimating total body fat and fat-free mass from skinfold thickness in adults with growth hormone deficiency. *Journal of Clinical Endocrinology and Metabolism*, **80**, 630-636.

Bird, Y.N., Waller, A.E., Marshall, S.W., Alsop, J.C., Chalmers, D.J. and Gerrard, D.F., 1998, The New Zealand rugby injury and performance project: V. Epidemiology of a season of rugby injury. *British Journal of Sports Medicine*, **32**, 319-325.

Chilibeck, P.D., Sale, D.G. and Webber, C.E., 1995, Exercise and bone mineral density. *Sports Medicine*, **19**, 103-122.

Conroy, B.P., Kraemer, W.J., Maresh, C.M., Fleck, S.J., Stone, M.H., Fry, A.C., Miller, P.D. and Dalsky, G.P., 1993, Bone mineral density in elite junior Olympic weightlifters. *Medicine and Science in Sports and Exercise*, **25**, 1103-1109.

Daniel, W.W., 1995, *Biostatistics: a Foundation for Analysis in the Health Sciences*, (Chichester: John Wiley & Sons).

Freeman, J.V., Cole, T.J., Chinn, S., Jones, P.R.M., White, E.M. and Preece, M.A., 1995, Cross-sectional stature and weight reference curves in the UK, 1990. *Archives of Disease in Childhood*, **73**, 17-24.

Hamdy, R.C., Anderson, J.S., Whalen, K.E. and Harvill, L.M., 1994, Regional differences in bone density of young men involved in different exercises. *Medicine and Science in Sports and Exercise*, **26**, 884-888.

Lohman, T.G., 1996, Dual-energy X-ray absorptiometry. In *Human Body Composition*, edited by Roche, A.F., Heymsfield, S.B. and Lohman, T.G. (Champaign: Human Kinetics), pp.63-78.

Lohman, T.G., Harris, M., Teixeira, P.J. and Weiss, L., 2000, Assessing body composition and changes in body composition: another look at dual-energy X-ray absorptiometry. In, *In vivo Body Composition Studies*, edited by Yasumura, S., Wang, J. and Pierson Jr, R.N. Annals New York Academy of Sciences, 94, pp 45-54.

McDougall, J.D., Webber, C.E., Martin, J., Ormerod, S., Chesley, A., Younglai E.V., Gordon, C.L. and Blimkie, C.J.R., 1992, Relationship among running mileage, bone density, and serum testosterone in male runners. *Journal of Applied Physiology*, **73**, 1165-1170.

Milburn, P.D., 1993, Biomechanics of rugby union scrummaging: technical and safety issues. Sports Medicine, **16**, 168-179.

Prentice, A., Parsons, T.J. and Cole, T.J., 1994, Uncritical use of bone mineral density in absorptiometry may lead to size-related artifacts in the identification of bone mineral determinants. *American Journal of Clinical Nutrition*, **60**, 837-842.

Smith, R. and Rutherford, O.M., 1993, Spine and total bone mineral density and serum testosterone levels in male athletes. *European Journal of Applied Physiology*, **67**, 330-334.

# 14   A Comparison of Musculoskeletal Function in Elite and Sub-elite English Soccer Players

N. Rahnama[1,2], T. Reilly[1], A. Lees[1] and P. Graham-Smith[1]
[1]Research Institute for Sport and Exercise Sciences, Liverpool
John Moores University, Henry Cotton Campus,
15-21 Webster Street, Liverpool, L3 2ET, UK
[2]Physical Education Department, Isfahan University, Isfahan, Iran

## 1. INTRODUCTION

Effective musculoskeletal function is important in soccer, both for enhancing performance and minimising injury. Impairment in muscle function is reflected in strength imbalance and insufficiency and poor flexibility in the lower extremities. These are influential in movements such as sprinting, jumping, tackling, changing direction and kicking, whereas during heading and tackling, strength in trunk and upper body muscles is also utilised.

Ekstrand and Gillquist (1983) indicated that an imbalance in muscle strength between limbs may predispose a player towards musculoskeletal injury. Bender *et al.* (1964) reported that 806 cadets who had differences greater than 10% in quadriceps strength between limbs were more likely than normal to get knee injuries in the weaker limb. Knapik *et al.* (1991) suggested that subjects with an imbalance of greater than 15% were 2.6 times more likely to suffer injury in the weaker leg. In a later study, Fowler and Reilly (1993) reported a 20% difference in muscle strength in professional soccer players prone to injury.

A gross imbalance in strength between the quadriceps and hamstrings muscle groups has also been suggested as a factor which leads to an increase in the susceptibility to joint as well as muscle injury (Coplin, 1971). The ratio between the strength of the knee flexors and knee extensors is of particular interest, a low ratio being associated with a risk of injury (Fowler and Reilly, 1993). The hamstring/quadriceps strength ratio varies between 50% and 62% in healthy people (Knapik and Ramos, 1980) while ratios for soccer players vary between 41% and 81% depending upon the angular velocity of movement. The agonist-antagonist relationship for knee flexion and extension may be better described by the more functional ratio of eccentric hamstring to concentric quadriceps, known as the dynamic control ratio (Aagaard *et al.*, 1998).

Besides this asymmetry in muscle strength, risk usually manifests itself as muscle weakness and poor co-ordination of muscle activation. Generally, it is the disproportionately weaker muscle group that is prone to injury (Burkett, 1970). Players who carry muscle weaknesses into competition are likely to experience situations where the muscle may fail and injury occurs (Reilly and Howe, 1996). Individuals with well-developed strength capabilities are less prone to musculoskeletal strain, sprain injuries and back fatigue than their weaker counterparts when placed in physically demanding activities (Chaffin *et al.*, 1978).

Muscular tightness which restricts the range of motion is also thought to predispose the muscle to injury and to impair performance in sports where flexibility is important. In soccer, around 17% of injuries have been attributed to muscle tightness (Ekstrand and Gillquist, 1983). The hamstring muscles (knee flexors and hip extensors) are one of the most commonly strained muscle groups in soccer: one of the possible causes of this injury is a lack of flexibility in the joints they act across. Athletes with a history of injury to the hamstrings have more tightness in those muscles than do their counterparts (Noonan *et al.*, 1994).

The assessment of muscle function has become increasingly important as it is realised that there is a large variation in this human attribute which is affected by both individual and environmental factors. The identification of asymmetric weakness or laxity within an individual player may be more important than comparison between team members (Reilly and Howe, 1996). Isokinetic dynamometry can be used to assess strength as it allows the comparison of hamstrings/quadriceps strength ratio, left/right leg ratio and fast-speed to slow-speed ratio to identify any muscle imbalance and deficit in specific muscle groups.

Elite players are likely to have elevated levels of muscle strength due to the requirements of a high performance level and freedom from injury. Yet in the course of their habitual training they may develop imbalances and tightness not evident in those playing at a lower level. The aim of this study therefore was to compare musculoskeletal function between elite and sub-elite soccer players. A subsidiary aim was to identify the influence of body size on this comparison.

## 2. MATERIALS AND METHODS

### 2.1 Participants

Twenty-eight soccer players (14 elite and 14 sub-elite) were studied. Elite players were classed as those who were signed for a professional club and played international soccer (full-time professional players with an English Premier League club). Sub-elite players were classed as those who were not signed for a professional club but were playing regularly for local and University teams.

Participants recruited were not injured or rehabilitating from injury at the time of testing. All participants were aged between 18-25 years. Informed consent was obtained from all subjects before data collection, and ethical approval for the study was obtained from the institution's Human Ethics Committee.

Participants were tested during the 2000-2001 English competitive soccer season. All the tests were scheduled for the same time of day (10:00 hours) to remove the effects of any circadian variation on the variables being measured (Reilly and Brooks, 1986). Measurements for each participant were in four categories: anthropometric (height and mass), muscle strength profiling, hamstrings flexibility, and vertical jump height. The procedures in each category are described in turn. Table 1 shows the descriptive statistics for age, height and mass of the participants.

**Table 1.** Mean (± SD) age, height and mass of elite and sub-elite soccer players.

| Groups | N | Age (years) | Height (m) | Mass (kg) |
|--------|---|-------------|------------|-----------|
| Elite | 14 | 23.7 (4.3) | 1.82 (0.06) | 85.5 (9.2) |
| Sub-elite | 14 | 23.1 (3.1) | 1.79 (0.06) | 75.2 (8.1) |

*Anthropometric profiling*

Each participant's body mass (kg) was determined using a calibrated precision weighing scales (Hotline, Hamburg, Germany). A cursor placed on the participant's head was used to help measure height (m) (Seca, MeB-und Wiegetechnik, Vogel and Halke, Hamburg, Germany).

*Muscle strength profiling*

Strength of knee flexors and extensors (dominant and non-dominant legs) was measured on an isokinetic dynamometer (Lido Active, Loredan, Davis, CA). Each subject visited the laboratory and was tested with the same protocol on two separate occasions. The first visit entailed familiarisation with the dynamometer and the experimental procedure.

A standardised warm-up was initially performed on a Monark cycle ergometer for 5 min with no resistance at 60 rev.min$^{-1}$ prior to the experimental protocol. This exercise was followed by 10 min of static stretching of the relevant muscle groups, which were concentrated on the lower extremities. The subject was then seated in the dynamometer in an adjustable chair; the upper body was stabilised with straps secured across the shoulder, chest and hips. A resistance pad was also positioned on the thigh, proximal to the knee joint to localise the quadriceps and hamstrings. The axis of rotation of the dynamometer shaft was aligned with the axis of rotation of the knee joint, mid-way between the lateral condyle of the tibia and the lateral condyle of the femur. The cuff of the dynamometer's lever arm was attached to the ankle, proximal to the malleoli. These positions were recorded for each subject and standardised for subsequent trials. Range of motion (ROM) was pre-set to 0 to 90°. The gravity compensation procedure required the subject to relax, while the leg was passively extended and flexed over the entire ROM.

The participant was instructed to grasp the handles adjacent to the chair during the tests and then perform two submaximal knee extension and flexion movements. Testing consisted of three maximal voluntary movements at angular velocities of 1.05, 2.09 and 5.23 rad.s$^{-1}$ (in concentric mode) and 2.09 $_{ecc}$ rad.s$^{-1}$ (in eccentric mode), first for the dominant and then for the non-dominant leg. This order of testing for the different angular velocities was standardised from the slowest to the highest. Each trial was separated by 1 min of passive recovery. Verbal instructions were also standardised and visual feedback was given. Gravity-corrected peak torque was selected from the strength indices as a measure of muscular performance. The test protocol is highlighted in Table 2.

**Table 2**. Test protocol used in isokinetic dynamometry (n = 28).

| Test | Muscle groups | Modes | Angular velocity (rad.s$^{-1}$) |
|---|---|---|---|
| 1 | Hamstrings & Quadriceps | Concentric | 1.05 |
| 2 | Hamstrings & Quadriceps | Concentric | 5.23 |
| 3 | Quadriceps | Concentric/Eccentric | 2.09 |
| 4 | Hamstrings | Concentric/Eccentric | 2.09 |

Data for 48 variables were recorded for each player. These included absolute quadriceps muscle strength for dominant and non-dominant legs at the four angular velocities (8 variables were included for the two legs and four tests), relative quadriceps muscle strength (peak torque/body mass) for dominant and non-dominant legs at different angular velocities (8 variables), absolute hamstrings muscle strength for dominant and non-dominant legs at different angular velocities (8 variables), relative hamstrings muscle strength (peak torque/body mass) for dominant and non-dominant legs at different angular velocities (8 variables), muscle balance (hamstrings/quadriceps ratio) for dominant and non-dominant legs at different angular velocities (8 variables), fast-speed to slow-speed ratio for dominant and non-dominant legs for quadriceps and hamstrings (4 variables). Finally, a bilateral comparison (left/right ratio) was made for quadriceps and hamstrings (4 variables). Dynamic control ratio (DCR) was expressed as eccentric hamstrings relative to concentric quadriceps strength at 2.09 $_{(ecc)}$ rad.s$^{-1}$.

*Flexibility*

The flexibility of the participant's hip joint (in flexion) was measured by means of a goniometer (MIE goniometer, Medical Research Limited, Leeds). The subject lay supine on the floor with the legs extended and the head on the floor. The quadriceps muscle on the right leg was palpated and the goniometer was placed half-way down the limb (from the hip to the knee). The goniometer was then altered so that the liquid inside was level at 0 degrees. The subject then slowly lifted the right leg, keeping the left leg on the floor. With the help of another person, the point when maximum hip flexion had been reached was determined. This point was decided by observing the tenseness in the muscle and by the player's subjective response. The reading on the goniometer was then recorded. This procedure was completed three times. This protocol was repeated on the opposite limb to assess flexibility of both dominant and non-dominant legs.

*Vertical jump*

An electronic timing mat was used to measure standing vertical jump height (Cranlea & Company, Bournville, Birmingham, England). The participant stood on the mat and placed his hands on his hips, to control the influence of the arms on the jump. The meter was reset and the subject performed three maximal vertical jumps, from which the highest distance jumped was recorded for analysis. The jump was recorded when the subject completed a full cycle of jumping, including preparation to jump, leaving from the mat and landing back on it.

## 2.2 Statistical analysis

The strength variables were categorised into seven groups for statistical analysis. These categories included quadriceps muscle strength (peak torque), relative quadriceps muscle strength (peak torque/ body mass), hamstring muscle strength (peak torque), relative hamstring muscle strength (peak torque/ body mass), muscle balance (hamstring/quadriceps ratio), fast to slow speed ratio (F/S Ratio) and bilateral comparison (left/right ratio). Each of these data sets was analysed using separate multivariate analyses of variance (MANOVA) in which "group" (elite, sub-elite) was the "between participant" variable. Follow-up univariate analysis of variance (ANOVA) tests were used where appropriate.

Those measures not included in this initial procedure were analysed using separate analyses of variance for independent samples. These measures included vertical jump height and hamstring flexibility. The level of significance on all tests was set at $p < 0.05$.

## 3. RESULTS

### 3.1 Anthropometric profiles

The MANOVA showed that there was a significant difference between the two groups of players with regard to body size measurement (mass and height) (Wilks' lambda = 0.716, $F_{2,25} = 4.95$, $p < 0.01$). The significant difference in body mass was confirmed by ANOVA ($F_{1,26} = 9.83$, $p < 0.005$). The difference in height between groups was non-significant.

## 3.2 Quadriceps muscle strength profile (peak torque)

The MANOVA showed there was a difference between the two groups of players when the eight quadriceps peak torque variables were considered as a whole (different angular velocities, dominant and non-dominant leg) (Wilks' lambda = 0.12, $F_{8,19} = 16.78$, $p < 0.001$).

For the dominant leg, univariate ANOVA showed significant differences in quadriceps peak torque between groups at 1.05 rad.s$^{-1}$ ($F_{1,26} = 7.42$, $p < 0.001$), 2.09 rad.s$^{-1}$ ($F_{1,26} = 11.38$, $p < 0.002$), 5.23 rad.s$^{-1}$ ($F_{1,26} = 13.18$, $p < 0.001$) and 2.09 $_{(ecc)}$ rad.s$^{-1}$ ($F_{1,26} = 28.66$, $p < 0.001$). At all angular velocities, the elite players were stronger than the sub-elite players (see Figure 1a).

For the non-dominant leg, univariate ANOVA showed significant differences in quadriceps muscle strength profile (peak torque) between groups at 1.05 rad.s$^{-1}$ ($F_{1,26} = 12.90$, $p < 0.001$), 2.09 rad.s$^{-1}$ ($F_{1,26} = 17.23$, $p < 0.001$), 5.23 rad.s$^{-1}$ ($F_{1,26} = 8.84$, $p < 0.006$) and 2.09 $_{(ecc)}$ rad.s$^{-1}$ ($F_{1,26} = 37.32$, $p < 0.001$). In all variables, the elite players were stronger than sub-elite players (Figure 1b).

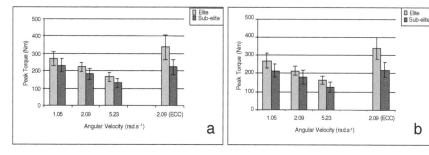

Figure 1. Comparison of quadriceps muscle strength (peak torque) between elite and sub-elite soccer players for the dominant leg (a) and non-dominant leg (b). Results are indicated for concentric mode at the three angular velocities and for eccentric mode at 2.09 rad.s$^{-1}$.

## 3.3 Relative muscle strength profile for the quadriceps group (peak torque/body mass)

The MANOVA showed a significant group difference in the quadriceps relative muscle strength, when corrected for body mass (Wilks' Lambda = 0.18, $F_{8,19} = 17.83$, $p < 0.001$). This finding corroborates the results of the comparison before data were normalised for body mass.

For the dominant leg, univariate ANOVA indicated significant differences in quadriceps relative muscle strength (peak torque normalised for body mass) between groups at 2.09 $_{(ecc)}$ rad.s$^{-1}$ ($F_{1,26} = 24.27$, $p < 0.001$) and 5.23 rad.s$^{-1}$ ($F_{1,26} = 4.57$, $p < 0.05$) with elite players being stronger than sub-elite players. No differences were apparent at 1.05 rad.s$^{-1}$ and 2.09 rad.s$^{-1}$ (see Figure 2a).

For the non-dominant leg, univariate ANOVA revealed significant differences in quadriceps relative muscle strength (peak torque normalised for body mass) between groups at 2.09 $_{(ecc)}$ rad.s$^{-1}$ ($F_{1,26}$ = 29.70, p < 0.001) and 5.23 rad.s$^{-1}$ ($F_{1,26}$ = 6.21, p < 0.02). No differences were apparent at 1.05 rad.s$^{-1}$ (p > 0.05) and 2.09 rad.s$^{-1}$ (p > 0.05). According to these data, the elite players had greater muscle strength at high velocities and in eccentric actions than the sub-elite players (see Figure 2b).

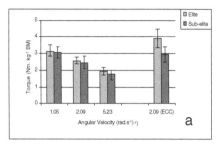 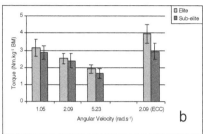

**Figure 2**. Comparison of quadriceps relative muscle strength (peak torque/body mass) between elite and sub-elite soccer players for the dominant leg (a) and non-dominant leg (b).

### 3.4 Hamstrings muscle strength (peak torque)

No significant differences between groups were indicated using MANOVA in analysing hamstrings muscle strength (peak torque) (Wilks' Lambda = 0.57, $F_{8,19}$ = 1.77, p > 0.05). Nevertheless, for the dominant leg, univariate ANOVA showed there was a significant difference in hamstrings muscle strength (peak torque) between groups at 1.05 rad.s$^{-1}$ ($F_{1,26}$ = 4.93, p < 0.03), and 2.09 $_{(ecc)}$ rad.s$^{-1}$ ($F_{1,26}$ = 12.42, p < 0.002) with elite players being stronger than sub-elite players. No differences were apparent at 2.09 rad.s$^{-1}$ and 5.23 rad.s$^{-1}$ (p > 0.05) (see Figure 3a).

For the non-dominant leg, univariate ANOVA indicated there was a significant difference between groups in muscle strength of the hamstrings (peak torque) at 1.05 rad.s$^{-1}$ ($F_{1,26}$ = 5.22, p < 0.03), 2.09 rad.s$^{-1}$ ($F_{1,26}$ = 4.69, p < 0.05), 5.23 rad.s$^{-1}$ ($F_{1,26}$ = 4.68, p < 0.05) and 2.09 $_{(ecc)}$ rad.s$^{-1}$ ($F_{1,26}$ = 12.50, p < 0.002). In all cases, elite players were stronger than sub-elite players (Figure 3b).

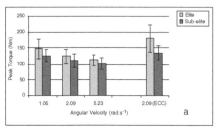
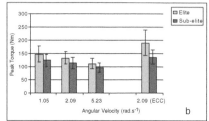

**Figure 3**. Comparison of hamstrings muscle strength (peak torque) between elite and sub-elite soccer players for the dominant leg (a) and non-dominant leg (b).

## 3.5 Relative muscle strength profile for the hamstring group (peak torque/body mass)

No significant differences between the groups were indicated using MANOVA (Wilks' Lambda = 0.56, $F_{8,19}$ = 1.83,  p > 0.05) when data were normalised for body mass. This finding corroborates the results of the comparison before data were corrected for body mass. Nevertheless, for the dominant leg, univariate ANOVA revealed a significant main difference in hamstrings relative muscle strength (peak torque/BM) between groups at 2.09 $_{(ecc)}$ rad.s$^{-1}$ ($F_{1,26}$ = 4.86,  p < 0.05). Again, the elite players showed the greater muscle strength (see Figure 4a).

For the non-dominant leg, univariate ANOVA revealed a significant main effect in relative muscle strength of the hamstrings (peak torque/BM) between groups at 2.09 $_{(ecc)}$ rad.s$^{-1}$ ($F_{1,26}$ = 4.86,  p < 0.05). The elite players showed the greater muscle strength (see Figure 4b).

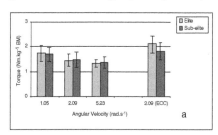
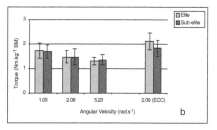

**Figure 4**. Comparison of hamstrings relative muscle strength (peak torque/body mass) between elite and sub-elite soccer players for the dominant leg (a) and the non-dominant leg (b).

### 3.6 Muscle balance (Hamstring/Quadriceps ratio)

There was no significant difference in muscle balance between the two groups of players (Wilks' Lambda = 0.39, $F_{8,19}$ = 3.73,  p > 0.05). Nevertheless, for the dominant leg, univariate ANOVA showed a significant difference between groups in hamstrings/quadriceps ratio for peak torque at 5.23 rad.s$^{-1}$ ($F_{1,26} = 7.34$, p < 0.01). The sub-elite players had a ratio closer to unity than the elite players. A higher dynamic control ratio (DCR) in the elite players was not significant (see Figure 5a).

For the non-dominant leg, univariate ANOVA showed a significant difference between groups in hamstring/quadriceps ratio (H/Q ratio of peak torque) at 5.23 rad.s$^{-1}$ ($F_{1,26} = 5.84$, p < 0.02). The sub-elite players had a ratio closer to unity than did the elite players. A higher DCR in the elite players was not significant (see Figure 5b).

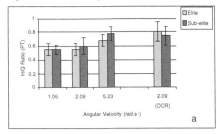 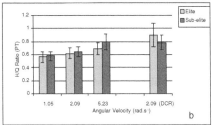

**Figure 5**. Comparison of H/Q ratio (peak torque) between elite and sub-elite soccer players for the dominant leg (a) and the non-dominant leg (b).

### 3.7 Fast/Slow-speed ratio

The fast-speed/slow-speed ratio (1.05 and 5.23 rad.s$^{-1}$ respectively) for quadriceps and hamstrings, showed no significant differences between the groups according to MANOVA (Wilks' Lambda = 0.78, $F_{8,19} = 1.61$). Nevertheless, for the dominant leg, univariate ANOVA showed that elite players had a higher fast-speed/slow-speed ratio in the quadriceps than the sub-elite players ($\overline{x} = 0.61 \pm 0.05$ vs. $0.56 \pm 0.09$ Nm, $F_{1,26} = 6.25$, p < 0.02). No significant difference was found between the groups in the ratio for the hamstrings ($\overline{x} = 0.76 \pm 0.06$ vs. $0.8 \pm 0.13$ Nm).

For the non-dominant leg, univariate ANOVA showed that there were no significant differences between groups in fast-speed/slow-speed ratio for peak torque in either quadriceps ($\overline{x} = 0.61 \pm 0.05$ vs. $0.58 \pm 0.06$ Nm) or hamstrings ($\overline{x} = 0.77 \pm 0.11$ vs. $0.79 \pm 0.1$ Nm) muscles.

### 3.8 Bilateral comparison (Left/Right ratio)

Regarding the bilateral comparison of peak torque using MANOVA, no significant differences were observed between the groups for either quadriceps or hamstrings muscles (Wilks' Lambda = 0.72, $F_{8,19} = 91$, p > 0.05). These findings are presented graphically in Figures 6a and b.

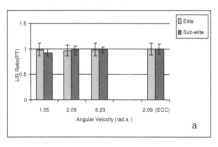
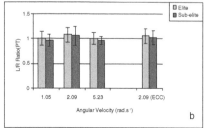

**Figure 6**. Comparison of left/right ratio (peak torque) between elite and sub-elite soccer players in the quadriceps (a) and hamstrings (b) muscles.

### 3.9 Flexibility of the hip joint

The MANOVA results showed a significant difference between groups in the flexibility of the hip joint (Wilks' Lambda = 0.57,   $F_{8,19}$ = 9.48,  p < 0.001). Univariate analyses indicated a significant difference for both the dominant leg ( $\overline{x}$ = 95 ± 11 vs. 81 ± 7 deg, $F_{1,26}$ = 17.38,  p < 0.001) and the non-dominant leg ( $\overline{x}$ = 97 ± 12 vs. 80 ± 8 deg, $F_{1,26}$ = 18.62,  p < 0.001). The elite players were the more flexible in both legs.

### 3.10 Vertical jump

Regarding the vertical jump, no significant difference between the elite and the sub-elite players ( $\overline{x}$ = 39 ± 5 cm vs. 36 ± 4 cm) was indicated using ANOVA.

### 4. DISCUSSION

In this study, important differences were noted between elite and sub-elite soccer players. The elite players had the higher values in (i) the peak torque levels of knee extensors, (ii) the peak torque levels of knee flexors, (iii) quadriceps strength relative to body size, (iv) hamstrings strength relative to body size in both dominant and non-dominant legs and in both contraction modes (concentric and eccentric), (v) hamstrings to quadriceps strength ratio in eccentric mode (both legs), (vi) fast-speed to slow-speed ratio in the quadriceps of the dominant leg and (vii) flexibility of the hip joint (both sides). The sub-elite players had a ratio closer to unity at high speed for both legs. No significant differences were found between these two groups of players for bilateral quadriceps and hamstrings strength ratio or vertical jump.

With respect to knee extensors and knee flexors, it is thought that the knee extensors play a main role in some soccer specific activities such as kicking the ball, jumping to head, sprinting (Fried and Lloyd, 1992) while the knee flexors have responsibility in stabilising the knee joint during some critical actions such as tackling, charging and changing pace, especially at high limb velocities. In the present study, the elite players were stronger in the quadriceps and hamstrings than the sub-elite, especially in eccentric actions. These findings confirm the results of Oberg *et al.* (1986) who found differences between Swedish soccer players in different divisions. Zakas *et al.* (1995) in Greek soccer players and Cometti *et al.* (2001) in French soccer players reported similar trends. It would seem that many years of soccer training increase quadriceps and hamstrings strength, as reflected in the superior strength values in the current professionals. This difference between elite and less skilled athletes is noted in other sports. Thorstensson *et al.* (1977) and Haymes and Dickinson (1980) reported similar differences in alpine skiers, jumpers, sprinters and skiing disciplines. It seems that the influence of specific soccer training is reflected in the strength differences between different levels of play.

The correction of peak torque values in flexors and extensors for body size did not change the findings substantially. This conclusion applied even though the professionals were on average 10 kg heavier than the other group.

An increase in the H/Q ratio with increasing velocity was observed in each limb, a finding which is consistent with previous research (Gilliam, 1979; Scudder, 1980; Davies *et al.*, 1981; Wyatt and Edward, 1981; Stafford and Grana, 1984; Oberg *et al.*, 1986). Although the sub-elite players had the higher H/Q strength ratio (but only at the higher angular velocity), the H/Q ratios of both groups were within the normal range (58%-80%) reported by Fowler and Reilly (1993). The H/Q ratio found in this study was 58% for both groups which is close to the ratio observed in US national and Asian soccer players (Mangine *et al.*, 1990; Chin *et al.*, 1994). Ratios for DCR of 81% (elite players) and 75% (sub-elite players) were observed. It is thought that this functional H/Q ratio is more suitable to recognise the ability of the knee flexors in stabilising the knee joint than the conventional ratio. Due to the high eccentric hamstring torque, the elite players had a marginally greater H/Q ratio than the sub-elite. In agreement with Cometti *et al.* (2001), due to the importance of the hamstring muscles in some specific soccer activities and the need for stabilisation of the knee joint during critical events, it is recommended that trainers should pay more attention to eccentric actions and strength training in their training sessions, in order to minimise the likelihood of injury occurrence. In soccer, the knee flexors are used concentrically to flex the knee and extend the hip in preparation for a kick and are used eccentrically to control knee extension and hip flexion towards the end of the kicking action (Clarys *et al.*, 1988). If the knee extensor strength greatly exceeds that of the hamstrings, the ability to resist knee extension is reduced which may result in a forced stretch of the hamstrings and consequent muscle damage (Fowler and Reilly, 1993).

Oberg *et al.* (1986) reported the relatively greater fast-speed/slow-speed ratio in national players compared to others. This study showed a higher fast-speed/slow-speed ratio in the quadriceps of the dominant leg in elite players than in sub-elite players which confirms the results of previous research. The greater fast-speed/slow-speed ratio indicates that a fast-speed capability is an important attribute in top-class soccer. Since some actions are performed at a high velocity (e.g. hard shots on goal), coaches should pay attention to fast actions in training.

With respect to bilateral quadriceps and hamstrings ratio, there was no difference between the groups. As limb symmetry was within the normal range (0.9-1.1), it seems that soccer strength training need not compromise the strength ratio between left and right limbs. Knapik *et al.* (1991) suggested that subjects with an imbalance exceeding 15% were 2.6 times more likely to suffer injury in the weaker leg. There was no such deficit observed among the players in this current study. This result is in agreement with studies by Oberg *et al.* (1986) and Goslin and Charteris (1979) who failed to observe differences in strength between the limbs.

With respect to flexibility of the hip joint, since we found that the elite players were more flexible than the sub-elite participants in both dominant and non-dominant legs, it seems that intensity of soccer training in top-class soccer improves the range of motion in the hip joint. If training programmes can be organised appropriately, the player can develop both muscle and joint flexibility. One of the major concerns of coaches in relation to strength training is that they believe it reduces flexibility whilst increasing muscle size but this is shown not to be the case. This point can be important if the hamstring muscles are to be protected from injury. Furthermore, the use of flexibility training to prevent muscle strain should not be neglected in the design of training and rehabilitation programmes for players. It would seem that muscle tightness, often observed in players, probably predisposes players to muscle injury.

Although the elite players demonstrated 3% better performance than the sub-elite in vertical-jumping ability, the difference was not significant. This observation confirms the results of Cometti *et al.* (2001). Thomas and Reilly (1979) reported that vertical-jump ability of English soccer players was constant throughout the competitive season. The lack of difference in vertical jump performance between players suggests that soccer training has more of an effect on peak torque than on explosive power. Therefore, trainers and players should pay more attention to specific plyometric training programmes during their training sessions to improve jumping ability and other dynamic activities.

## 5. CONCLUSIONS

In conclusion, this research has revealed that elite soccer players differ from sub-elite soccer players in terms of most muscle functional variables; the elite players demonstrated greater absolute strength and also greater strength relative to body mass and greater flexibility. They tended to have the better values in the DCR ratio and fast-speed/slow-speed ratio which suggests they are less at risk of injury than less skilled players. It is thought that several years of soccer training and match-play at a high level improve the strength of knee extensors and knee flexors, irrespective of body size, and also flexibility in elite players. This investigation has also established a comprehensive isokinetic strength reference database for English soccer players.

**Acknowledgements**

Nader Rahnama is supported by a research grant from the Ministry of Sciences, Research and Technology of Iran and also by Isfahan University.

# REFERENCES

Aagaard, P., Simonsen, E.B., Magnusson, S.P., Larsson, B. and Dyhre-Poulsen, P., 1998, A new concept for isokinetic hamstring: quadriceps muscle strength ratio. *American Journal of Sports Medicine*, **26**, 231-237.

Bender, J.A., Pierson, J.K., Kaplan, H.D. and Johnson, A.J., 1964, Factors affecting the occurrence of knee injuries. *Journal of American Medical Association,* **18**, 130-134.

Burkett, L.S., 1970, Causative factors in hamstring strains. *Medicine and Science in Sports*, **2**, 39-42.

Chaffin, D.B., Herrin, G.D. and Keyserling, W.M., 1978, Preemployment strength testing: an updated position. *Journal of Occupation and Medicine*, **20**, 403-408.

Chin, M.K., So, R.C.H., Yuan, Y.W.Y., LI, R.C.T. and Wong A.S.K., 1994, Cardiorespiratory fitness and isokinetic muscle strength of elite Asian junior soccer players. *Journal of Sports Medicine and Physical Fitness,* **34**, 250-257.

Clarys, J.P., Bollens, E., Cabri, J. and Dufour, W., 1988, Muscle activity in the soccer kick. *In Science and Football*, edited by Reilly, T., Lees, A., Davids, K. and Murphy, W. (London: E and F.N. Spon), pp. 434-440.

Cometti, G., Maffiuletti, N.A., Pousson, M., Chatard, J.C. and Maffulli, N., 2001, Isokinetic strength and anaerobic power of elite, subelite and amateur French soccer players. *International Journal of Sports Medicine*, **22**, 45-51.

Coplin, T.H., 1971, Isokinetic exercise: Clinical usage. *National Athletic Trainers Association*, **6**, 110-114.

Davies, G.J., Kirkendall, D.T., Leigh, D.H., Lui, M.L., Reinbold, T.R. and Wilson, P.K, 1981, Isokinetic characteristics of professional football players: normative relationship between quadriceps and hamstrings muscle groups and relative to body weight (abstract). *Medicine and Science in Sports and Exercise*, **13**, 76-77.

Ekstrand, J. and Gillquist J., 1983, Soccer injuries and their mechanisms. *Medicine and Science in Sports and Exercise*, **15**, 267-270.

Fowler, N.E. and Reilly, T., 1993, Assessment of muscle strength asymmetry in soccer players. *In Contemporary Ergonomics*, edited by Lovesey, E.J. (London: Taylor and Francis), pp. 327-332.

Fried, T. and Lloyd, G.J., 1992, An overview of common soccer injuries. Management and prevention. *Sports Medicine*, **14**, 269-275.

Gilliam, T.H., 1979, Isokinetic torque levels for high school football players. *Archives of Physical Medicine and Rehabilitation*, **60**, 110-114.

Goslin, B.R. and Charteris, J., 1979, Isokinetic dynamometry: normative data for clinical use in lower extremity (knee) cases. *Scandinavian Journal of Rehabilitation and Medicine*, **11**, 105-109.

Haymes, E. M. and Dickinson, A.I., 1980, Characteristics of elite male and female ski racers. *Medicine and Science in Sports and Exercise*, **12**, 153-158.

Knapik, J. and Ramos, M., 1980, Isokinetic and isometric torque relationship in the human body. *Archives of Physical Medicine and Rehabilitation*, **61**, 64-67.

Knapik, J.J., Baumann, C.L., Jones, B.H., Harris, J.M. and Vaughan, L., 1991, Pre-season strength and flexibility imbalances associated with athletic injuries in female collegiate athletes. *American Journal of Sports Medicine*, **19**, 76-81.

Mangine, R.E., Noyes, F.R., Mullen, M.P. and Barber, S., 1990, A physiological profile of the elite soccer athlete. *Journal of Orthopaedic and Sports Physical Therapy*, **12**, 147-152.

Noonan, T.J., Best, T.M., Seaber, A.V. and Garrett, W.E., 1994, Identification of a threshold for skeletal muscle injury. *American Journal of Sports Medicine*, **22**, 257-261.

Oberg, B., Moller, M., Gillquist, J. and Ekstrand, J., 1986, Isokinetic torque levels for knee extensors and knee flexors in soccer players. *International Journal of Sports Medicine*, **17**, 50-53.

Reilly, T. and Brooks, G.A., 1986, Exercise and the circadian variation in body temperature measures. *International Journal of Sports Medicine*, **7**, 358-368.

Reilly, T. and Howe, T., 1996, Injury prevention and rehabilitation. *In Science and Soccer*, edited by Reilly, T. (London: E. and F.N. Spon), pp. 161-162.

Scudder, N.G., 1980, Torque curves produced of the knee during isometric and isokinetic exercise. *Archives of Physical Medicine and Rehabilitation*, **61**, 68-72.

Stafford, M.G. and Grana, W.A., 1984, Hamstring/quadriceps ratios in college football players: A high velocity evaluation. *American Journal of Sports Medicine*, **12**, 209-211.

Thomas, V. and Reilly, T., 1979, Fitness assessment of English League players through the competitive season. *British Journal of Sports Medicine*, **13**, 103-109.

Thorstensson, A., Larsson, L., Tesch, P. and Karlsson, J., 1977, Muscle strength and fibre composition in  athletes and sedentary men. *Medicine and Science in Sports,* **9**, 26-30.

Wyatt, M.P. and Edward, A.M., 1981, Comparison of quadriceps and hamstrings torque values during isokinetic exercise. *Journal of  Orthopaedic and Sports Physical Therapy,* **3**, 48-56.

Zakas, A., Mandroukas, K., Vamvakoudis, E., Christoulas, K. and Aggelopoulou, N., 1995, Peak torque of quadriceps and hamstring muscles in basketball and soccer players of different divisions. *Journal of Sports Medicine and Physical Fitness,* **35**, 199-205.

# 15    The Ratio of 2$^{nd}$ and 4$^{th}$ Digit Length: A Prenatal Correlate of Ability in Sport

J.T. Manning[1], P.E. Bundred[2] and R. Taylor[3]
[1]School of Biological Sciences, [2]Department of Primary Care, and
[3]Football Industry Group, University of Liverpool, Liverpool,
L69 3BX, UK

## 1. INTRODUCTION

What are the major factors which come together to make a good athlete? Here we suggest that foetal "programming", and in particular the organisational effects of prenatal testosterone, is important in the aetiology of athletic ability. "Programming" describes the processes whereby influences during critical periods of early development permanently change the structure and function of the body. One important organisational influence on the foetus is that of sex steroids such as testosterone and oestrogen. The uterine environment is difficult to access and it is not possible to measure directly an adult's exposure to prenatal sex hormones. What is required is a "window" into foetal sex hormone concentrations. The ratio between the length of the 2$^{nd}$ (index finger) digit and 4$^{th}$ (ring finger) digit (the 2D:4D ratio) may provide such a window (Manning, 2002).

The formation of the gonads (and therefore the early production of sex steroids) and the differentiation of the fingers are both influenced by *Homeobox* (*Hox*) genes. In particular, mutations in *Hoxa* and *Hoxd* genes result in defects in the digits and urinogenital system (Kondo *et al.*, 1977). These observations led Manning *et al.* (1998) to suggest that patterns of finger formation may reflect prenatal gonad function and sex steroid production. One obvious candidate for an association between foetal sex hormones and fingers is the 2D:4D ratio. Thus [i] mean values of 2D:4D are lower for males than females i.e. males tend to have longer 4$^{th}$ digits relative to 2$^{nd}$ digits than do females (Phelps, 1952; Manning *et al.*, 1998) [ii] sex differences in 2D:4D are present as early as two years and do not appear to change at puberty (Manning *et al.*, 1998) [iii] 2D:4D shows considerable geographical and ethnic variation but the sex difference remains robust across populations (Manning *et al.*, 2000) [iv] mothers with a high waist:hip ratio, a positive correlate of testosterone, tend to have children with low or masculinised 2D:4D ratios (Manning *et al.*, 1999) and [v] the amniotic fluid of mothers with a masculinised 2D:4D ratio has high concentrations of foetal testosterone (Manning, 2002).

Low 2D:4D ratio may therefore be a correlate of high prenatal testosterone and low prenatal oestrogen. It has been suggested that this type of foetal environment is associated with the formation of an efficient male cardiovascular system and high athletic ability (Manning and Bundred, 2000; Manning and Bundred, 2001; Manning and Taylor, 2001). In support of this suggestion, data are presented which show associations in men between low 2D:4D and running speed and soccer ability, and high 2D:4D and early presentation of heart disease.

## 2. 2D:4D AND RUNNING SPEED

Manning and Taylor (2001) considered the relationship between self-reported sporting attainment and 2D:4D in a sample of 128 men. The preferred sport of the participants included running (45% of subjects). The 2D:4D of the right hand (but not the left) was negatively associated with sporting ability independent of age, experience and type of preferred sport. Participants with lower right 2D:4D compared to left (Dr-l) also reported high sporting attainment. Similarly a sample of 47 middle distance runners also showed significant negative correlations between right 2D:4D and Dr-l and the mean of their last three times in 800 m and 1500 m races (Manning, 2002). Here two further studies concerning 2D:4D and running speed are reported.

### 2.1 Self-reported personal best times in middle-distance athletes

There were 118 male subjects in this sample. All athletes were participants in winter cross-country races. Measurements of $2^{nd}$ and $4^{th}$ digit length were made of the right and left hands before races. Fifty hands from 50 subjects were measured twice (for measurement protocol see Manning *et al.*, 1998). Height and weight were measured, and age and current number of training sessions per week were recorded. Athletes reported their personal best 800 m (n=97) and 1500 m times (n=67). Finger measurements were made blind to personal bests which were reported after measurement. The descriptive statistics (means and SDs) of the sample were: 2D:4D right and left $0.98 \pm 0.03$, age $23.45 \pm 4.79$ years, height $1.72 \pm 0.062$ m, mass $84.69 \pm 10.34$ kg, training frequency $2.5 \pm 0.85$ per week, best 800 m time $139.96 \pm 21.59$ s and 1500 m $255.97 \pm 20.25$ s. Intra-class correlation coefficients indicated high repeatability for 2D:4D ratio measurements (right $r_l = 0.94$; left $r_l = 0.89$) and repeated measures ANOVA analyses gave significantly higher values for between-subject variation in 2D:4D compared to measurement error (right $F = 29.96$, $p = 0.0001$; left $F = 17.72$, $p = 0.0001$). Therefore our calculated 2D:4D ratios represented real differences between individuals.

Table 1 shows that athletes with low right hand 2D:4D ratios reported faster personal bests for both 800 m and 1500 m than athletes with high 2D:4D ($p = 0.0001$ and $p = 0.008$ respectively). This was also the case for those participants with low 2D:4D in their right hand compared to left (Dr-1 = right 2D:4D – left 2D:4D). After Bonferroni adjustment for multiple tests, the right 2D:4D relationship with 800-m best time remained significant (p = 0.001). Older athletes reported faster 800 m times (p = 0.003) and this remained significant after Bonferroni adjustment (p = 0.04). Presumably this result reflected a longer opportunity to record a low personal best. Current training frequencies per week were not significantly related to personal bests, but this may have been because times were recorded some time before the measurements. Partial correlation coefficient analysis showed that right 2D:4D was significantly related to best time over 800 m ($r = 0.38$, p = 0.0008) independent of the influence of age ($r = -0.30$, p = 0.001).

**Table 1.** Pearson Product Moment Correlation Coefficients between seven variables and 800-m and 1500-m self-reported personal best times.

| Trait | 800 m (n = 97) | | 1500 m  (n = 67) | |
|---|---|---|---|---|
| | *r* | *p* | *r* | *p* |
| 2D:4D Right | 0.39 | 0.0001 | 0.32 | 0.008 |
| 2D:4D Left | 0.13 | 0.20 | 0.05 | 0.67 |
| D r-l | 0.26 | 0.009 | 0.29 | 0.02 |
| Age | -0.30 | 0.003 | -0.27 | 0.03 |
| Height | -0.16 | 0.31 | -0.13 | 0.32 |
| Weight | -0.07 | 0.63 | 0.03 | 0.71 |
| Training Frequency | -0.003 | 0.98 | -0.21 | 0.07 |

## 2.2 Running speed in long-distance athletes

The sample consisted of 47 male students competing in a 6-mile Inter-university cross-country race in Edinburgh, UK. As in the middle-distance sample, 2nd and 4th digits of the right and left hands were measured and 30 right and left hands were measured twice. Age and training frequency were recorded. The athletes' times were obtained some weeks after the race and finger measurements were therefore made blind to running speed. Descriptive statistics (means and SDs) of the sample were: 2D:4D right $0.97 \pm 0.02$ and left $0.98 \pm 0.02$, age $20.58 \pm 1.32$ years, weekly training frequency $3.73 \pm 1.38$, race time $2421.75 \pm 268.90$ s. The intra-class correlation coefficients for 2D:4D were high (right $r_1 = 0.99$; left $r_1 = 0.98$) and repeated measures ANOVA tests showed between-subject variation to be significantly higher than measurement error (right $F = 307.75$, p = 0.0001; left $F = 141.15$, p = 0.0001). Therefore measurement error was low.

Table 2 shows that right and left 2D:4D were positively correlated with race times ($r = 0.52$ and 0.51 respectively). That is men with low 2D:4D ran faster than men with high 2D:4D. Values for Dr-l did not correlate significantly with race times. This sample of long-distance runners reported higher mean weekly frequencies of training (3.73) than the middle-distance athletes (2.50). Training frequency was strongly correlated with race time ($r=-0.76$). A partial correlation analysis (Table 3) showed that training frequency was significantly associated with race times independent of 2D:4D and age. The 2D:4D ratio was no longer significantly correlated with race times ($r=0.16$) but was negatively and significantly related to training frequency ($r=-0.32$).

**Table 2.**   Product Moment Correlation Coefficients between five variables and time recorded in a 6-mile cross-country race.

|  | Race Time | |
|---|---|---|
| Trait | $r$ | $p$ |
| 2D:4D Right | 0.52 | 0.0002 |
| 2D:4D Left | 0.51 | 0.0002 |
| D r-l | -0.03 | 0.85 |
| Age | -0.10 | 0.85 |
| Training Frequency | -0.76 | 0.0001 |

**Table 3.**  Partial Correlation Coefficients between four variables recorded in a 6-mile cross-country race.

| Trait | 2D:4DR | Age | Training Freq. | Race time |
|---|---|---|---|---|
| 2D:4D Right | – | | | |
| Age | -0.01 | – | | |
| Training Frequency | -0.32* | 0.13 | – | |
| Race Time | 0.16 | 0.04 | -0.66** | – |

*$p=0.03$, **$p=0.0001$

## 3. 2D:4D AND FOOTBALL ABILITY

It has been suggested that low 2D:4D is related to good football ability in men (Manning and Taylor, 2001; Manning, 2002). In support of this view, 2D:4D ratios measured in players from the English leagues have shown (i) lower ratios in professional players compared to controls (ii) $1^{st}$ team players had lower ratios than reserves while youth team players had intermediate values of 2D:4D and (iii) players who have represented their country had lower 2D:4D than players who had not played at international level.

We consider data from two samples of players:

### 3.1 2D:4D and football ability in English amateur players

The sample consisted of 108 amateur male football players. The participants played on an infrequent (not every week, n = 37) or frequent (every week, n = 71) basis in Winter local and University leagues in the Liverpool area. The $2^{nd}$ and $4^{th}$ digits were measured in the right and left hands, all measurements were made twice and were blind to ratings of ability. Height and weight were measured and age was recorded. Participants reported an estimate of their football ability on a scale from 1 to 10 (1 = low ability, plays infrequently to 10 = very high ability, has played at national level). In addition the ability of subjects who played frequently was rated on the same scale by five of their fellow players. Descriptive statistics of the complete sample (n = 108) were as follows: 2D:4D right 0.97 ± 0.01, left 0.96 ± 0.01; age 18.88 ± 1.67 years; height 1.81 ± 0.064 m; mass 73.91 ± 6.50 kg. Mean self-rated ability was 7.08 ± 1.90 and mean rating by fellow-players was 7.19 ± 0.94. Self-rating and fellow player rating were significantly correlated ($r = 0.72$, p = 0.0001). Intra-class correlation coefficients of the first and second measurements of 2D:4D were high (right $r_1 = 0.90$, left $r_1 = 0.88$), and $F$ values showed significantly higher between-individual differences in 2D:4D compared to measurement error (repeated measures ANOVA, right $F = 18.84$, p = 0.0001; left $F = 16.24$, p = 0.0001). Therefore the calculated 2D:4D ratios reflected real differences between subjects.

Table 4 shows that 2D:4D right and left ratio were negatively and significantly correlated with football ability which is both self-rated and rated by fellow players. That is low 2D:4D was predictive of good football ability. However, unlike running speed the left hand ratio was the strongest correlate of ability. Those players with lower left hand 2D:4D compared to right hand 2D:4D (positive Dr-l) reported high football ability. Again this differed from the findings regarding running speed where negative Dr-l was predictive of fast running speed.

**Table 4.** Pearson Product Moment Correlation Coefficients between self-rated football ability and other-player rated ability, and 2D:4D, Dr-l, age, height and weight.

| Trait | Self-rated ability | | Other players rating | |
|---|---|---|---|---|
| | r | p | r | p |
| 2D:4D Right | -0.33 | 0.0005 | -0.37 | 0.002 |
| 2D:4D Left | -0.56 | 0.0001 | -0.34 | 0.004 |
| D r-l | 0.22 | 0.02 | -0.06 | 0.64 |
| Age | -0.10 | 0.29 | -0.13 | 0.27 |
| Height | 0.05 | 0.61 | 0.22 | 0.054 |
| Weight | 0.02 | 0.87 | 0.002 | 0.99 |

### 3.2  2D:4D and football ability in elite Brazilian professional players

This sample consisted of 33 professional footballers from the Brazilian $1^{st}$ Division club Internacional of Porto Alegre. Two measurements were made of the $2^{nd}$ and $4^{th}$ digits of the right and left hands. The measurements were made blind to the status of the players. After measurements were made the senior coach divided the players into a "first team squad" (n = 20) and a group of reserves (n = 13).

Intra-class correlation coefficients were high for both right ($r_l = 0.97$) and left 2D:4D ($r_l = 0.98$). Repeated measures ANOVA analyses showed between-subject variation in 2D:4D was higher than measurement error, indicating the calculated 2D:4D ratios reflected real differences between subjects (right $F = 27.21$, p = 0.0001; left $F = 29.70$, p = 0.0001). We concluded that measurement error was small compared to between-subject differences in 2D:4D ratio.

In the complete sample the mean 2D:4D ratios were right hand $0.94 \pm 0.03$ and left hand $0.93 \pm 0.03$. Players in the first team squad had significantly lower 2D:4D ratios  than the reserves and the difference was strongest for the left hand (right hand $1^{st}$ team $0.93 \pm 0.03$, reserves $0.96 \pm 0.03$, t = 3.11, p = 0.004; left hand $1^{st}$ team $0.92 \pm 0.03$, $0.96 \pm 0.02$, t = 4.54, p = 0.0001).

### 3.3  2D:4D and age at first myocardial infarction in men

There is evidence that prenatal and adult testosterone is protective against heart disease in males (Manning and Bundred, 2000; Rosano, 2000). A negative relationship between 2D:4D ratio and age at first myocardial infarction (MI) has been reported by Manning and Bundred (2001) in a sample of 151 men. Here we present data from a new sample of 277 men from the Wirral area of NW England. The participants had experienced a MI, and all were measured at the Wirral

Cardiac Rehabilitation Unit, St Catherine's Hospital, Birkenhead. The Wirral Research Ethics Committee approved the study and the patients gave signed informed consent. The length of the 2nd and 4th digits was measured in right and left hands. A hundred right and left hands were measured twice. Height and weight were also measured and age at first MI and smoking habits in the six months before the MI were recorded.

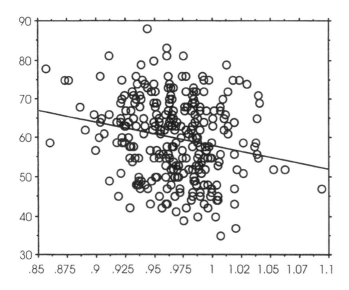

**Figure 1.** The relationship between 2D:4D of the right hand and age at first MI in 277 men.

The intra-class correlation coefficients for 2D:4D were high for right ($r_I$ = 0.97) and left ($r_I$ = 0.95) hands. Repeated measures ANOVA analyses showed between-individual differences in 2D:4D were significantly greater than measurement error (right $F$ = 58.20, p = 0.0001; left $F$ = 5.49, p = 0.0001). We concluded our values of 2D:4D reflected real differences between subjects. Descriptive statistics of the sample (means and SDs) were: age 63.59 ± 10.07 years, age at first MI 59.77 ± 10.47, height 1.74 ± 0.07 m, mass 79.54 ± 13.06 kg. There were 107 patients who smoked in the six months prior to their MI and 170 who did not.

There were negative relationships between 2D:4D and age at first MI. That is men with high values of 2D:4D were younger at first MI than men with low 2D:4D ratio. As in the study by Manning and Bundred (2001) the associations were stronger for the right hand ($r$ = -0.21, p = 0.0005, Figure 1) than the left ($r$ = -0.12, p = 0.047). There was a trend for participants with higher 2D:4D in the right hand to be younger at MI than subjects with low Dr-1 but this was not significant ($r = -0.09$, p = 0.14). Partial correlation analysis showed that right 2D:4D remained significantly negatively correlated with age at MI ($r = -0.18$, p = 0.004), independent of age ($r = 0.79$, p = 0.0001), height ($r = 0.09$, p = 0.14), weight ($r = -0.14$, p = 0.03), smoking habits (yes = 1, no = 2; $r = 0.16$, p = 0.009). We concluded that men with high values of 2D:4D ratio tended to be younger at first MI than men with low 2D:4D ratio. Smoking and weight were positively and independently related to early MI.

## 4. CONCLUSIONS

We have the following results. Firstly low 2D:4D ratio in male runners was associated with fast running times. This was the case when speed was measured by self-reported personal bests in a sample of middle-distance athletes and for times in a long-distance race. In the latter sample, training frequency was the most important correlate of running speed but 2D:4D correlated with training frequency. There was evidence in the middle-distance sample that 2D:4D of the right hand was the strongest correlate of running speed. Overall these data suggest that 2D:4D is an important correlate of running speed and/or the ability to maintain a heavy training schedule. Secondly low 2D:4D ratio was correlated with high ability in football. This was the case for amateur football players when ability was self-reported or assessed by fellow players. It was also found to be so in Brazilian professional players when coaches assessed ability. For football ability there is some evidence that the left hand 2D:4D ratio is the stronger predictor of performance. Thirdly, and finally, we found that men with high values of 2D:4D ratio were younger at first MI than men with low 2D:4D. This result was independent of age, height, weight and smoking habits and was strongest for the right 2D:4D ratio.

It is not yet clear whether right 2D:4D ratio rather than left is the strongest correlate of running speed and heart disease, and left rather than right 2D:4D the better predictor of football ability. Stronger associations with right hand rather than left 2D:4D have been found for testosterone, sperm counts, hand preference, waist:hip ratios, verbal fluency, running speed and heart disease. Left 2D:4D has been found to be the better correlate of football ability and age at presentation of breast cancer (Manning, 2002). There is some evidence that the male form of sexually dimorphic traits is most intensely expressed on the right side (Tanner, 1990). It has also been suggested that lower 2D:4D ratio in the right hand compared to the left is a correlate of high prenatal and adult testosterone (Manning, 2002). In support of this waist:hip ratio and left-handedness (there is evidence that both are proxies for high testosterone) are negatively related to Dr-1 (Manning, 2002).

Why should prenatal sex steroids influence male athletic ability? An explanation couched in Darwinian terms may be found in sexual selection theory (Darwin, 1871). Males and females of many species show different variances in offspring number. The difference arises from the cost of sperm and egg production.

The cost of a single sperm is vanishingly low, males produce very large numbers, and they are therefore capable of fathering many offspring. As a result the limiting factor of male reproductive success is in obtaining females, and males can have high variance in offspring number. In other words successful males may father many children while unsuccessful males will remain childless. Females are limited in their ability to produce large families because the cost of eggs, pregnancy, and lactation are high. Repeated matings with many males are unlikely to increase female fecundity, therefore the variance in female family size is lower than that of males. This means that sexual selection favours adaptations in men which increase their physical competitiveness and favour individuals in male-male competition. Speed, strength and visuo-spatial perception are therefore likely to be highly developed in males, and the appropriate organisational changes in the cardiovascular system and the brain may occur as a response to levels of foetal testosterone. There is evidence that low 2D:4D is a proxy for high foetal androgen and a correlate of running speed, football ability and visuo-spatial perception. Low 2D:4D ratio may also be a marker for a slow progression of age-dependent deterioration in the heart and blood vessels.

## REFERENCES

Darwin, C., 1871, *The Descent of Man, and Selection in Relation to Sex*, (London: Raven Press).

Kondo, T., Zakany, J., Innis, J., and Duboule, D., 1997, Of fingers, toes and penises. *Nature*, **390**, 29.

Manning, J.T., 2002, *Digit Ratio: a Pointer to Fertility, Behavior and Health*, (New Jersey: Rutgers University Press).

Manning, J.T., Barley, L., Lewis-Jones, I., Walton, J., Trivers, R.L., Thornhill, R., Singh, D., Rhode, P., Bereckzei, T., Henzi, P., Soler, M. and Sved, A., 2000, The $2^{nd}$ to $4^{th}$ digit ratio, sexual dimorphism, population differences and reproductive success: evidence for sexually antagonistic genes. *Evolution and Human Behavior*, **21**, 163-183.

Manning, J.T. and Bundred, P.E. 2000, The ratio of $2^{nd}$ to $4^{th}$ digit length: a new predictor of disease predisposition? *Medical Hypotheses*, **54**, 855-857.

Manning, J.T. and Bundred, P.E., 2001, The ratio of second to fourth digit length and age at first myocardial infarction in men: a link with testosterone? *British Journal of Cardiology*, **8**, 720-723.

Manning, J.T., Scutt, D., Wilson, J. and Lewis-Jones, D.I., 1998, The ratio of $2^{nd}$ to $4^{th}$ digit length: a predictor of sperm numbers and levels of testosterone, LH and oestrogen. *Human Reproduction*, **13**, 3000-3004.

Manning, J.T. and Taylor, R.P., 2001, $2^{nd}$ to $4^{th}$ digit ratio and male ability in sport: implications for sexual selection in humans. *Evolution and Human Behavior*, **22**, 61-69.

Manning, J.T., Trivers, R.L., Singh, D. and Thornhill, R., 1999, The mystery of female beauty. *Nature*, **399**, 214-215.

Phelps, V.R., 1952, Relative index finger length as a sex-influenced trait in man. *American Journal of Human Genetics*, **4**, 72-89.

Rosano, G.M.C., 2000, Androgens and coronary artery disease: a sex specific effect of sex-hormones? *European Heart Journal*, **21**, 868-871.

Tanner, J.M., 1990, *Foetus into Man: Physical Growth from Conception into Maturity*, (Cambridge, Mass: Harvard University Press).

# 16    Maximum Grip Width Regulations in Powerlifting Discriminate against Larger Athletes

Gareth Gilbert and Adrian Lees

Research Institute for Sport and Exercise Sciences, Liverpool John Moores University, Henry Cotton Campus, 15-21 Webster Street, Liverpool, L3 2ET, UK

## 1. INTRODUCTION

The bench press is a popular weight-training exercise among recreational weightlifters and is a competitive event in powerlifting. The exercise is easily adjusted and is considered by strength trainers to be relatively safe for individuals to use. The bench press is often used in exercise programmes designed to develop upper-body strength.

Adjustment of the incline of the bench brings about selective development of the upper and lower chest (Glass and Armstrong, 1997), and grip width has been shown to affect the contribution of upper-body muscle groups to the exercise (Clemons and Aaron, 1997). For example the discus thrower is able to develop the pectoral area by employing a wider grip width which increases the contribution of the pectoral muscle group and the shot putter is able to develop triceps strength by using a narrower grip width and forcing a greater contribution from the triceps (Wagner *et al.*, 1992).

During the preparation phases of their competitive year, it is common for field event athletes to participate in power and weightlifting competitions to fulfil goals and to help maintain motivation. In preparation for powerlifting competition, field event athletes may deviate from the grip width that they normally use in their event training in order to maximise their single repetition maximum (IRM). However, that deviation is restricted in competition to a maximum width of 81 cm under Bench Press technical rule 5 of the International Powerlifting Federation (IPF), the international governing body for this sport.

Clemons and Aaron (1997) suggested a grip width of between 190 and 200% of the biacromial breadth (BB) as optimal for maximal bench press performance. The implication of their findings is that athletes with a biacromial breadth greater than 42.6 cm may well not be able to perform to their maximum in an IPF competition as they would be required to use a grip width of less than the recommended optimum.

The aim of the study therefore was to investigate the relationships between biacromial breadth, grip width and IRM bench press in order to assess whether the maximum grip width regulation in powerlifting discriminates against larger athletes.

## 2. METHODS

### 2.1 Participants

Eight male weightlifters gave verbal informed consent to participate in the study. All participants had at least two years experience in performing a maximal bench press. The physical characteristics (mean ± SD) of the participants can be found in Table 1.

Table 1. Subject physical and bench press performance characteristics (mean ± SD).

| Age (yrs) | Mass (kg) | Height (m) |
|-----------|-----------|------------|
| 24.5 (1.1) | 103.9 (10.7) | 1.84 (0.07) |

### 2.2 Assessment of 1RM and preferred grip width

Prior to testing, single repetition maximum (1RM) for the bench press was assessed on two separate occasions. All attempts were conducted according to IPF regulations. Subjects gave their estimated 1RM value and a load of 80% of estimated 1RM was used as the start point for establishing the true 1RM. Participants used their preferred grip width during assessment of 1RM. Participants used chalk on the hands whilst establishing true 1RM and the distance between the chalk residue on the bar as made by the forefingers was measured. The bar was wiped clean after each lift. If a subject was judged to be unsuccessful on three consecutive lifts with any given load, the load used in the previous successful lift was taken as the true 1RM.

### 2.3 Assessment of biacromial breadth

Biacromial breadth was assessed using a standard sliding scale anthropometer. Participants stood in the anatomical position and the measurement was taken from behind the subject. The lateral borders of the acromial processes were palpated and the distance between the lateral borders was measured.

### 2.4 Warm up

Due to the strenuous nature of the testing procedure participants were allowed to perform their own individual warm up, but were also asked to minimise the number of lifts performed prior to testing.

### 2.5 Test protocol

Eight grip widths were used in the assessment of maximal strength. Participants were tested on 6 separate occasions with at least 3 days of rest between each session. Participants were required to perform no upper-body weight training exercise outside the test sessions for the duration of their participation in the study. Grip width was selected randomly based on percentages of the subject's biacromial breadth (grip width range – 90 to 230% of biacromial breadth). Following discussion between subjects and the lifting judge the starting weights were set in terms of percentages of the true 1RM. (See Table 2.)

**Table 2.** Starting loads for maximal bench press exercise expressed as a percentage of true 1RM. Biacromial breadth is denoted by BB whilst GW refers to grip width.

|  | GW 1 | GW2 | GW3 | GW 4 | GW 5 | GW 6 | GW 7 | GW 8 |
|---|---|---|---|---|---|---|---|---|
| Grip Width % BB | 90 | 110 | 130 | 150 | 170 | 190 | 210 | 230 |
| Load (% 1RM) | 50 | 55 | 60 | 65 | 70 | 75 | 70 | 65 |

All bench press attempts were judged by a certified powerlifting referee. Subjects lay supine on a horizontal bench, with the shoulders and buttock maintaining contact with the bench, and the soles of the feet maintaining contact with the floor, throughout the lift. For each attempt the bar was received from two spotters, one on each side of the subject. The bar was then lowered to the chest until the referee signalled that the upward phase could begin. The bar was then pressed symmetrically until both elbows were fully extended and the bar was stationary. Following a second signal from the referee, the bar was returned to the stands with the help of the spotters. Subjects were not informed of the performances of other subjects until the end of the study.

### 2.6 Data analysis

Analysis of the effect of grip width on maximal bench press performance was performed with a two-way analysis of variance using MINITAB for Windows$^©$. A value of $p<0.05$ was used to determine significant differences.

### 3. RESULTS

No significant differences were found between estimated and true maximal bench press strength values, and first and second assessments of true maximal bench press load. Limits of agreement set at 2 SD (Atkinson and Nevill, 1999) for tests one and two were calculated to be 126.8–159.2 kg

Test-retest scores were found to be within limits of agreement. Pre-test and post-test 1 RM scores were also found not to be significantly different (see Table 3).

**Table 3.** Estimated, test-retest and post-test scores for maximal
bench press load at preferred grip width.

|  | Mean | SD |
|---|---|---|
| Estimated 1RM | 143.4 | 17.4 |
| 1 RM Test 1 | 143.0 | 16.2 |
| 1 RM Test 2 | 143.0 | 15.7 |
| Post-Test 1RM | 143.2 | 15.4 |

Figure 1 shows the mean 1RM for the subject group at different grip widths. It can
be seen that bench press performance was greatest at a grip width of 190% of the
biacromial breadth and that performance at narrower and wider grip widths was
reduced.

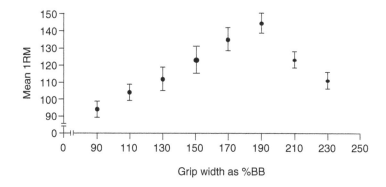

**Figure 1.** Mean 1 RM for bench press at different grip widths
expressed as a percentage of biacromial breadth.

**Table 4.** Details of individual biacromial breadth, preferred grip width, grip width as a percentage of
biacromial breadth, and predicted optimal grip width based on data shown in Figure 1.

| Subject No. | 1 | 2 | 3 | 4 | 5 | 6 | 7 | 8 |
|---|---|---|---|---|---|---|---|---|
| BB (cm) | 43 | 44 | 42 | 41 | 39 | 41 | 41 | 46 |
| Preferred GW(cm) | 78 | 85 * | 76 | 82 * | 75 | 84 * | 80 | 87 * |
| Grip width as % BB | 181.4 | 193.2 | 181.0 | 200.0 | 192.3 | 204.9 | 195.1 | 189.1 |

* Indicates a GW greater than the 81cm maximum stipulated in IPF regulations

From a two-way ANOVA significant differences ($F_{7,7}$ = 28.26, p<0.05) were found between mean 1RM at different grip widths. Mean 1RM was greatest at 190% biacromial breadth, which corresponds to a grip width of 79.99 cm for the participants.

## 4. DISCUSSION

Madsen and McLaughlin (1985) suggested that a wide grip was advantageous to the athlete. They highlighted an inverse relationship between grip width and the distance that the bar must travel, thus reducing the work required to raise the bar.

As stated previously, Clemons and Aaron (1997) suggested that the optimal grip lies between 190 and 200% of the biacromial breadth. The results of this study, suggest an optimal grip width of 190%.

**Table 5**. The suggested range of optimal grip widths for participating subjects.

| Subject No. | BB (cm) | 190 % BB |
|---|---|---|
| 1 | 43 | 81.7 |
| 2 | 44 | 83.6 |
| 3 | 42 | 79.8 |
| 4 | 41 | 77.9 |
| 5 | 39 | 74.1 |
| 6 | 41 | 77.9 |
| 7 | 41 | 77.9 |
| 8 | 46 | 87.4 |

When considering this finding and the range of biacromial breadths of subjects participating in this study, it is evident that the IPF restriction of a maximum grip width to 81 cm could prevent athletes from competing at their optimal levels. Table 5 shows the predicted optimal grip widths based on this study and that of Clemons and Aaron (1997). Although five of the eight subjects in our study would be allowed to compete using their optimal grip width, three would not, a clear implication that larger athletes are restricted from competing at their optimal grip width and are hence penalised by their size.   ed

Madsen and McLaughlin (1995) suggested  that the maximum grip width exists to prevent athletes from using a wider grip to minimise the length of travel of the bar during the bench press. The results of the present study and those of Clemons and Aaron (1997) would suggest that as maximal bench press performance drops substantially when using a grip width of 210% biacromial breadth then there is no advantage to using an overly-wide grip anyway. Therefore defining and enforcing an absolute maximum is a redundant exercise which the IPF should consider scrapping.

Further investigation is now needed to establish whether a specific value for optimal grip width expressed in terms of the biacromial breadth, rather than a range. There is also a need to establish the extent of the increase in performance for larger athletes that may result following a revision of the absolute maximum grip width to a maximum expressed in terms of biacromial breadth.

## REFERENCES

Clemons, J.M. and Aaron, C., 1997, Effect of grip width on the myoelectric activity of prime movers in the bench press. *Journal of Strength and Conditioning Research*, **11**(2), 82-87.

Glass, S.C. and Armstrong, T., 1997, Electromyographical activity of the pectoralis muscle during incline and decline bench presses. *Journal of Strength and Conditioning Research*, **11**(3), 163-167.

International Powerlifting Federation, 2002, *The International Powerlifting Federation Technical Rules Book*, pp. 15.

Madsen, N.H. and McLaughlin, T.M., 1985, Kinematic factors influencing performance and injury risk in the bench press exercise. *Medicine and Science in Sports and Exercise,* **16**, 376-381.

Wagner, L.L., Evans, S.A., Weir, J.P., Housh, T.J. and Johnson, D.B., 1992, The effect of grip width on bench press performance. *International Journal of Sports Biomechanics*, **8**, 1-10.

# 17 Kinanthropometric and Performance Characteristics of Gaelic Games Players

Dominic A. Doran, John Paul Donnelly and Thomas Reilly
Research Institute for Sport and Exercise Sciences, Liverpool John Moores University, UK

## 1. INTRODUCTION

Recently there has been an emphasis on examining the factors that influence performance in Gaelic games. Reilly and Doran (2001) have recently reviewed the current sports science literature as applied to Gaelic football. The diversity in scientific information specific to Gaelic football has not been mirrored in the other main Gaelic field sport of hurling. Hurling is a team game played on a pitch ~137 m x ~82 m using a 15-player team; it is similar to hockey in that it is played with a small leather ball (sliothar) and a curved wooden stick (camán). The ball can be stuck while on the ground, or played in the air. A significant amount of play occurs in the air, especially above head height (Figure 1). Unlike hockey, the ball can be picked up with the camán and carried for four steps. The ball then must either be bounced on the camán and back to the hand, or carried with the ball balanced on the camán. Similarly, Gaelic football, consists of 15 players on the field at any one time but the pitch is about 40% longer than a soccer pitch. The ball can be played with the hands or with the feet, long or short. The ball is round like a soccer ball: the skills employed in playing it include high catching, long distance kicking for accuracy, passing and moving the ball, solo-running by kicking the ball to oneself and collecting it before it bounces, and blocking an opponent's kick or hand pass. It is common tactical practice in both codes to follow a person-to-person marking strategy. The team configuration consists of a goalkeeper, two defensive lines each of three players, each line in turn being confronted by a corresponding trio of forwards. The remaining two players take up the centre-field positions. The roles of individual players vary according to playing position and positional changes are common for tactical purposes. Matches consist of two 30-min halves. Time is increased to 70 min in inter-county (elite) championship games. The ball is rarely out of play for long periods, especially since new rules were introduced in 1990, which allowed players fewer respites during a match. The players are required to run repeatedly, with or without the ball or to give or receive a pass. To score, in both codes the ball must pass over or under the crossbar for a point or goal respectively, the latter being the equivalent of three points. Players can physically contest possession of the ball with shoulder-to-shoulder charges or blocking with either the camán or the body; therefore both Gaelic game codes are highly physical (Figure 1).

Areas of previous research into hurling have included the analysis of physical work capacity (Watson, 1977), analysis of injuries (O'Donoghue and Condon, 1979; Watson, 1993; Watson, 1996; Watson, 1999), the simulated physiological cost of carrying a camán (Fenton, 1996) and the suggested endurance demands of hurling (Reilly, 2000).   However, there has been no direct research into the physiological and anthropometric characteristics of elite and non-elite senior hurling players. By examining the kinanthropometric and physiological capacity of both elite and non-elite players it is possible to formulate an understanding of the physical demands of the game; such strategies have occurred for other intermittent field games (Reilly, 1990; Reilly and Borrie, 1992; Bell *et al.*, 1993; Bangsbo and Michalsik, 2002). The physiological demands of Gaelic football have been suggested to resemble those of hurling (Reilly, 2000).   Therefore, by comparing results, or borrowing from the pool of scientific information on Gaelic football it may be useful to examine the similarities and differences between both codes of Gaelic games (Douge, 1988).   The aim of this study was to characterise the kinanthropometric and performance profiles of elite and non-elite Gaelic games players.

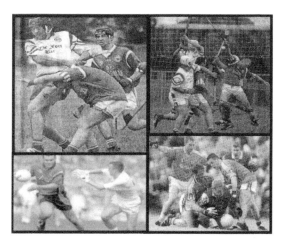

**Figure 1.** Representation of Gaelic games, Hurling (above) and Gaelic football (below).

## 2. METHODS

### 2.1 Subjects

Participants in this study were 7 senior male inter-county hurling players, 14 club-level senior hurling players, and 33 inter-county Gaelic footballers. The inter-county and club hurlers were drawn from the same successful Northern Ireland Hurling County. The Gaelic footballers were members of the Mayo squad who successfully competed in the 1999 All-Ireland Gaelic football championship. After being informed of the nature and methodology of the study, written informed consent was obtained in accordance with the institutional ethical procedures. Sample characteristics are presented in Table 1.

### 2.2 Anthropometric measurements

Anthropometric characteristics were determined from standard anthropometric techniques as described by Lohman *et al.* (1991). The technical error of measurement was calculated for all anthropometric measurements and was less than approximately 2% which is within acceptable measurement error. In addition to age, a total of 11 anthropometric measures were determined on the right hand side of the body. Each participant's height was measured in the Frankfort plane to the nearest 0.01 (cm) with a portable stadiometer (Seca, Menheimn, Germany). Body mass (kg) was determined to the nearest 0.1 kg on balance beam scales (Seca, Menheimn, Germany). Subcutaneous adipose tissue was measured at five skinfold sites (mm), (biceps, triceps, subscapular and suprailiac and medical calf utilising Harpenden calipers (British Indicators LTD, Luton). Furthermore two diameters – biepicondylar humerus and biepicondylar femur – and two circumferences – maximal calf and upper arm circumference – were also recorded. These directly determined anthropometric variables were utilised to permit the calculation of a series of derived measurements. These included the somatotype ratings for ectomorphy, mesomorphy, and endomorphy according to the technique of Carter and Honeyman-Heath (1990). Fat Free Mass Index (FFMI) $(kg.m^2)$ (Kouri *et al.*, 1995) was also calculated. Body density was determined utilising the sum of four skinfold sites: biceps, triceps, subscapular and suprailliac (Durnin and Womersley, 1974). Body fat % was calculated based upon the equation of Siri (1956).

### 2.3 Performance analysis

A series of field based performance tests were carried out in order to characterise the physical performance of the Gaelic games players. Such an approach is widespread in research and applied support scenarios given the specificity of testing protocols to game demands (Reilly and Doran, 2003). Maximal oxygen uptake was estimated ($\dot{V}O_{2\,max}$) from performance on the 20-m shuttle test

(Ramsbottom *et al.*, 1988).    Maximal running speed and repeated sprint performance were determined using a 7 × 30-m sprint test with a 15-s active recovery. Electronic timing lights (Eleiko, Halmstad Sweden) were placed at 10 and 30 m to determine sprint performance. All subjects were instructed to provide a maximal effort on each sprint. Sprint performances over 10 and 30 m and fatigue index profiles (FI%), which incorporated the % decline in time from the fastest to slowest of seven repeated sprints over both the 10-m and 30-m sprints were calculated (Wilkinson and Moore, 1995). Vertical jump was determined using the elevation in the centre of mass using a electronic jumping mat (Eleiko Sport, Halmstad, Sweden). Flexibility of the hamstrings, the lower middle and upper paraspinals and calf muscles was determined using the sit-and-reach test. Leg-and-back strength was measured using a back and leg dynamometer (Cranlea, Birmingham) following the procedure outlined by Heyward (1998).

### 2.4 Data analysis

Data were expressed as mean (±SD). Data were checked for normal distribution using the Anderson-Darling technique. All variables were analysed using one-way analysis of variance to test for differences between groups. Where a significant F ratio was indicated, a Tukey post hoc analysis was applied to assess its occurrence. The $p<0.05$ level of confidence was chosen as the minimal level for acceptance of statistical significance.

### 3. RESULTS

The Gaelic football players were significantly taller, heavier and expressed higher muscularity ratings than both the elite and non-elite hurlers ($p<0.05$). No differences in these parameters were evident between the elite and non-elite hurlers.   Adiposity ratings expressed as sum of 4 skinfolds or % body fat demonstrated no significant differences between groups.

Significant differences were apparent between the groups on all physical parameters, except for flexibility.   On the majority of tests the elite Gaelic footballer and hurlers outperformed the non-elite club players ($p<0.05$). Significant differences between the elite footballers and hurlers were only apparent on the fatigue index over the repeated 10-m and 30-m sprints ($p<0.05$).

**Table 1**. Anthropometric and somatotype characteristics of elite and non-elite Gaelic games players. Data are mean (± SD).

| Variables | Hurlers (Elite Inter-county) | Hurlers (Non-elite) | Gaelic football (Elite Inter-county) |
|---|---|---|---|
| Stature (m) | $1.743 \pm 0.052$ | $1.773 \pm 0.057$ | $1.79 \pm 0.07^{\#}$ |
| Body Mass (kg) | $73.4 \pm 7.7$ | $73.8 \pm 8.2$ | $79.2 \pm 8.2^{\blacktriangle}$ |
| FFMI (kg.m$^2$) | $21.1 \pm 1.3$ | $20.1 \pm 1.3$ | $23.9 \pm 2.1^{\blacktriangle}$ |
| Body fat (%) | $13.1 \pm 1.4$ | $14.1 \pm 3.1$ | $12.3 \pm 2.9$ |
| Σ 4 skinfolds | $30.6 \pm 3.15$ | $33.9 \pm 7.20$ | $26.8 \pm 6.6$ |
| Endomorphy | $2.5 \pm 0.4$ | $2.7 \pm 0.67$ | $2.7 \pm 0.5$ |
| Mesomorphy | $4.6 \pm 0.5$ | $3.8 \pm 1.3$ | $5.7 \pm 0.8^{\blacktriangle}$ |
| Ectomorphy | $1.8 \pm 0.5$ | $2.4 \pm 0.9$ | $1.9 \pm 0.6$ |
| SAM | 0.76 | 1.49 | 1.17 |
| $S^2_A$ | 0.07 | 1.01 | 0.36 |
| $S_A$ | 0.25 | 1.00 | 0.60 |

$^{\blacktriangle}$ Gaelic footballers > than both elite and non-elite hurlers (p<0.05).
$^{\#}$ Gaelic footballers > elite hurlers (p<0.05)


**Table 2**. Performance characteristics of elite and non-elite Gaelic games players. Data are mean (± SD). Where differences exist between cohorts, this is indicated by appropriate annotation.

| Variable | Hurlers (Elite Inter-county) | Hurlers (Non-elite) | Gaelic football (Elite Inter-county) |
|---|---|---|---|
| $\dot{V}O_{2\,max}$ (ml.kg$^{-1}$.min$^{-1}$) | $58.9 \pm 4.8^{\$}$ | $53.8 \pm 4.0$ | $58.8 \pm 3.8^{*}$ |
| Sprint speed 10 m (s) | $1.78 \pm 0.08^{\$}$ | $1.94 \pm 0.12$ | $1.76 \pm 0.08^{*}$ |
| Sprint speed 30 m (s) | $4.43 \pm 0.17^{\$}$ | $4.72 \pm 0.35$ | $4.41 \pm 0.16^{*}$ |
| Fatigue index 10m (%) | $5.84 \pm 2.8^{£}$ | $10.7 \pm 2.7$ | $10.5 \pm 5.28$ |
| Fatigue index 30m (%) | $4.41 \pm 2.8^{£}$ | $9.36 \pm 1.7$ | $9.7 \pm 4.29$ |
| Vertical jump (cm) | $40.8 \pm 4.5^{\$}$ | $33.0 \pm 2.7$ | $58.3 \pm 6.31^{\blacktriangle}$ |
| Flexibility: Sit and reach (cm) | $24.6 \pm 7.3$ | $21.7 \pm 3.2$ | $21.9 \pm 7.2$ |
| Leg-and-back strength (kg) | $192.4 \pm 31.9^{\$}$ | $163.9 \pm 22.8$ | - |

$^{\blacktriangle}$ Gaelic footballers >elite and non-elite hurlers (p<0.05).
£ Elite hurlers > elite Gaelic footballers and non-elite hurlers (p<0.05).
$ Elite hurlers > non-elite hurlers (p<0.05).
* Gaelic footballers > non-elite hurlers (p<0.05).

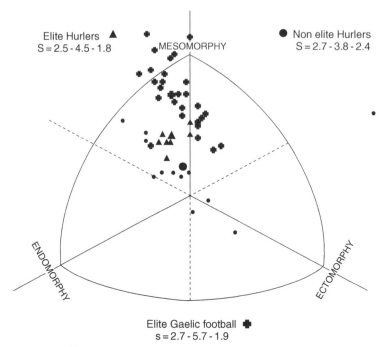

Figure 2. Somatoplot of elite and non-elite Gaelic games players.

## 4. DISCUSSION

The present study examined the anthropometric and performance characteristics of elite and non-elite Gaelic games players. Examination of the physical and anthropometric characteristics of elite performers in these codes can facilitate a better understanding of the particular requirements these field sports impose on their participants.   Comparisons have been made between soccer and Gaelic football (Strudwick *et al.*, 2002). Such comparisons are important particularly in Gaelic games as players compete in both activities at recreation and elite level. Senior-level inter-county matches generally represent the highest level of attainment in hurling as no international competition takes place given the indigenous nature of the sport. Gaelic football generally mirrors this situation although international matches between Ireland and Australia take place in a hybrid competition that mixes Gaelic football and Australian rules football.

Gaelic football players were taller, heavier and more muscular than both hurling cohorts (Table 1). Successful Gaelic games players' teams tend to be taller and heavier than their less successful opponents (Keane *et al.*, 1997; Watson, 1977). Such data may indicate that to compete in Gaelic football at elite level the requirements of being heavier and taller are necessary within the caveat of positional restraints. Fenton (1996) observed body mass values of 83.3 ± 8.5 (kg) in ten elite hurling players, which exceed those presented in the current study. The body mass ranges indicate that elite and non-elite Gaelic games players are relatively heterogeneous with respect to body size. The smaller stature and lower body mass of the elite hurlers may be an artefact of a positional bias toward recruitment of players from the full and half forward line. Nevertheless, small stature is not necessarily a bar to success in Gaelic games (Reilly, 2000). Hurlers can utilise the camán to field the ball, effectively extending their reach, ensuring that height may not be as strong a determining factor in performance success. Those players that are the taller and heavier individuals tend to be found in the midfield and central attacking and defensive roles, forming a link between full-back and full-forward, the smaller players being dispersed on the wings and most notably in attack.

The somatotype ratings noted agree with the mean somatotype of 2.6-5.6-3.1 reported by Watson (1995) for Gaelic football. The ratings observed for the club and elite hurlers are comparable to those reported by Florida-James and Reilly (1995) of 2.4-4.2-2.4 for under-21 English based club Gaelic players and values reported for international Rugby Union "sevens" players (Reilly *et al.*, 2000). The non-elite hurling players were either balanced mesomorphs or endo-mesomorphs while the elite senior players were characterised as balanced mesomorphs (Figure 2). Mesomorphy ratings in the elite and non-elite hurlers are lower than in the Gaelic football players. Endomorphy and ectomorphy are similar between groups and are supported by the adiposity data (Table 1). These findings for Gaelic footballers, and elite hurlers suggest that lower endomorphy and increased mesomorphy are integral to competition at an inter-county level. Fat Free Mass Index has also been used to provide an indication of muscularity development and supports the view regarding the importance of muscularity Normative values of 20 $kg.m^2$ indicate a moderate muscularity rating while values above 22 $kg.m^2$ indicate a high level of muscularity (Kouri *et al.*, 1995). The Gaelic players expressed a significantly higher degree of muscularity than that presented by the hurlers, particularly the non-elite group. In intermittent field games were body mass must be rapidly accelerated during sprints or jumps, low levels of adiposity are desirable and where body fat is elevated performance can be compromised (Strudwick *et al.*, 2002). Reilly and Doran (2001) reported that players with a low percentage of body fat would be expected to be more mobile around the field of play due to carrying less redundant weight. As the elite hurling and Gaelic football players had a lower % of body fat in comparison to the non-elite players, their ability to contest possession in the air or on the ground should be superior. Fenton (1996) has reported values of 16.9 (± 3.1%) for ten inter-county hurling players which exceed that reported for the elite and non-elite hurling and Gaelic football players in this study.

The elite Gaelic football and hurling players attained significantly higher maximal oxygen uptake ($\dot{V}O_{2\,max}$) estimates than the non-elite players. This most likely reflects the higher work-rate achieved during competition and preparation for competition. According to Reilly and Doran (2001) elite Gaelic teams that reach a high level of endurance fitness participate in highly systematic training programmes at inter-county level, something that may not be replicated at the non-elite club level. Fenton (1996) reported $\dot{V}O_{2\,max}$ values of 56.8 (± 4.9) $ml.kg^{-1}.min^{-1}$ for ten inter-county level hurling players, which compare favourably with those noted in both elite cohorts. The values reported for the non-elite hurlers are comparable to those of English based club Gaelic football players ($52.6 \pm 4.0$ $ml.kg^{-1}.min^{-1}$) observed by Florida-James and Reilly (1995). The 37 inter-county players studied by Keane *et al.* (1997) had values of 54.1 (3.2) $ml\cdot kg^{-1}\cdot min^{-1}$ compared to the 51.4 ($\pm 5.8$) $ml\cdot kg^{-1}\cdot min^{-1}$ observed for 40 senior club players. In soccer the $\dot{V}O_2$ max reported for elite male outfield players range from 56 to 69 $ml.kg^{-1}.min^{-1}$ (Bangsbo and Michalsik, 2002). The values obtained for elite Gaelic football and hurling players are within this range. Positional variations in $\dot{V}O_2$ max are commonly reported in soccer and other intermittent field sports; it would be unexpected that such positional variations in aerobic power would not be replicated in Gaelic games players. In soccer a threshold for $\dot{V}O_{2\,max}$ would seem to exist around 60 $ml.kg^{-1}.min^{-1}$ that differentiates the elite from non-elite players. Nevertheless, the values reported for elite hurling and Gaelic football players exceed expectations when the amateur status of the players is considered. Gaelic games players at the elite level of hurling and Gaelic football require an aerobic power comparable to professional soccer players, even though matches are approximately 20 minutes shorter.

The physical nature of both Gaelic football and hurling, combined with the multifactoral technical and physical skills base, requires the players to contest balls on the ground, in the air as well as accelerating to intercept crosses and players. The ability to produce this key component of match-play is expressed in terms of absolute sprinting speed, sprint fatigue resistance and muscular power. Both elite groups had faster sprint speeds over 10 m and 30 m than the non-elite hurlers. Acceleration over an initial 10-m distance would seem to be a prerequisite to successful elite performance in Gaelic games. Any deficits in this acceleration capability from a standing start would disadvantage individuals in either code when contesting either aerial or ground play. Comparable data in professional rugby league backs for 10-m acceleration sprints of $1.79 \pm 0.09$ s have been reported (O'Connor, 1995). Speed over 30-m did not differ between the elite players, again reflecting the need to move forward with attacking play and track back to quickly re-establish defensive cover.

Fatigue index, was utilised to represent the ability of the players to maintain acceleration and speed on a repeated basis with increasing fatigue. The elite hurlers presented a significantly lower fatigue index (%) over 10 m and 30 m compared to either the elite Gaelic footballers or the non-elite group. Smaros (1980) has reported that $\dot{V}O_{2\,max}$ influences the amount of sprints and sprinting ability that players were able to attempt within a soccer match. In relation to the present study the 7 x 30-m repeated sprints place significant demand on glycolytic and oxidative energy pathways. Those players with higher aerobic capacities should be able to maintain sprint speed more effectively over the test duration than those with lower $\dot{V}O_{2\,max}$. This is not the case between the elite Gaelic football and hurlers where significant difference in fatigue index were found(Table 2). Explanation may lie in the heterogeneous nature of the Gaelic football group which comprised players from all positions, including goalkeepers. This contrasts with the elite hurlers who were predominately forward and centre-half forward players where fatigue resistance during repeated sprints is a desirable quality.

Substantial differences in vertical jump performance between the elite hurlers and footballers was evident, that may reflect differences in training emphasis. Reilly and Thomas (1977) reported where there is an emphasis on aerobic conditioning, vertical jump performance may be restrained. In both codes strong jumping ability is essential for aerial fielding, sub-optimal jumping ability will compromise performance.

## 5. CONCLUSIONS

Profiling the anthropometric and performance characteristics of elite and non-elite Gaelic games players is still evolving. The present study suggests the physical requirements to compete at an elite level do not differ significantly between Gaelic games codes at an elite level. Identifying what characteristics are expressed at this level of competition provides information indirectly on the demands of both codes, particularly hurling. If such information can be determined, the profiles should be used to inform the development and implementation of conditioning programmes.

## REFERENCES

Bangsbo, J. and Michalsik, L., 2002, Assessment of the physiological capacity of elite soccer players. In *Science and Football IV* edited by Spinks, W., Reilly, T. and Murphy, A. (London: E. and F. N. Spon), pp. 53-62.

Bell, W., Cobner, D., Cooper, S.M. and Phillips, S.J.,1993. Anaerobic performance and body composition of international rugby union players. In *Science and Football II,* edited by Reilly, T., Clarys, J. and Stibbe, A., (London: E. and F.N. Spon), pp. 40-42.

Carter, J.E.L. and Honeyman-Heath, B., 1990, *Somatotyping: Developments and Applications*, (Cambridge University Press).

Douge, B., 1988, Football: the common threads between the games. In *Science and Football*, edited by Reilly, T., Lees, A., Davids, K. and Murphy, W.J., (London: E. and F.N. Spon), pp. 3-19.

Durnin, J.V.G.A. and Womersley, J., 1974, Body fat assessed from total body density and its estimation from skinfold thickness: measurements on 481 men and women aged from 16 to 72 years. *British Journal of Nutrition*, **32**, 77-97.

Fenton, C., 1996, A comparison in hurling of the physiological cost between carrying and not carrying a hurley. *Journal of Sports Sciences*, **14**, 81-82.

Florida-James, G. and Reilly, T., 1995, The physiological demands of Gaelic football. *British Journal of Sports Medicine*, **29**, 41-45.

Heyward, V.H., 1998, *Advanced Fitness Assessment and Exercise Prescription*. Champaign Illinois: Human Kinetics Publishers.

Keane, S., Reilly, T. and Borrie, A., 1997, A comparison of fitness characteristics of elite and non-elite Gaelic football players. In *Science and Football III*, edited by Reilly, T., Bangsbo, J. and Hughes, M., (London: E. and F.N. Spon), pp. 3-6.

Kouri, E.M., Pope, H.G., Katz, D.L. and Oliva, P., 1995, Fat free mass index in users and nonusers of anabolic-androgenic steroids. *Clinical Journal of Sports Medicine*, **5**, 223-238.

Lohman, T.G., Roche, A.F., Martorell, R., 1991, *Anthropometric Standardisation Reference Manual.* (Champaign Illnois: Human Kinetic Books).

O'Connor, D., 1995, Fitness profile of professional Rugby League players. In *Science and Football III* edited by Reilly, T., Bangsbo, J. and Hughes, M., (London: E. and F.N. Spon), pp. 21-27.

O'Donoghue, J. and Condon, K.C., 1979, Facial injuries to hurlers. *Irish Medical Association*, **10**, 448-449.

Ramsbottom, R., Brewer, J. and Williams, C., 1988, A progressive shuttle run to estimate maximal oxygen uptake. *British Journal of Sports Medicine*, **22**, 141-144.

Reilly, T., 1990, Football. In *Physiology of Sports*, edited by Reilly, T. Secher, N. Snell, P. and Williams, C., (London: E. and F.N. Spon), pp. 371-425.

Reilly, T., 2000, Endurance aspects of soccer and other field games. In *Endurance in Sport*, edited by Shephard, R.J. and Åstrand, P.O., (Oxford: Blackwell Science Ltd), pp. 900-930.

Reilly, T. and Borrie, A., 1992, Physiology applied to field hockey. *Sports Medicine*, **14**, 10-26.

Reilly, T., and Doran, D., 2001, Science and Gaelic football: A review. *Journal of Sports Sciences*, **19**, 181-193.

Reilly, T., and Doran, D. (2003). Fitness assessment. In *Science and Soccer 2$^{nd}$ Edition,* edited by Reilly, T. and Williams, A.M., (London: E. and F.N. Spon), pp. 21-46.

Reilly, T. and Thomas, V., 1977, Application of multivariate analysis to the fitness assessment of soccer players. *British Journal of Sports Medicine*, **11**,183-184.

Reilly, T., Rienzi, E. and Doran, D. 2000. Kinanthropometric profiles of elite players in three football codes. *Communication to VII European College of Sports Science Conference* (Jyvaskyla, Finland).

Siri, W.E., 1956, Gross composition of the body. In *Advances in Biological and Medical Physics*, edited by Lawerence, J.H. and Tobais, C.A., (New York: Academic Press, Inc).

Smaros, G., 1980, Energy usage during a football match. In *Proceeding of the 1$^{st}$ International Congress on Sports Medicine Applied to Football*, Rome, edited by Vecchiet, L., pp. 795-801.

Strudwick, T., Reilly, T. and Doran D., 2002, Anthropometric and fitness profiles of elite players in two football codes. *Journal of Sports Medicine and Physical Fitness*, **42**, 239-242.

Watson, A.W.S., 1977, A study of the physical working capacity of Gaelic football and hurlers. *British Journal of Sports Medicine*, **11**, 133-137.

Watson, A.W.S., 1993, Incidence and nature of sports injuries in Ireland: Analysis of four types of sport. *American Journal of Sports Medicine*, **21**, 137-143.

Watson, A.W.S., 1996, Sports injuries in the game of hurling a one-year prospective study. *American Journal of Sports Medicine*, **3**, 323-328.

Watson, A.W.S., 1999, Ankle sprains in players of field-games Gaelic football and hurling. *Journal of Sports Medicine and Physical Fitness*, **39**, 66-70.

Wilkinson, D. and Moore, P., 1995, *Measuring Performance: A Guide to Field based fitness testing*, (Leeds: National Coaching Foundation).

# Part IV

# FEMALES AND EXERCISE

# 18 Anthropometric Fat Patterning in Male and Female Subjects

Arthur D. Stewart

Department of Biomedical Sciences, University of Aberdeen, King's College, Aberdeen, AB24 3FX, UK

## 1. INTRODUCTION

Human fat has traditionally been partitioned between *essential* and *excess* components, with females requiring greater essential levels than males to maintain optimal function and general health. The sum of these two components is commonly expressed as a percentage of total body mass, and is estimated by various levels of approach and methods of differing complexity and cost (Hawes and Martin, 2001). Adipose tissue is the storage depot for excess fat on the body, and follows a series of checks and balances between energy intake, energy expenditure through basal metabolism and movement, and thermodynamic considerations between individuals and their environment (Stewart, 2002).

Fat patterning refers to the distribution of fat throughout an individual. It can be assessed as differential distribution between compartments such as visceral and subcutaneous, or variable distribution within a compartment. While level of fatness relates to health risk, fat patterning possibly does so to a greater extent, and avoids the assumptions required to convert measurements into a percentage. Examination of an individual's fat pattern may employ medical imaging techniques such as magnetic resonance imaging or computed tomography, but the expense of these largely limits their utility to clinical study. Regional fat distribution has been described with the use of dual X-ray absorptiometry (Stewart and Hannan, 2000a) and this technique holds promise as facilities become more widespread. Of the other methods available which examine the subcutaneous compartment, ultrasound has proved useful in estimating segmental fat (Eston *et al.*, 1994) yet such studies remain relatively rare, and while infra-red interactance has appeal, it has yet to be widely accepted.

Surface anthropometry is probably the most convenient technique for assessing fat patterning, as it is relatively inexpensive, and non-invasive. Circumferences are used to provide the waist to hip ratio, or, in conjunction with height and mass, the conicity index (Valdez, 1991). However, skinfolds enable a far more complete picture of fat patterning to be created within and between individuals, because there are so many recognised sites for measurement. Standardisation of protocols and equipment, together with error quantification has extended the validity and utility of skinfold measures, without conversion to % fat (Marfell-Jones, 2001).

The subcutaneous fat on the body is not a veneer of uniform thickness but a variable 'topography' modelled by independent but concurrent influences of gender, age, level of adiposity, ethnicity and exercise (Malina, 1996; Nindl *et al.*, 1996).

In addition, pregnancy, lactation and clinical conditions such as the metabolic syndrome or Cushing's syndrome may further complicate an already complex pattern. Age-related centralisation and differential lipolysis of adipose tissue arising from exercise combine to produce wide individual variation in fat pattern, and simultaneously limit the validity of generalised formulae to predict fat content of an individual. Therefore the purpose of this study was to investigate fat patterning using various derived skinfold ratios, and explore their stability across gender, and ranges of age, adiposity and exercise.

## 2. METHODS

A total of 139 male and 64 female healthy and Caucasian adults participated in the study. All were measured for skinfold thickness by the same experienced anthropometrist. Of these, 106 males and 33 females were athletes, as defined by competition at University level or above, and training for a minimum of three hours per week averaged over the previous year. The male athletes were part of a previous study of body composition (Stewart and Hannan, 2000b), which quantified the intra-tester technical error of measurement for each skinfold site which averaged 3.8% (range 2.1–6.5%). Physical characteristics of the sample are summarised in Table 1.

Each subject presented either fasted or having eaten only lightly on the day of measurement, having refrained from exercise on the day of measurement. Each was measured wearing shorts and training vest with Harpenden calipers (British Indicators, Luton, UK) using a 41 – measurement protocol (Hawes and Soucie, 1993) by the same experienced anthropometrist. Measurements included body mass, heights, eight bone breadths, nine circumferences and 19 skinfolds. Skinfolds were measured on the right side of the body at the following sites: cheek, chin, pectoral, triceps, subscapular, thorax, supraspinale, abdominal, thigh (patella), mid-thigh, proximal calf, mid-calf, biceps, forearm (anterior), forearm (radial), medial calf, suprailium, axilla and iliac crest. Measurements followed procedures endorsed by the International Society for the Advancement of Kinanthropometry (ISAK). Female subjects were measured with another female present. Each subject was questioned on participation in physical activity and sport, in terms of years of participation, standard, and training hours each week, averaged over the previous year. Data were analysed using SPSS version 8. Local ethical permission was obtained for the measurements, and level of statistical significance was set at $p < 0.05$.

One novel and two previously established skinfold ratios were calculated to describe fat patterning within the subcutaneous compartment. Established ratios were the subscapular:triceps ratio (ST) (Malina, 1996), and the trunk : extremity ratio (TE) which is the ratio of the sum of abdominal + subscapular + iliac crest to the sum of biceps + triceps + medial calf (Malina and Bouchard, 1988). The proposed new ratio was the abdominal : medial calf ratio (AMC).

## 3. RESULTS

**Table 1**. Physical characteristics of subjects.

|  | Males (n = 139) | | Females (n = 65) | |
| --- | --- | --- | --- | --- |
| Age (years) | 27.9 | 7.7 | 26.9 | 8.7 |
| Height (m) | 1.80 | 0.07 | 1.67 | 0.06 |
| Mass (kg) | 77.5 | 9.7 | 60.34 | 9.7 |
| Endomorphy | 3.00 | 1.09 | 3.77 | 1.64 |
| Mesomorphy | 4.98 | 1.23 | 3.83 | 1.12 |
| Ectomorphy | 2.51 | 1.08 | 2.84 | 1.28 |
| Σ19 skinfolds (mm) | 207.3 | 46.7 | 222.7 | 90.3 |
| Exercise (h.week$^{-1}$) | 8.3 | 5.2 | 6.4 | 4.9 |

Males were of similar age to females (p>0.05) but were taller and had greater mass (p<0.001). Males were higher in mesomorphy (p<0.001) and lower in endomorphy (p<0.01) than females.   There was no difference in age and ectomorphy between the groups (p>0.05). Males had similar Σ19 skinfold totals to females (p>0.05) but exercised for an average of 1.9 hours more per week (p<0.05).   Men had greater ST, AMC and TE skinfold ratios than women (p<0.001), as shown in Figure 1.

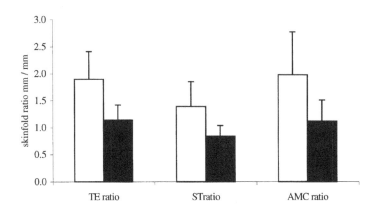

**Figure 1**.  Skinfold ratios of male (light) and female (dark) subjects.

Correlation coefficients for the relationships between these variables are provided in Table 2.

Table 2. Correlation coefficients of age, exercise and skinfolds.

| Males | Exercise (h.week$^{-1}$) | ST ratio | AMC ratio | TE ratio | Σ19 skinfolds |
|---|---|---|---|---|---|
| Age (years) | -0.16 | 0.24** | 0.25** | 0.27** | 0.18* |
| Exercise (h.week$^{-1}$) | | -0.07 | -0.13 | -0.25** | -0.30** |
| ST ratio | | | 0.48** | 0.67** | 0.18 |
| AMC ratio | | | | 0.86** | 0.15 |
| TE ratio | | | | | 0.32** |
| | | | | | |
| Females | | | | | |
| Age (years) | -0.26* | 0.35** | 0.42** | 0.37** | 0.25* |
| Exercise (h.week$^{-1}$) | | 0.16 | -0.21 | -0.17 | -0.58** |
| ST ratio | | | 0.37** | 0.66** | 0.11 |
| AMC ratio | | | | 0.82** | 0.33** |
| TE ratio | | | | | 0.42** |

$p < 0.05$; **$p < 0.01$

Stepwise regression analysis was used using a probability of F to enter of ≤ 0.05, and F to remove of ≥ 0.10 to estimate the extent to which skinfold ratios were independently explained by age, exercise hours and skinfold total in males and females. The regressions produced are summarised in Table 3.

Table 3. Regression analysis of age, Σ19 skinfolds and hours of exercise against skinfold ratios.

| Dependent variable | TE | AMC | ST | Constant | $R^2$ | SEE | p |
|---|---|---|---|---|---|---|---|
| Males | | | | | | | |
| Age (years) | 4.11 | * | * | 20.1 | 0.08 | 7.4 | = 0.001 |
| Σ19 skinfolds (mm) | 111.9 | -40.1 | -48.5 | 141.3 | 0.28 | 39.9 | < 0.001 |
| hours | -8.0 | 2.8 | 2.9 | 13.9 | 0.12 | 4.9 | < 0.001 |
| Females | | | | | | | |
| Age (Years) | * | 8.97 | * | 16.9 | 0.16 | 8.0 | = 0.001 |
| Σ19 | 204.0 | * | -139.1 | 108.2 | 0.24 | 80.2 | < 0.001 |

* excluded variables

Significant regressions were produced in all the analyses with the exception of hours of exercise in females. In males, regression of both hours and skinfold total selected all three ratios as predictors, while regression of age selected only the TE ratio. In females, regression of age selected only the AMC ratio, while regression of skinfold total selected the TE and ST ratios.

# 4. DISCUSSION

These data suggest male and females display highly significant differences in fat patterning depicted by skinfold ratios, despite no difference in skinfold total. Of all the variables, gender would appear to exert the most powerful influence over fat distribution, involving preferential storage on peripheral regions. By contrast, male storage favoured torso sites. Independent t-tests comparing males and females showed that of the 19 skinfolds measured, only five (the subscapular, thorax, supraspinale, abdominal and iliac crest) failed to show significant differences between the sexes (p>0.05). While it could be argued that this could be partly attributed to the fact that males exercised for longer than females, this effect does not appear strong by comparison with gender. Further, self-reported exercise may not be a particularly good indicator of metabolic cost of exercise, whose intensity will vary between activities. On one hand, there may be a trade-off between intensity and duration of exercise which could reduce the difference exercise hours exerts on lipolysis, while on the other, variation in physiological cost, levels of fitness and perceived exertion between individuals may influence exercise duration.

Excess adiposity would appear to be the next strongest influence on fat patterning, as suggested by the explained variance of the regression analysis. Higher levels of excess adiposity are associated with a centralisation of the fat and adjustment of the skinfold ratios. The TE ratio appears to be the most sensitive, perhaps not surprisingly as it profiles six locations on the body rather than two, which can accommodate individual differences. The ST and AMC ratios could both conceivably influence the TE ratio due to co-linearity, but the stepwise regression selected both as separate predictors in males and the ST ratio in females. While some of the subjects in this study were overweight, none were clinically obese. Raising a skinfold on obese subjects may present more difficulties for the anthropometrist, as this may require two hands, may fail to have parallel sides, or may exceed the jaw aperture of the calipers.

Age had a weak but significant effect in both males and females in this sample, with increasing age associated with greater centralisation of excess fat on the torso. While this is in agreement with other studies (Malina, 1996), this sample was predominantly active, and because exercise would appear to oppose the centralising effect of age, a greater age effect would probably prevail in a less active or sedentary sample.

The data show self-reported exercise to have an effect on TE ratio in males, but not females. This may be due to the difficulty in relating self-reported exercise to a true physiological cost, or the fact that the effect size is weaker in females, and this study had too few females to detect such an effect. However, magnetic resonance imaging studies of female adolescents showed that level of physical activity had an influence on fat patterning, and that skinfolds correlated highly with adipose tissue from MRI (Eliakim *et al.*, 1997). A recent study of a group of 557 men and women aged 16–65 exposed to 20 weeks intervention of endurance training further emphasised the altered fat pattern asssociated with exercise (Wilmore *et al.*, 1999). There appeared differences in training response by race and gender, but not age, providing further evidence that activity opposes the centralising effect on fat patterning.

These findings suggest that fat patterning does alter according to gender, adiposity, age and self-reported exercise, and that different skinfold ratios are required to explain these effects. The TE appears to be the most discriminating of the ratios, although the traditional ST and the new AMC ratios are also of utility for describing variation in fat topography in this sample. As the Western world faces increasing health threats from obesity and physical inactivity, the use of skinfold ratios as markers of trends over time, or for comparison between groups is set to increase in future studies in this field.

## REFERENCES

Eliakim, A., Burke, G.S. and Coper, D.M., 1997, Fitness, fatness and the effect of training assessed by magnetic resonance imaging and skinfold thickness measurements in healthy adolescent females. *American Journal of Clinical Nutrition*, **66**, 223-231.

Eston, R., Evans, R. and Fu, F., 1994, Estimation of body composition in Chinese adults. *British Journal of Sports Medicine*, **28**, 9-13.

Hawes, M.R. and Martin, A.D., 2001, Human body composition. In *Kinanthropometry and Exercise Physiology Manual: Tests, Procedures and Data. 2nd ed., Vol 1: Anthropometry*, edited by Eston, R.G. and Reilly, T. (London: Routledge), pp. 7-46.

Hawes, M.R. and Soucie, A., 1993, *Anthropometric Definer* software, Athletic Computer Systems, Calgary, Canada.

Malina, R.M., 1996, Regional body composition: Age, sex and ethnic variation. In *Human Body Composition*, edited by Roche, A.F., Heymsfield, S.B. and Lohman, T.G. (Champaign, IL: Human Kinetics), pp. 217–255.

Malina, R.M. and Bouchard, C., 1988, Subcutaneous fat distribution during growth. In *Fat Distribution During Growth and Later Health Outcomes*, edited by Bouchard, C. and Johnston, F.E. (New York: Plenum), pp. 63-84.

Marfell-Jones, M., 2001, The value of the skinfold – background, assumptions, cautions and recommendations on taking and interpreting skinfold measurements. *Proceedings of the Seoul International Sports Science Congress*, 313-323.

Nindl, B.C., Friedl, K.E., Marchitelli, L.J., Shippee, R.L., Thomas, C.D. and Patton, J.F., 1996, Regional fat placement in physically fit males and changes with weight loss. *Medicine and Science in Sports and Exercise*, **28**, 786-793.

Stewart, A.D., 2001, Assessing body composition in athletes. *Nutrition*, **17**, 694-695.

Stewart, A.D., 2002, Fat patterning – Indicators and implications. *Nutrition* – in press.

Stewart, A.D. and Hannan, J., 2000a, Sub-regional tissue morphometry in male athletes and controlls using DXA. *International Journal of Sport Nutrition and Exercise Metabolism,* **10**, 157–169.

Stewart, A.D. and Hannan, W.J., 2000b, Body composition prediction in male athletes using dual X-ray absorptiometry as the reference method. *Journal of Sports Sciences*, **18**, 263-274.

Valdez, R., 1991, A simple model-based index of abdominal adiposity. *Journal of Clinical Epidemiology*, **44**, 955-956.

Wilmore, J.H., Despres, J.P., Stanforth, P.R., Mandel, S., Rice, T., Gagnon, J., Leon, A.S., Rao, D.C., Skinner, J.S. and Bouchard, C., 1999, Alterations in body weight and composition consequent to 20 wk of endurance training: the HERITAGE family study. *American Journal of Clinical Nutrition*, **70**, 346-352.

# 19    Mass Fractionation in Male and Female Athletes

Arthur D. Stewart

Department of Biomedical Sciences, University of Aberdeen,
King's College, Aberdeen, AB24 3FX, UK

## 1. INTRODUCTION

While an interest in human structure and composition can be traced back to the ancient Greeks, a fractional approach to mass fractionation into different components was pioneered by Jindrich Matiegka, based on anatomical dissection (Matiegka, 1921) and is still used today. In this landmark study, total mass was subdivided into bone, muscle, subcutaneous adipose tissue + skin and residual mass comprising the organs and viscera. Extensive anthropometry was performed on a limited number of subjects, using cadaver dissection as the reference method. Equations were constructed to enable bone mass to be predicted from skeletal breadths, muscle mass from corrected girths, and subcutaneous adipose tissue (plus skin) mass from skinfolds. Residual mass was obtained by subtracting these components from total mass. This methodology was applied to the Brussels cadaver study of the 1980s, and Matiegka's original equations tested and others derived for 18 cadavers (Drinkwater et al., 1986). These studies are among a very few to relate anthropometry to dissection anatomy, which is the absolute against which other body composition methods are judged.

An alternative approach to mass fractionation uses a theoretical unisex phantom (Drinkwater and Ross, 1980), with the results scaled to the subject's size. A z-score is calculated for each constituent of total mass by averaging the z scores of the anthropometric measurements within each subset.

$$M_{adj} = z(mean).s + p$$

Where $M_{adj}$ is the fractional mass at phantom size, $s$ is the phantom standard deviation for the mass, and $p$ is the phantom mean mass. The mass of the constituent components can then be calculated independently as

$$Mass\ (kg) = M_{adj}\ [h.170.18.^{-1}]^3$$

Since the late 1980s, dual X-ray absorptiometry (DXA) has been capable of measuring total and regional bone mineral, fat and fat-free soft tissue masses by differential absorption of low energy X-rays. It is a technique which has been validated on the carcasses of pigs subjected to chemical analysis (Mitchell et al., 1996), and has proved more accurate than densitometry for predicting fat content in athletes (Prior et al., 1997). Scan output provides total and regional tissue masses for bone mineral, fat and fat-free soft tissue components. The attractiveness of the technology has prompted some investigators to attempt to derive a muscle mass from the fat-free soft tissue mass by assumptions which relate to the distribution of each in different regions of the body (Hansen *et al.*, 1999). The cadaver evidence upon which this assumption is based (cited in Snyder *et al.*, 1975) suggests that 75% of skeletal muscle mass is situated on the limbs.

This study compared anthropometric mass fractionation with the DXA model, and further investigated the stability of muscle mass predictions relative to the validated cadaver model in a group of male and female athletes.

## 2. METHODS

One hundred and five male and 30 female subjects participated in the study. Each was a University, National or International level athlete, had competed for a minimum of three years at his/her selected sports, and trained for a minimum of three hours per week, averaged over the calendar year. Physical characteristics of the subject are summarised in Table 1.

Each presented fasted and underwent a whole body scan (Hologic QDR 1000W, Bedford, MA, software version 5.5) and 41 anthropometric measurements (Hawes and Soucie, 1993) including total, sitting, supraspinale and suprasternale heights, eight bone breadths, nine girths and 19 skinfolds by the same experienced anthropometrist. Measurements followed procedures endorsed by the International Society for the Advancement of Kinanthropometry (ISAK). Male athletes were part of a previous study of body composition (Stewart and Hannan, 2000a and b), which quantified the intra-tester technical error of measurement for each skinfold site which averaged 3.8% (range 2.1–6.5%). Female athletes were measured with another female present.

Data were analysed using SPSS version 8. Local ethical permission was obtained for the measurements, and level of statistical significance was set at $p < 0.05$.

## 3. RESULTS

Male athletes tended to be older than their female counterparts (28.4 v 25.6 years, $p = 0.06$), but there was no difference in the hours of training (9.1 for both groups, $p < 0.0001$).

With male and female subjects pooled, there was high correlation between the scale mass and the fractionated mass and DXA scan mass ($r = 0.969$ and $r = 0.998$ respectively; $p < 0.0001$), as summarised in Figure 1. However, scale mass was underestimated by a mean of 2.0 kg and 0.8 kg by fractionated mass and DXA scan mass respectively ($p < 0.001$).

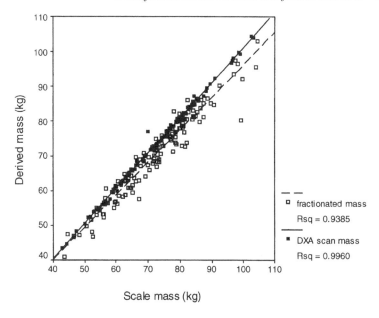

**Figure 1.** Comparison of scale mass with fractionated and DXA scan mass (male and female subjects pooled).

Those individuals whose fractionated mass departed markedly from scale mass tended to be more strength trained. The disparity between scale and fractionated mass was positively correlated with endomorphy and mesomorphy, and negatively correlated with ectomorphy (p<0.01). Indices of conicity of the limbs, defined as corrected upper arm to forearm, and corrected thigh to corrected calf girth and also corrected chest girth divided by stature were significantly correlated with the disparity (p < 0.01). Scale, Fractionated and DXA mass results are summarised separately for males and females in Table 1.

**Table 1.** DXA and anthropometric mass fractions for male and female athletes.

|  | Males | SD | Females | SD |
|---|---|---|---|---|
| Scale mass | 77.4 | 9.7 | 56.6 | 7.3 |
| Fat mass | 7.9 | 2.1 | 7.6 | 2.4 |
| Muscle mass | 34.8 | 4.8 | 23.6 | 3.0 |
| Bone mass | 12.9 | 1.8 | 9.0 | 1.4 |
| Residual mass | 19.9 | 2.4 | 14.6 | 1.4 |
| Fractionated total mass | 75.4 | 9.2 | 54.8 | 6.2 |
| DXA fat mass | 8.4 | 4.3 | 9.7 | 4.4 |
| DXA fat-free soft tissue | 64.9 | 7.9 | 44.3 | 5.1 |
| DXA bone mineral | 3.2 | 0.5 | 2.2 | 7.3 |
| DXA scan mass | 76.5 | 9.6 | 56.3 | 7.4 |

All mass measurements in kg; mean ± 1SD

There were significant differences in all tissue masses between male and female athletes (p < 0.001) except for absolute fat mass both by fractionated mass and DXA (p > 0.05). Fractionated fat mass became significant when adjusted to the phantom dimensions (p < 0.05).

Muscle mass estimates were compared using mass fractionation, validated cadaver and DXA models. The DXA approach uses limb fat-free soft tissue mass is multiplied by 4/3 (Hansen *et al.*, 1999). Results for male and female athletes are illustrated in Figure 2.

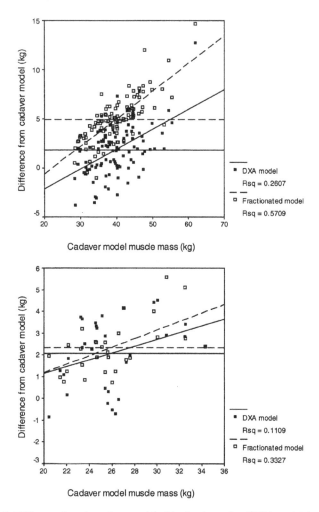

**Figure 2**. Difference from the cadaver model of the fractionated and DXA models in male (upper) and female (lower) athletes.

In males, the cadaver muscle mass was underestimated by 4.9 kg and 1.8 kg by the fractionated and DXA models respectively (p < 0.001). In females, the equivalent values were 2.3 kg and 2.1 kg respectively (p < 0.001).

With male and female data pooled, regression analysis of the total of limb fat free soft tissue against the cadaver muscle mass produced the following equation:

$$Muscle\ mass\ (kg) = 1.348.(DXA\ limb\ FFST) + 1.518$$

$$R^2 = 0.92;\ SEE = 2.35;\ p < 0.001$$

Where FFST is fat-free soft tissue mass

The equivalent equation for males was as follows:

$$Muscle\ mass\ (kg) = 1.412.(DXA\ limb\ FFST) - 0.404$$

$$R^2 = 0.84;\ SEE = 2.50;\ p < 0.001$$

The equivalent equation for females was as follows:

$$Muscle\ mass\ (kg) = 1.241.(DXA\ limb\ FFST) + 3.727$$

$$R^2 = 0.79;\ SEE = 1.64;\ p < 0.001$$

## 4. DISCUSSION

Perhaps it is not surprising that two methods for predicting total mass independently of gravity show disparity with scale mass. The stability of the fractionated model is slightly poorer than the DXA model, perhaps because the density of body tissues is altered in response to the conditioning programmes athletes follow. The increase in bone density which is a common result of chronic exercise is accommodated by DXA measurements, which are primarily concerned with detection of osteoporosis, rather than body composition.

The close proximity of the coefficient for DXA limb fat-free soft tissue to 4/3 for pooled data could lead investigators to believe that the assumed muscle distribution is valid. However, separate treatment of males and females suggests that disparities occur in a gender specific, and most probably a sport specific way. While postural muscles of the upper and lower leg may be common to all activities, strength training triggers adaptations including hypertrophy and force velocity characteristics according to movement and activity type according to the principle of specificity (American College of Sports Medicine, 2002). Thus the relative contribution of arm fat-free soft tissue to the total for arms + legs would differ between sports which emphasise the upper body and lower body, respectively.

In addition to regional muscle development, it is likely that variability in symmetry and proportionality may also account for these differences. The calculation of fractionated muscle mass is affected by equal weighting to the $z$-scores derived from forearm and corrected upper arm, chest, thigh and calf girths. A weighting of the calculated average $z$-score in proportion to the magnitude of the measurements would eliminate much of the difference seen in the disparity between the fractionated and validated cadaver methods. A disparity of 12.05 kg was observed in one Olympic weightlifter, whose excessive chest, thigh and upper arm measurements were compensated for by relatively small calf and forearm measurements.

While cadaver dissection is the criterion against which other body composition methods are judged, the absence of cadaver-validated data on athletes is a strategic weakness in research in this field. The assumed distribution of skeletal muscle between limbs and torso may not apply to athletes, whose specific exercise patterns govern muscle morphology in a site-specific way. DXA is an appealing technology which overcomes some of these limitations and it is increasingly seen as a reference method in itself. However, for muscle, further work with other techniques such as magnetic resonance imaging may enable future muscle mass models to be constructed with greater validity.

## REFERENCES

American College of Sports Medicine (ACSM) 2002, Position stand on progression models in resistance training for healthy adults. *Medicine and Science in Sports and Exercise*, **34**, 364–380.

Drinkwater, D. and Ross, W.D., 1980, Anthropometric fractionation of body mass. In *Kinanthropometry II*, edited by Ostyn, W., Beunen, G. and Simons, J. (Baltimore: University Park Press), pp. 177–188.

Drinkwater, D.T., Martin, A.D., Ross, W.D. and Clarys, J.P., 1986, Validation by cadaver dissection of Matiegka's equations for the anthropometric estimation of anatomical body composition in adult humans. In *The 1984 Olympic Scientific Congress Proceedings: Perspectives in Kinanthropometry* edited by Day, J.A.P., (Champaign, IL: Human Kinetics), pp. 221–227.

Hansen, R.D., Raja, C., Aslani, A., Smith, R.C. and Allen, B.J., 1999, Determination of skeletal muscle and fat-free mass by nuclear and dual energy x-ray methods in men and women aged 51 to 84. *American Journal of Clinical Nutrition*, **70**, 228–233.

Hawes, M.R. and Soucie, A., 1993, *Anthropometric Definer* software, Athletic Computer Systems, Calgary, Canada.

Matiegka, J., 1921, The testing of physical efficiency. *American Journal of Physical Anthropology*, **4**, 223–230.

Mitchell, A.D., Conway, J.M. and Potts, W.J.E. (1996). Body composition analysis of pigs by dual-energy X-ray absorptiometry. *Journal of Animal Science*, **74**, 2663–2671.

Prior, B.M., Cureton, K.J., Modelsky, C.M., Evans, E.M., Slonogeer, M.A., Saunders, M. and Lewis, R.D., 1997, In vivo validation of whole body composition estimates from dual-energy X-ray absorptiometry. *Journal of Applied Physiology*, **83**, 623–630.

Snyder, W.S., Cook, M.J., Nasset, E.S., Karhausen, L.R. Parry Howells, G. and Tipton, I.H. 1975, *International Commission on Radiological Protection Report of the task group on Reference Man*, (Oxford: Pergamon Press).

Stewart, A.D. and Hannan, W.J., 2000a, Body composition prediction in male athletes using dual X-ray absorptiometry as the reference method. *Journal of Sports Sciences*, **18**, 263–274.

Stewart, A.D. and Hannan, J., 2000b, Sub-regional tissue morphometry in male athletes and controls using DXA. *International Journal of Sport Nutrition and Exercise Metabolism*, **10**, 157–169.

# 20 Relation Between Body Mass, Body Composition and Muscular Strength, and Bone Mass and Bone Density in Premenarcheal Girls

Leen Van Langendonck, Albrecht L. Claessens and Gaston Beunen
Department of Sport and Movement Sciences
Faculty of Physical Education and Physiotherapy
K.U. Lcuven, Tervuursevest 101, B-3001 Leuven, Belgium

## 1. INTRODUCTION

Osteoporosis is an increasing health-care concern especially in the industrialised countries as populations age. Enhancement of bone mineral acquisition during growth may be useful in the prevention of osteoporosis. Because bone mass is an important determinant of bone strength and fracture risk (Hui *et al.*, 1989; Cummings *et al.*, 1990), identifying factors that influence bone mineral has important implications in the design of appropriate strategies to prevent or slow down the rate of bone loss and thereby potentially reduce the risk for fracture.

Body mass has been found to be an important determinant of bone mass (Vico *et al.*, 1992; Kröger *et al.*, 1994). Nevertheless, there is still discussion about the relative importance of lean mass and fat mass. Moreover, the question can be asked whether lean mass or rather muscle strength is important for bone health. Only a few studies addressed the question of the importance of lean and fat mass and strength as determinants of bone mass in prepubertal children. In most of these studies a clear relationship between lean mass/muscle area and bone mass was demonstrated (Young *et al.*, 1995; Schoenau *et al.*, 2000; Heinonen *et al.*, 2001).

In the present study the relation between on the one hand bone mass and bone mineral density and on the other hand body composition and strength was investigated in prepubertal girls.

## 2. METHODS

### 2.1 Subjects

Twenty one prepubertal girls of 8.7 (SD 0.7) years of age were included in this study. Information about the menstrual status was assessed by questionnaire and breast stage was monitored during the anthropometric measurements. None of the subjects had a known disease that might affect bone metabolism.

## 2.2 Bone mineral density (BMD)

Bone mineral density was assessed by dual-energy X-ray absorptiometry (DXA: Hologic QDR-4500A). A total body scan (TB) and a scan of the lumbar spine (LS=L1-L4) were taken. All scans were taken by the same experienced radiographer. The in vivo precision of DXA in the University Hospital is approximately 1% for BMD of the lumbar spine and less than 1% for total body BMD.

## 2.3 Skeletal maturity

Radiographs in a standardised position of the right hand of the premenarcheal girls were taken at an exposure of 1.0 s at 30 mA and 70 kV to assess skeletal maturity (TW2 age) using the Tanner-Whitehouse technique as described by Tanner *et al.* (1983).

## 2.4 Anthropometry and body composition

A set of 28 anthropometric dimensions was measured; body mass, 7 length, 6 width, 8 girth measurements and 6 skinfolds. The measurements were made by experienced trainees following the instructions described by Renson *et al.* (1986) and Claessens *et al.* (2000).

The sum of the 6 skinfolds (biceps SF + triceps SF + subscapular SF + suprailiac SF + thigh SF + calf medial SF) and several muscle indices [AMAG $(cm^2)$ = (upper arm girth relaxed – $\pi$ triceps $SF)^2/4\ \pi$ (Gurney and Jelliffe, 1973); CMAG $(cm^2)$ = (calf girth – $\pi$ calf medial $SF)^2/4\ \pi$ (Gurney and Jelliffe; 1973)] were calculated.

Lean mass, fat mass and percent fat of the total body were taken from the DXA scan of the total body. The coefficients of variation (CV) are respectively 0.6%, 1.5% and 1.3%.

## 2.5 Muscle strength

Peak torque of the flexors and extensors of the knee, the trunk and the elbow was measured using the Cybex isokinetic dynamometers (NORM, TEF, 350). Prior to testing the subjects were familiarised with the test procedure. The subjects performed 2 sets of 3 repetitions on 60°/s (1.05 rad.s$^{-1}$) and 1 set of 5 repetitions on 120°/s (2.09 rad.s$^{-1}$). Prior to each test set the subjects performed a practice trial.

Knee flexion-extension was performed from 100° flexion to full extension. Trunk flexion-extension was performed in the upright position over a range of motion of 60°, from 0° extension till 60° flexion. Elbow flexion-extension was performed lying with the right arm slightly abducted. Range of motion was 100°, from full extension to 100° flexion.

Also several field tests were used to assess muscular strength. Hand grip, arm pull, standing broad jump, leg lifts, bent arm hang and sit ups were measured following the instructions described by Claessens *et al.* (1990).

## 2.6 Statistical analysis

Descriptive statistics were calculated for chronological and skeletal age, the strength measurements, body composition and bone mineral.

The relation between bone mineral on the one hand, and body mass, body composition and strength on the other hand was analyzed using Pearson correlation coefficients for normal distributed variables and using Spearman correlation coefficients for variables not normally distributed.

Stepwise multiple regression analysis was used to determine independent predictors of bone mineral. Significance level for entrance was set at $\alpha=0.05$.

All statistical analyses were executed using the SAS package (SAS institute Inc).

## 3. RESULTS

The descriptive statistics of BMC and BMD, body composition and strength are presented in Table 1.

The correlation analysis showed that BMC LS and BMC TB were correlated significantly with most of the body composition measurements (r between 0.38 and 0.93) and with several strength measurements (r between -0.24 and 0.79) (Table 2). There was a significant correlation between BMD LS and some body composition measurements (body mass 0.44, sum skinfolds 0.43, fat mass 0.44 and arm muscle area 0.44) but not with the strength measurements. The BMD TB correlated significantly with body mass, fat and with only two strength indices (trunk extension 1.05 rad.s-1 and standing broad jump).

**Table 1**. Descriptive statistics of BMC and BMD, body composition and strength characteristics (n=21).

|  | Mean | SD |
|---|---|---|
| Age (year) | 8.7 | 0.7 |
| Skeletal age (year) | 9.5 | 1.0 |
| Body mass (kg) | 28.8 | 4.5 |
| Height (m) | 1.32 | 0.06 |
| Lean mass (kg) | 20.8 | 2.5 |
| Fat mass (kg) | 7.6 | 2.4 |
| % Fat | 25.4 | 4.8 |
| Sum skinfolds (mm) | 63.3 | 19.3 |
| Arm muscle area (cm$^2$) | 19.5 | 3.3 |
| Calf muscle area (cm$^2$) | 41.1 | 6.2 |
| Knee flexion peak torque 1.05 rad.s$^{-1}$ (Nm) | 29.1 | 9.9 |
| Knee flexion peak torque 2.09 rad.s$^{-1}$ (Nm) | 24.4 | 8.8 |
| Knee extension peak torque 1.05 rad.s$^{-1}$ (Nm) | 49.9 | 12.9 |
| Knee extension peak torque 2.09 rad.s$^{-1}$ (Nm) | 39.7 | 11.3 |
| Trunk flexion peak torque 1.05 rad.s$^{-1}$ (Nm) | 31.4 | 10.1 |
| Trunk flexion peak torque 2.09 rad.s$^{-1}$ (Nm) | 22.9 | 8.0 |
| Trunk extension peak torque 1.05 rad.s$^{-1}$ (Nm) | 69.5 | 23.4 |
| Trunk extension peak torque 2.09 rad.s$^{-1}$ (Nm) | 52.0 | 14.2 |
| Elbow flexion peak torque 1.05 rad.s$^{-1}$ (Nm) | 11.2 | 4.5 |
| Elbow flexion peak torque 2.09 rad.s$^{-1}$ (Nm) | 9.9 | 3.9 |
| Elbow extension peak torque 1.05 rad.s$^{-1}$ (Nm) | 15.4 | 5.6 |
| Elbow extension peak torque 2.09 rad.s$^{-1}$ (Nm) | 13.5 | 4.5 |
| Hand grip (kg) | 13.3 | 3.6 |
| Arm pull (kg) | 20.1 | 3.0 |
| Standing broad jump (cm) | 123.3 | 18.9 |
| Leg lifts (n/20 s) | 14.6 | 3.1 |
| Bent arm hang (s) | 7.3 | 7.3 |
| Sit ups (n/20 s) | 12.1 | 2.8 |
| BMC Lumbar spine (g) | 21.6 | 2.5 |
| BMD Lumbar spine (g/cm$^2$) | 0.58 | 0.07 |
| BMC Total body (g) | 918.9 | 137.9 |
| BMD Total body (g/cm$^2$) | 0.85 | 0.03 |

**Table 2**. Correlation coefficients between BMD-BMC and body composition and strength (n=21).

| | | BMC | | BMD | |
|---|---|---|---|---|---|
| | | LS | TB | LS | TB |
| Body composition | Height | 0.71** | 0.69** | 0.24 | 0.17 |
| | Weight | 0.82** | 0.93** | 0.44* | 0.48* |
| | Sum sfinfolds | 0.57** | 0.63** | 0.43* | 0.48* |
| | % fat | 0.60** | 0.66** | 0.37 | 0.45* |
| | Fat mass | 0.76** | 0.84** | 0.44* | 0.48* |
| | Lean mass | 0.77** | 0.88** | 0.38 | 0.41 |
| | Arm muscle area | 0.67** | 0.77** | 0.44* | 0.36 |
| | Calf muscle area | 0.38 | 0.61** | 0.02 | 0.25 |
| Strength measurement | | | | | |
| Cybex | Knee flex 1.05 rad.s$^{-1}$ | 0.28 | 0.55** | 0.04 | 0.27 |
| | Knee ext 1.05 rad.s$^{-1}$ | 0.32 | 0.60** | -0.01 | 0.21 |
| | Knee flex 2.09 rad.s$^{-1}$ | 0.49* | 0.69** | 0.10 | 0.38 |
| | Knee ext 2.09 rad.s$^{-1}$ | 0.58** | 0.76** | 0.16 | 0.31 |
| | Trunk flex 1.05 rad.s$^{-1}$ | 0.75** | 0.77** | 0.35 | 0.19 |
| | Trunk ext 1.05 rad.s$^{-1}$ | 0.57** | 0.79** | 0.23 | 0.44* |
| | Trunk flex 2.09 rad.s$^{-1}$ | 0.37 | 0.49* | 0.31 | 0.17 |
| | Trunk ext 2.09 rad.s$^{-1}$ | 0.06 | 0.42 | -0.08 | 0.24 |
| | Elbow flex 1.05 rad.s$^{-1}$ | 0.31 | 0.42 | 0.04 | 0.04 |
| | Elbow ext 1.05 rad.s$^{-1}$ | 0.40 | 0.46* | 0.07 | 0.14 |
| | Elbow flex 2.09 rad.s$^{-1}$ | 0.41 | 0.50* | 0.15 | 0.07 |
| | Elbow ext 2.09 rad.s$^{-1}$ | 0.47* | 0.56** | 0.14 | 0.16 |
| Field tests | Hand grip | 0.37 | 0.53** | 0.20 | 0.12 |
| | Arm pull | 0.41 | 0.59** | 0.32 | 0.31 |
| | Standing broad jump | 0.34 | 0.55** | 0.32 | 0.44* |
| | Leg lifts | -0.13 | -0.16 | 0.14 | 0.10 |
| | Bent arm hang | -0.24 | 0.10 | 0.12 | 0.16 |
| | Sit ups | 0.26 | 0.19 | 0.13 | 0.12 |

* p<0.05
** p<0.01

Explained variances of 0.94 (BMC LS), 0.91 (BMC TB), 0.20 (BMD LS) and 0.23 (BMD TB) were found. Standard errors of estimate were respectively 0.72, 42.79, 0.06 and 0.03. The best explaining variables were body mass or fat mass for BMD TB and BMD LS, and body mass for BMC TB and BMC LS.

## 4. DISCUSSION

In this study the relation between bone mineral and body composition (lean and fat mass) and strength was investigated. Except for calf muscle area, significant moderate to high correlation coefficients were observed between the body composition components and BMC (r varying from 0.38 to 0.93). Rather low to moderate correlation coefficients could be observed for BMD (r varying from 0.02 to 0.48). Lean mass and fat mass had comparable correlation coefficients with BMD lumbar spine and total body. It seems that in premenarcheal children mass is the important determinant regardless of whether it is fat mass or lean mass. Young *et al.* (1995) on the contrary found in premenarcheal twins that lean mass and not fat mass was an independent predictor of BMD. Witzke and Snow (1999) also found in adolescent girls higher correlation coefficients between BMD and lean mass (r=0.50 LS, 0.60 FN and 0.77 TB) than between BMD and fat mass (r=0.33 LS, 0.35 FN and 0.60 TB) and concluded also that lean mass or muscle power but not fat mass were independent predictors of BMD. Snow *et al.* (2000) concluded in a study on gymnasts, runners and controls that the relationship between bone and lean mass may be mediated by IGF-I. An explanation for the relation between lean mass and bone mass has been suggested by Seeman *et al.* (1996). They deemed that the association between lean mass and BMD is likely to be determined by genes regulating size. They found that genetic factors account for 60-80% of the individual variances of both BMD FN and lean mass, and more than 50% of their covariance. This is in contrast with the findings of Nguygen *et al.* (1998) who concluded that lean mass and BMD have little common genetic factors and that the association between lean mass and BMD appears to be mediated principally via common environmental influences.

In the present study also significant moderate correlation coefficients were found between several strength measurements and BMC. However, except for trunk extension at 2.09 rad.s$^{-1}$ and standing broad jump, no significant correlations were observed between the strength measurements and BMD.

Higher correlation coefficients were found between BMC and the body composition and strength measurements than between BMD and these characteristics. This finding suggests that in prepubertal girls the association between bone and body composition and strength is indeed size-related.

It can be concluded that in prepubertal girls body mass is strongly related to BMC and BMD of the lumbar spine and the total body. This relationship is due to both fat mass and lean mass. Muscle strength is not a strong determinant of BMD of the lumbar spine or the total body.

## REFERENCES

Claessens, A.L.M., Vanden Eynde, B., Renson, R. and Van Gerven, D., 1990, The description of tests and measurements. In *Growth and Fitness of Flemish Girls: the Leuven Growth Study*, edited by Simons, J., Beunen, G., Renson, R., Claessens, A.L.M., Vanreusel, B. and Lefevre, J. (Champaign: Human Kinetics), pp. 21-39.

Claessens, A.L., Beunen, G. and Malina, R.M., 2000, Anthropometry, physique, body composition and maturity. In: *Paediatric Exercise Science and Medicine*, edited by Armstrong, N. and Van Mechelen, W. (Oxford: Oxford University Press), pp. 11-22.

Cummings, S.R., Black, D.M., Nevitt, M.C., Browner, W.S., Cauley, J.A., Genant, H.K., Mascioli, S.R., Scott, J.C., Seeley, D.G., Steiger, P. and Vogt, T.M., 1990, Appendicular bone density and age predict hip fracture in women. *Journal of the American Medical Association*, **263**, 665-668.

Gurney, J.M. and Jelliffe, D.B., 1973, Arm anthropometry in nutritional assessment: nomogram for rapid calculation of muscle circumference and cross-sectional muscle and fat areas. *American Journal of Clinical Nutrition*, **26**, 912-915.

Heinonen, A., McKay, H.A., Whittall, K.P., Forster, B.B. and Khan, K.M., 2001, Muscle cross-sectional area is associated with specific site of bone in prepubertal girls: a quantitative magnetic resonance imaging study. *Bone*, **29**, 388-392.

Hui, S.L., Slemenda, C.W. and Johnston, C.C., 1989, Baseline measurement of bone mass predicts fracture in white women. *Annals of Internal Medicine*, **111**, 355-361.

Kröger, H., Tuppurainen, M., Honkanen, R., Alhava, E. and Saarikoski, S., 1994, Bone mineral density and risk factors for osteoporosis: a population-based study of 1600 perimenopausal women. *Calcified Tissue International*, **55**, 1-7.

Nguyen, T.V., Howard, G.M., Kelly, P.J. and Eisman, J.A., 1998, Bone mass, lean mass, and fat mass: same genes or same environments? *American Journal of Epidemiology*, **147**, 3-16.

Renson, R., Beunen, G., Van Gerven, D., Simons, J. and Ostyn, M., 1986, Description of motor ability tests and anthropometric measurements. In *Somatic and Motor Development of Belgian Secondary Schoolboys: Norms and Standards*, edited by Ostyn, M., Simons, J., Beunen, G., Renson, R. and Van Gerven, D. (Leuven: Leuven University Press), pp. 24-44.

Schoenau, E., Neu, C.M., Mokov, E., Wassmer, G. and Manz, F., 2000, Influence of puberty on muscle area and cortical bone area of the forearm in boys and girls. *Journal of Clinical Endocrinology and Metabolism*, **85**, 1095-1098.

Seeman, E., Hopper, J.L., Young, N.R., Formica, C., Goss, P. and Tsalamandris, C., 1996, Do genetic factors explain associations between muscle strength, lean mass, and bone density? A twin study. *American Journal of Physiology*, **270**, E320-E327.

Snow, C.M., Rosen, C.J. and Robinson, T.L., 2000, Serum IGF-I is higher in gymnasts than runners and predicts bone and lean mass. *Medicine and Science in Sports and Exercise*, **32**, 1902-1907.

Tanner, J.M., Whitehouse, R.H., Cameron, N., Marshall, W.A., Healy, M.J.R. and Goldstein, H., 1983, *Assessment of Skeletal Maturity and Prediction of Adult Height (TW2 method)*, 2nd ed., (London: Academic Press), pp. 1-108.

Vico, L., Prallet, B., Chappard, D., Pallot-Prades, B., Pupier, R. and Alexandre, C., 1992, Contributions of chronological age, age at menarche and menopause and of anthropometric parameters to axial and peripheral bone densities. *Osteoporosis International*, **2**, 153-158.

Witzke, K.A. and Snow, C.M., 1999, Lean body mass and leg power best predict bone mineral density in adolescent girls. *Medicine and Science in Sports and Exercise*, **31**, 1558-1563.

Young, D., Hopper, J.L., Nowson, C.A., Green, R.M., Sherwin, A.J., Kaymakci, B., Smid, M., Guest, C.S., Larkins, R.G. and Wark, J.D., 1995, Determinants of bone mass in 10- to 26-year-old females: a twin study. *Journal of Bone and Mineral Research*, **10**, 558-567.

# 21 Menstrual Dysfunction in Elite Ice Hockey Players Preparing for the 2002 Winter Olympics

E. Egan[1], M. Giacomoni[2], T. Reilly[1], N.T. Cable[1] and G. Whyte[3]
[1]Research Institute for Sport and Exercise Sciences,
Liverpool John Moores University,
[2]Laboratoire Ergonomie Sportive et Performance,
Université de Toulon-Var, France,
[3]British Olympic Medical Centre, Middlesex, UK

## 1. INTRODUCTION

Research relating to reproductive health in women over the past twenty years has highlighted the implications of amenorrhoea, oligomenorrhoea and delayed menarche on psychological wellbeing, injury susceptibility, fertility and future health. Associations between reduced hormone levels and impaired muscle phosphocreatine recovery rates (Harber *et al.*, 1998) and lowered basal metabolic rates also suggest possible implications for sports performance. To date, exercise-induced menstrual dysfunction is largely unexplored in 'winter sports' athletes. Altered training seasons and colder training conditions in countries with altered light/dark cycles (i.e. shorter days) may have an effect on the complex endocrine system which controls the menstrual cycle.

Surveys of Olympic athletes at the summer games show between 7.5% and 59% menstrual disruption depending on definitions used (Zaharieva, 1965; Webb *et al.*, 1979). Irregularity and delayed menarche were most often reported in gymnasts, swimmers, rowers, runners and volleyball players (Zaharieva, 1965; Malina *et al.*, 1979; Webb *et al.*, 1979).

Higher incidences of hypothalamic amenorrhoea in athletic populations may be related to competitive stress, body composition, nutrient intake and energy imbalance and alterations of the complex endocrine control of the hypothalamic-pituitary-ovarian axis resulting from physiological responses to the exercise itself. Athletes involved in sports where low body weight/lean body mass is emphasised, appear more susceptible, but factors such as age, prior menstrual dysfunction, age at menarche, nulliparity, and lifestyle factors also play a role.

The aims of this study were to examine the incidence of menstrual dysfunction among elite female winter sports athletes and to assess some of the factors contributing to increased risk of menstrual dysfunction.

## 2.   METHODS

### 2.1  Subjects

Athletes who were preparing for the 2002 Winter Olympic Games were considered elite and thus eligible for participation in this study.  Players from the Swedish (n = 22), American (n = 17) and Canadian (n = 4) ice hockey teams volunteered to complete the questionnaire. Questionnaires were completed 5 months (Swedish and Canadian teams) and 1 month (American team) prior to the Games and prior to selection in the case of the former two.  Athletes' characteristics (mean ± SD) were 23.5 ± 2.0 years, 1.68 ± 0.14 m and 68.2 ± 5.7 kg.

### 2.2  Questionnaire

The questionnaire, approved by the Human Ethics Committee at Liverpool John Moores University, was piloted for ease of understanding and accuracy among a sample of active individuals within the university.  Questions on each of the following were included in the questionnaire:

Anthropometric data:  Athletes were asked to record their height (cm), mass (kg), date of birth and body fat (%) if known and the method by which it was obtained.  Body mass index (BMI, $kg.m^{-2}$) was calculated.

Training:  Athletes were asked to describe their typical training week, including information on intensity, frequency, duration and timing of training sessions, to outline their training year and to give details of their sports participation outside ice hockey.

Reproductive history and menstrual status:  Athletes were asked to report age at menarche (the first menstrual period), whether or not they were involved in vigorous training for a sport prior to this event, the type of sports and the level of competition.  The athletes were asked how many children they had and if they had ever been diagnosed with any gynaecological dysfunction.  Perimenstrual symptoms were assessed using Moos' (1985) Menstrual Distress Questionnaire. Questions on past and present oral contraceptive use were also included.  Athletes were asked to indicate if they considered their menstrual cycle to be regular, how often they experienced menstrual dysfunction and what type of menstrual dysfunction they experience(d) according to the following criteria:

- Frequently long cycles (35-45 days)
- Frequently short cycles (less than 21 days)
- Oligomenorrhoea (cycles of between 45-90 days)
- Amenorrhoea (3 or less menstruations per year)
- Intermenstrual bleeding (small blood loss between real periods)

Lifestyle: Lifestyle questions included frequency of smoking and alcohol use, frequency and type of medication and occurrence of sleep disturbances.  Athletes reported past and present vegetarianism, described their typical dietary patterns and indicated the degree to which they controlled their diet with respect to type of food and energy intake. An open-ended question assessing the role of body image and pressures to maintain a low body weight was also included.

## 2.3 Statistical analysis

Results are expressed as mean ± SE. Statistical analysis was carried out using SPSS version 10. Independent samples t-tests and one-way ANOVAs were used to analyse group differences of parametric data and Mann-Whitney and Kruskal-Wallis tests were applied to non-parametric data (age at menarche and mass). When significance was found, a Tukey post-hoc test was performed. A Spearman's non-parametric two-tailed correlation was applied to correlation data. Statistical significance was accepted at a confidence level of $p<0.05$.

## 3. RESULTS

### 3.1 Anthropometry

Athletes did not differ in age or height with nationality ($p>0.05$), but the Canadian athletes were heavier ($p<0.01$) and had a greater body mass index (BMI, $p<0.05$) than the Swedish and American athletes. Body fat data, as measured by skinfold thickness, were only available for the American athletes. Values ranged from 10.5% to 21% with a mean value of $15.2 \pm 0.7\%$.

**Table 1.** Anthropometric values (mean ± SE) for each nationality and for the group as a whole.

|  | Age (yrs) | Mass (kg) | Height (m) | BMI (kg.m$^{-2}$) | Body fat (%) |
|---|---|---|---|---|---|
| Americans | 25.3 (1.6) | 68.5 (1.7) | 1.67 (0.01) | 24.7 (0.6) | 15.2 (0.7) |
| Canadians | 22.2 (1.4) | 80.8 (3.5) | 1.74 (0.02) | 26.8 (1.4) | - |
| Swedish | 23.0 (1.3) | 65.6 (0.9) | 1.68 (0.01) | 23.4 (0.4) | - |
| Group | 23.5 (4.8) | 68.2 (1.2) | 1.68 (0.01) | 24.1 (0.4) | 15.2 (0.7) |

Current body mass index was negatively correlated with age at menarche ($r=-0.41$, $p<0.05$). The relationship was significant even when controlled for current age. The age at which the athlete started playing ice hockey was not related to any of their current anthropometric characteristics ($p>0.05$).

### 3.2 Training

Twenty two (51%) of the players had previously competed at an Olympic Games and an average of $15.1 \pm 0.8$ years experience at ice hockey identified an experienced sample. Nine of the athletes played other sports, seven in other team sports (football and softball) and two in individual pursuits (orienteering, golf, water-skiing). Half the athletes (n=22) participated in psychological training and/or relaxation sessions.   Training sessions per week ranged from 6 to 11 with a mean of 8.1 ± 1.8 sessions.  The competitive season lasted 6.5 ±1.0 months.

### 3.3 Age at menarche

All the athletes reported having reached menarche.  Age at menarche was reported to the nearest month by 13 (30%) of the athletes, in whole years by 26 of the athletes and was not reported by 4 of the athletes.  Age at menarche was 13.3 ± 0.2 years but values ranged from 9.5 to 15 years.  Median and modal values were 13.0 and 14.0 years respectively.  The distribution of age at menarche was negatively skewed, 47% of the sample not reaching menarche until after their 14th birthday.

Participation in vigorous prepubertal training appears to delay menarche by 0.5 years though this was not significant ($p = 0.24$) (Table 1).  Level of competition prior to menarche did not affect age at menarche ($p > 0.05$).

Table 2. Mean values for age at menarche (years).

|  | n | Mean | SE | Range |
|---|---|---|---|---|
| Prepubertal training |  |  |  |  |
| Vigorous training | 17 | 13.6 | 0.3 | 12–15 |
| No vigorous training | 22 | 13.1 | 0.3 | 9.5–15 |
| Competition level |  |  |  |  |
| None | 1 | 14 |  | 14 |
| Local | 10 | 12.7 | 0.5 | 9.5–15 |
| County/regional | 15 | 13.7 | 0.3 | 12–15 |
| National | 11 | 13.3 | 0.4 | 11–15 |
| International | 2 | 13 | 1.0 | 12–14 |
| Total | 39 | 13.3 | 0.2 | 9.5–15 |

The sports in which the athlete participated and competed prior to menarche were analysed to assess trends and to determine if participation in certain sports resulted in delayed menarche.  This analysis was difficult since the athletes competed in and trained for a number of individual and team sports.  Twenty-six (60.5%) of the athletes competed in more than one sport and only one athlete did not participate in any sport prior to menarche.  Thirty-nine (90%) of the athletes competed in at least one team sport and 13 (30%) competed in at least one individual sport.   Seventeen athletes trained vigorously for a sport prior to menarche, 9 did so for more than one sport. There was no difference in age at menarche with either number of sports (1, 2, 3 or more) in which the athlete participated or the type of sports participated in (individual only, team only, or both team and individual sports). Thirty-one of the athletes competed in ice hockey prior to menarche and 12 of these trained vigorously for the sport prior to menarche.  The negative correlation between the age at which participating in ice hockey began and age at menarche was not significant ($r=-0.395$, $p=0.332$).

Table 3. Types of sports participated in prior to menarche.

|  | Participated in | Trained vigorously for |
|---|---|---|
| ≥1 Individual sport | 13 (30%) | 3 (7%) |
| ≥1 Team sport | 39 (91%) | 15 (35%) |
| Ice Hockey | 31 (72%) | 12 (28%) |
| 1 Sport | 42 (98%) | 17 (40%) |
| >1 Sport | 26 (60%) | 6 (14%) |

In total the athletes competed in 17 different sports including endurance events (triathlon, orienteering), indoor games (table tennis), court games (tennis, basket ball), field games (hockey, football), batting games (baseball, softball), aesthetic sports (gymnastics) and other winter sports (snowboarding). These sports cover a variety of skills, physiques and physiological abilities though ice hockey and football were the most popular.   With one exception, an athlete who participated in tetrathlon, those who competed at a national or international level prior to menarche (n=14) did so only for ice hockey and/or football.

### 3.4 Pill use

Fifteen (34.9%) of the athletes were using oral contraceptives, varying in type and brand (see Table 4). A higher proportion of Canadians and Americans were using the pill compared with Swedish athletes (50%, 47.1% and 22.7% respectively).

Oral contraceptives were used for contraceptive reasons only in 7 of the athletes, while 8 used them for regulation of the cycle and control of menstrual symptoms.  A further 8 athletes (18.6%) had previously used oral contraceptives. Reasons for termination of use included contraceptive reasons (4), impaired sports performance (2) and impracticalities (1).

Table 4. Pill use among the athletes, number and percentage of athletes using each brand of pill.

|  | Type |  | No. | % |
|---|---|---|---|---|
| None |  |  | 28 | 65.1 |
| Pill users | Phasic | Trionette 28 | 3 | 6.9 |
|  |  | Ortho try-cyclen | 3 | 6.9 |
|  | Total |  | 6 | 14.0 |
|  | Combined | Restovar | 1 | 2.3 |
|  |  | Diane 35 | 1 | 2.3 |
|  |  | Alesse 21 | 1 | 2.3 |
|  |  | Levlen | 1 | 2.3 |
|  |  | Loestrin | 2 | 4.7 |
|  | Total |  | 6 | 14.0 |
|  | Not specified |  | 3 | 6.9 |
| **Total** |  |  | 15 | 34.9 |

### 3.5 Menstrual function

Five athletes considered themselves to have irregular cycles, one athlete had regular cycles which lasted less than 21 days and the remainder of the athletes reported usual regular cycle length of 21-35 days. This did not take into account pill use, past menstrual history and minor disruptions and irregularities.

One of the athletes suffered from an underlying gynaecological dysfunction (hirsutism and polycystic ovary syndrome) and experienced seven years amenorrhoea prior to taking the pill. Two more of the pill users previously had amenorrhoea and one had oligomenorrhoea. One athlete also had oligomenorrhoea prior to having a child.

Two (4.7%) athletes reported 'often' experiencing oligomenorrhoea. Minor menstrual disturbances such as cycles outside the 'normal' 21-35 day range and intermenstrual bleeding, were 'rarely' or 'sometimes' experienced by 24 of the athletes (57.1%). There was a particularly high incidence of intermenstrual bleeding among pill users (21.4%). Ten (23.8%) of the athletes reported never experiencing any form of menstrual dysfunction. This experience was higher in those who did not use the pill than those who did (28.5% compared with 21.4%).

In those not using oral contraceptives, no significant relationship was found between BMI, body mass, age, gynaecological age, number of years experience at their sport or age at menarche and the severity of menstrual dysfunction (p values >0.05). Trends can, however, be seen between the severity of menstrual dysfunction and age and gynaecological age (Figure 1).

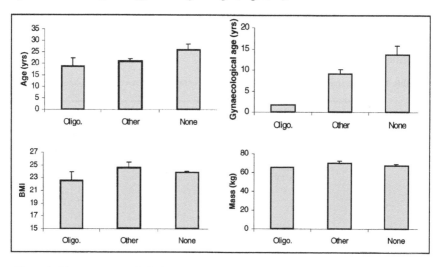

**Figure 1**. Mean age, gynaecological age, mass and BMI for athletes grouped according to severity of menstrual dysfunction. The groups are 1) oligomenorrhoeic (oligo.), 2) athletes with minor menstrual dysfunction such as frequently long or short cycles or intermenstrual bleeding (other) and 3) athletes who never experience any form of menstrual dysfunction (none).

The athletes were asked to consider a list of factors associated with menstrual dysfunction and to indicate which ones they associated with their own menstrual dysfunction. A breakdown of the results is given in Table 5. Factors relating to training were most often reported (increased training volume and increased training intensity), followed by pressure-related factors.  Fifty-two percent of the athletes who experienced menstrual dysfunction related their state to at least one training-related factor, 35% indicated some form of stress and 16% associated menstrual dysfunction with an eating/weight-related factor. Those who experienced severe menstrual dysfunction (amenorrhoea/oligomenorrhoea) either currently or in the past, all indicated a training factor and 80% related it to an eating-related factor also, with the exception of the individual whose menstrual dysfunction was explained by hirsutism and polycystic ovary syndrome.

**Table 5**. Factors associated by the athletes with menstrual dysfunction. No. represents the number of athletes indicating each response and % is calculated as percent of those who experience menstrual dysfunction (n=31)

| Factor | No. | % |
|---|---|---|
| Increased training volume | 14 | 45.1 |
| Increased training intensity | 12 | 38.7 |
| Increased pressure from competition | 6 | 19.4 |
| Increased pressure from work | 5 | 16.1 |
| Increased pressure from family friends | 3 | 9.7 |
| Changes in body composition | 3 | 9.7 |
| Increased competition frequency | 2 | 6.5 |
| Changes in dietary pattern | 2 | 6.5 |
| Caloric restriction | 2 | 6.5 |
| Long haul flights | 2 | 6.5 |
| Injury | 1 | 3.2 |
| Rapid weight loss | 1 | 3.2 |
| A particular time of year | 1 | 3.2 |
| Sleep deprivation | 1 | 3.2 |
| New female company | 1 | 3.2 |
| Underlying gynaecological dysfunction | 1 | 3.2 |

## 3.6 Perimenstrual symptoms

Athletes appear to experience increased perceptions of pain, water retention and negative affect during the menstrual and premenstrual phases of the menstrual cycle. Symptoms during the menstrual phases appeared worse in those who did not use hormonal contraceptives compared with those who did with the exception of water retention. This was significant only for pain ($p<0.05$) (Figure 2a). There did not appear to be any difference in any of the symptoms between pill users and non-users during the premenstrual phase (Figure 2b).

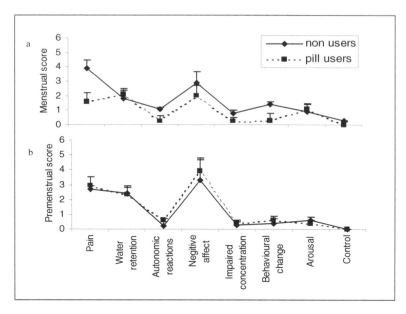

**Figure 2**. Reported subjective menstrual (a) and premenstrual (b) symptoms grouped according to hormonal contraceptive status. Results are presented as group means ± SE.  * denotes p<0.05.

Since side-effects and menstrual symptoms may differ depending on the type and dosage of pill used, menstrual and premenstrual symptoms were compared according to pill type (phasic or combined) and on whether the pill contained a low (20 mg) or medium (21-35 mg) oestrogen component.   The only significant difference was in negative affect symptoms (e.g. anxiety, mood swings, irritability and tension) during the menstrual phase with a higher mean score for those who used combined type compared with phasic type pill (p < 0.05, Figure 3). Combined pills also had increased negative symptoms during the premenstrual phase though these were not significant.

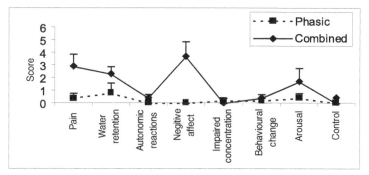

**Figure 3**. Reported subjective menstrual symptoms grouped according to type of contraceptive. Results are graphed as group means ± SE.  * denotes p<0.05.

**3.7 Diet**

The athletes' subjective view of how much they control their diet is given in Figure 4. A larger percentage of the athletes appeared to be moderately or less controlling for calorie intake than for type of food (68% compared with 32%). Conversely 68% reported 'often' or 'always' controlling their diet with respect to type of food.

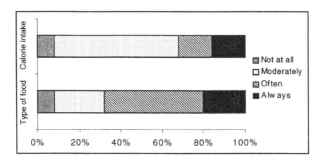

**Figure 4**. Percentages of athletes controlling their diet with respect to calorie intake and type of food.

Responses of the athletes to the question; 'In your opinion does body image play an important role in your sport? Is there pressure within your sport (from coaches, other people, spectators) to maintain a low body weight/lean body composition? Describe', are summarised in Table 6. Over 50% had no comment.

**Table 6**. Attitudes of the athletes on the role that body image plays in ice hockey.

| Comment | No. of Respondents |
| --- | --- |
| No comment | 23 |
| Played no part | 11 |
| Important | 2 |
| Under pressure to gain weight | 1 |
| Good body mass essential for ice hockey | 3 |
| Energy requirements important | 1 |
| Competition among athletes for leanest body physique | 1 |
| Physique not important because of full clothing | 1 |

## 4. DISCUSSION

In order to assess the vulnerability of ice hockey players to health-related complications associated with delayed menarche and menstrual dysfunction, it is necessary to assess the extent of such conditions within the sport and to examine factors such as nutrition, body composition, training and lifestyle factors which may predispose an athlete to such conditions.

Mean values for the onset of menarche are slightly higher than expected results for American (12.8 years) and Canadian (13.1 years) populations reported by Malina (1983). A large proportion did not reach menarche until 14 years. A two-part hypothesis with respect to delayed menarche in athletes has been proposed (Malina, 1983). The first part is that participation in sporting events and in vigorous training delays menarche by altering hormone secretion patterns, increasing stress levels and by reducing body fat. Participation in vigorous training appears to delay the onset of menarche (Frisch *et al.*, 1981; Casey *et al.*, 1984), though it was not significant here. Unfortunately no details on the volume/intensity of training or the age at which the athlete started vigorous training was available.

The second part of the theory is that athletes are more suited to sport because of leaner physiques and longer limb length associated with delayed menarche. Thus those who now compete at an elite level experienced delayed menarche. Extreme delay in menarche may mean that athletes are more suited to sports where a lean physique is desirable e.g. figure skating and gymnastics, while moderate delay of menstruation as seen in this sample is sufficient for sports where a higher body weight is desirable. Sharma *et al.* (1988) reported more height for weight and lower body fat in girls who reach menarche later. In this sample current body mass index was negatively correlated with age at menarche.

This group of athletes participated in a number of sports covering a wide range of skills, physiques and physiological characteristics, prior to menarche. Those who competed at national and international level did so only for team sports (ice hockey and football), suggesting that they were always more suited to this type of event rather than selecting it because relatively early attainment of menarche (compared with gymnasts, track and field athletes, speed skaters, figure skaters) made them more suitable to this type of exercise.

Body mass, body fat, weight loss and nutritional factors have previously been associated with menstrual dysfunction. A previous suggestion that a critical percent body fat is necessary to commence and maintain menstruation (Frisch *et al.*, 1973; Frisch and McArthur, 1974), has since been questioned (Trussell, 1980, Scott and Johnston, 1982). Unfortunately body fat values were only available for a small number of this group. Body mass index or body mass did not seem to affect menstrual function. Canadian players appear to be heavier and have a greater body mass index than players from either of the other two countries, suggesting possible genetic or physique differences which may affect menstrual dysfunction between nations. However, analysis of data available from internet sources (www.saltlake2002.com, www.canadianhockey.ca) for the entire teams competing at the Olympic Games shows no significant difference between the teams.

Factors appearing to affect menstrual function are age and gynaecological age (Vollman, 1977). The first few years of menstruation have been associated with irregular cycles in non-athletes and younger athletes have previously been found more susceptible to menstrual dysfunction (Gray and Dale, 1983). Athletes most often reported that increased training volume and intensity and increased psychological pressure caused their menstrual dysfunction.

Body image concerns do not appear pronounced in ice hockey, due in part to the fact that full clothing is worn by the athletes in competition. A high number of athletes controlled their diet for type of food. Controlling for calorie intake did not appear so pronounced. This may be due in part to nutritional education of the athletes as they attempt to maximise energy availability.

In summary, menarche was not severely delayed in these athletes. Menstrual dysfunction levels were not higher than expected and were reversed by pill use in those with severe dysfunction. It remains to be answered if pill use provides the same protection of health as normal regular menstruation. Age but not any physique parameter was associated with menstrual dysfunction. There is little alarm for body image concern or energy restriction among the sample, though it should always be remembered that one of the characteristics of disordered eating is often denial by the athletes themselves of such practices.

## Acknowledgements

The work is supported by a Pfizer grant in association with the International Olympic Committee's Medical Commission. The authors are very grateful to Murray Costello at the International Ice Hockey Federation and the Swedish, Canadian and American teams for their co-operation and participation.

## REFERENCES

Casey, J.C., Jones, E.C., Foster, C., Pollock, M.L. and DuBois, J.A., (1984), Effect of the onset and intensity of training on menarchal age and menstrual irregularity among elite speed skaters. In *Sport and Elite Performers – The 1984 Olympic Scientific Congress Proceedings*, Vol. 3, edited by Landers, D.M. (Champaign: Human Kinetics), pp. 33–44.

Frisch R.E. and McArthur, J.W., 1974, Menstrual cycles: Fatness as a determinant of minimum weight for height necessary for their maintenance or onset. *Science*, **185**, 949–951.

Frisch, R.E., Gotx-Welbergen, A.V., McArthur, J.W., Albright, T., Witchi, J., Bullen, B., Birnholz, J., Reed, R.B. and Hermann, H., 1981, Delayed menarche and amenorrhoea of college athletes in relation to age of onset of training. *Journal of the American Medical Association*, **246**, 1559–1563.

Frisch, R.E., Revelle, R. and Cook, S., 1973, Components of weight at menarche and the initiation of the adolescent growth spurt in girls: estimated total water, lean body weight and fat. *Human Biology*, **45**, 469–483.

Gray, D.P. and Dale, E., 1983, Variables associated with secondary amenorrhea in women runners. *Journal of Sports Sciences*, **1**, 55-67.

Harber, V.J., Petersen, S.R. and Chilibeck, P.D., 1998, Thyroid hormone concentrations and muscle metabolism in amenorrheic and eumenorrheic athletes. *Canadian Journal of Applied Physiology*, **3**, 293–306.

http://www.canadianhockey.ca, 15/04/2002.

http://www.saltlake2002.com, 21/02/2002.

Malina, R.M., 1983, Menarche in athletes: a synthesis and hypothesis. *Annals of Human Biology*, **10**, 1–24.

Malina, R.M., Bouchard, C., Shoup, R.F., Demirjian, A. and Lariviere, G., 1979, Age at menarche, family size, and birth order in athletes at the Montreal Olympic Games. *Medicine and Science in Sports and Exercise*, **11**, 354–358.

Moos, R.H., 1985, *Perimenstrual symptoms: A manual and overview of research with the menstrual distress questionnaire.* Social Ecology Laboratory, Department of Psychiatry & Behavioral Sciences, Stanford University School of Medicine and Vererans Administration Medical Centers, Palo Alto.

Scott, E.C. and Johnston, F.E., 1982, Critical fat, menarche and the maintenance of menstrual cycles; a critical review. *Journal of Adolescent Health Care*, **2**, 249–260.

Sharma, K., Talwar, I. and Sharma, N., 1988, Age at menarche in relation to adult body size and physique. *Annals of Human Biology*, **15**, 431–434.

Trussell, J., 1980, Stastical flaws in evidence for the Frisch hypothesis that fatness triggers menarche. *Human Biology*, **52**, 711–720.

Vollman, R., 1977, *The Menstrual Cycle*, (Philadelphia: W.B. Saunders).

Webb, J.L., Millan, D.L. and Stolz, C.J., 1979, Gynecological survey of American female athletes competing at the Montreal Olympic Games. *Journal of Sports Medicine and Physical Fitness*, **12**, 405–412.

Zaharieva, E., 1965, Survey of sports women at the Tokyo Olympics. *Journal of Sports Medicine and Physical Fitness*, **5**, 215–219.

# 22   Interaction Effects of Time of Day and Menstrual Cycle on Muscle Strength

E. Bambaeichi[1,2], N.T. Cable [1], T. Reilly [1] and M. Giacomoni [3]
[1]Research Institute for Sport and Exercise Sciences, Liverpool John Moores University, 15-21 Webster Street, Liverpool, L3 2ET, UK
[2] Physical Education Department, Isfahan University, Isfahan, Iran
[3] Laboratoire Ergonomie Sportive et Performance, UFR STAPS, Université de Toulon-Var, France

## 1. INTRODUCTION

Numerous studies have established that there is a circadian rhythm in muscle strength in males, measured in both isometric and dynamic conditions and in many muscle groups. Diurnal rhythms have also been apparent in neuromotor performance, and gross motor function when limited measurements per day have been conducted (Reilly, 1990). Isokinetic muscle strength consistently peaks in the early evening, regardless of the muscle groups tested or the speed of contraction (Atkinson and Reilly, 1996). The circadian rhythm in muscle strength has been shown to be in phase with that of core body temperature (Reilly *et al.*, 1997).

Variations in muscular performance during the menstrual cycle have been widely documented in the literature. Circamensal rhythms in isometric strength have been reported for quadriceps (Sarwar *et al.*, 1996; Greeves, 1997), handgrip (Sarwar *et al.*, 1996) and the adductor pollicis (Phillips *et al.*, 1996). Greeves *et al.* (1997) observed the highest isometric and dynamic strength of the quadriceps during the mid-luteal phase and reported a negative relationship between strength and the ratio of oestrogen to progesterone concentration.

Until more recently, rarely have investigators studied circadian rhythms in females. There are many unknowns relating to potential effects of circamensal variations on human circadian rhythms. Very few studies are available on the effect of the menstrual cycle on the circadian rhythm of core body temperature (Kattapong *et al.*, 1995; Cagnacci *et al.*, 1996). These studies have demonstrated a decrease in the amplitude of the circadian rhythm in body temperature during the luteal phase of the menstrual cycle. However, there is a lack of data regarding interaction of circadian and circamensal rhythms on muscle performance. Giacomoni and Garnett (2002) failed to show any interaction between time of day and menstrual cycle phase on different indices of maximal muscle performance. These authors used only two time points during the day (07:00 and 19:00 h), which make the result difficult to interpret in terms of circadian rhythm modification. Therefore the present aim was to investigate the combined effects of six times of day (i.e. number of equidistant points necessary in the modelling of circadian rhythms) and two phases of the menstrual cycle (follicular and luteal) on muscle strength in eumenorrhoeic young females.

## 2. MATERIALS AND METHODS

### 2.1 Subjects

Subjects were 8 healthy women with regular menstrual cycles (25-31 days). None had used any form of oral contraceptives for at least 4 months before entering the study. They were all free from any musculoskeletal injury of the lower limb for at least three years before recruitment. Informed consent was obtained from all subjects, and the Human Ethics Committee of Liverpool John Moores University approved the protocol. All subjects were asked to keep their activity level constant during the experimental period. The participants' characteristics were:- age 28 ± 4 years, height 1.61 ± 0.08 m and body mass 59.9 ± 5.6 kg.

### 2.2 Procedures

All subjects underwent two familiarisation sessions in order to minimize learning effects. Menstrual cycle history, chronotype (Smith *et al.*, 1989) and habitual physical activity were assessed from questionnaires completed during the first familiarisation session. At each session, on arrival at the laboratory, body mass (calibrated precision weighing scales; Hotline, Hamburg, Germany) and height (Seca, MeB-und Wiegetechnik, Vogel and Halke, Hamburg, Germany) were measured and a 5-ml venous blood sample was taken following a 5-min rest from the antecubital vein to confirm levels of oestrogen, progesterone and testosterone. Before each test, subjects completed questionnaires about menstrual distress (Moos, 1985), physical activity, musculoskeletal injury, sleep patterns and fatigue (Edwards *et al.*, 2002).

Before each test, rectal temperature was recorded during a 30-min period using a rectal probe inserted to a depth of 14 cm beyond the external anal sphincter, in the standard position (i.e. lying supine and awake). The data were recorded continuously through a Squirrel 1000 data logger (Grant Instruments LTD, Shepreth, UK) and the mean value of the last 5-min period was kept for analysis.

The experimental procedures were conducted twice in both the mid-follicular (days 7, 8, 9) and the mid-luteal (days 19, 20, 21) phases of the menstrual cycle. Basal body temperature (BBT) was used to determine the cycle phases which were later confirmed by hormonal assays. Subjects were asked to take their sub-lingual temperature (Omron MC-63B, Wegalaan, Europe B.V) for one month prior to the test, every morning on awaking before getting up, in order to get an idea of occurrence of ovulation (0.3 °C rise in temperature). Subjects confirmed occurrence of ovulation using a home ovulation test (Clearplan, Unipath Ltd., Bedford, UK). Subjects were asked to eat a light meal at least 3 hours prior to attending the laboratory tests. They were also asked to refrain from consuming drinks containing caffeine.

*Muscle strength measurement*

Maximal isometric and isokinetic strength of quadriceps and hamstrings muscle groups for the dominant leg were measured at 02:00, 06:00, 10:00, 14:00, 18:00 and 22:00 hours in the two phases of the menstrual cycle, in a random order to counterbalance any learning/fatigue effects. At least 12 hours separated each session to allow for recovery.

A standardised 5-min warm up was performed on a Monark cycle ergometer before muscle strength was assessed. The workload (80 < power < 120 W) was established for each subject in proportion to the body mass and the physical fitness level.

All the strength measurements were performed using the Lido Active isokinetic dynamometer (Loredan, Davis, CA). Subjects were asked to perform at maximal effort, and visual feedback and consistent encouragement were provided to ensure maximal effort.

The appropriate dynamometer position was set during the familiarisation and kept for all the test sessions. The lateral femoral condyle was aligned with the axis of rotation of the dynamometer. Subjects were secured to the back-seat by seat belts. The dominant leg was stabilised with a strap above the knee.

Maximal voluntary dynamic movements of knee extensors and flexors were made at angular velocities of 1.05 and 3.14 $rad.s^{-1}$ (90° range of motion). For each contraction mode, 3 submaximal efforts were performed with a 3-min passive recovery before 3 maximal efforts performed as hard as possible. Each maximal effort was followed by 3 min of passive recovery. The best of the three performances was kept for statistical analysis. A 3-min recovery separated measurements between each angular velocity and each contraction mode (isokinetic, isometric).

Maximal voluntary isometric contraction of the knee extensors (MVCext) and knee flexors (MVCflex) was measured at 60° of knee flexion. Before each MVC measurement, subjects performed 3 submaximal contractions, followed by 3 min of passive recovery. Subjects were asked to push as fast and as hard as possible against the measuring device for 5 s. The same procedure was used for MVCflex measurement by pulling back the leg as fast and as hard as possible for 5 s. Three maximum trials were completed for each contraction (MVCext, MVCflex), repeated after a 3-min rest. The highest value was retained for analysis.

*Electrostimulation*

Three more MVCext efforts were performed after a 5-min recovery with super-imposed electrical twitches. Two surface electrodes (7.6 cm × 12.7 cm, Chattanooga, Bicester, UK) were positioned on the proximal and medial anterolateral side of the thigh of the dominant leg. Three MVCext trials were performed, separated by 3 min of passive recovery while electrical impulses were applied to the musculocutaneous nerves of the quadriceps. Electrical impulses (50 HZ) were delivered through the electrodes at 250 volts with a pulse width of 200 μs using a computer driven stimulator (model DS7, Digitimer Ltd, Welwyn Garden City, UK). Force output was channelled through an amplifier, interfaced with a data acquisition system (Biopac MP100WS, Santa Barbara, CA). The best of the three trials was used for analysis.

## 2.3 Statistical analysis

The Statistical Package for the Social Sciences (SPSS) and Excel (windows version) were used for data analysis. Two-way repeated measures ANOVA (time of day × cycle phase) was used to examine the effect of time of day and phases of the menstrual cycle. A paired-sample t-test was used to compare circadian acrophases and amplitudes between the two phases of the menstrual cycle.

Data for rectal temperature and muscle strength were subjected to cosinor analysis using COSINOR (Nelson *et al.*, 1979). This program derives characteristics of circadian rhythms (mesor, amplitude, acrophase). In addition, further analysis was performed to reduce the error due to individual differences by comparing the percentage change from minimum peak torque across times of day (the relative change in the six values across the solar day). Statistical significance was set at $p < 0.05$ for all analyses.

## 3. RESULTS

### 3.1 Anthropometric profiles

There was no significant effect of time of day, menstrual cycle nor any interaction effects on body mass.

### 3.2 Rectal temperature

A significant circadian variation in rectal temperature was found in both phases of the cycle ($F_{5,7} = 18.3$, $p < 0.05$). There were significant differences in rectal temperature between 02:00 h and 06:00 h, 14:00 h, 18:00 h, 22:00 h, between 06:00 h and 10:00 h, 14:00 h, 18:00 h, 22:00 h and between 10:00 h and 14:00 h, 18:00 h. In addition, there were significant differences in the mesor of rectal temperature between follicular and luteal phases ($\overline{x} = 36.8 \pm 0.95$ vs $37.0 \pm 0.10$ °C), of the menstrual cycle ($F_{1,7} = 8.3$, $p < 0.05$). A significant interaction effect ($F_{5,7} = 5.9$, $p < 0.05$) was also found between time of day and the two cycle phases for rectal temperature (Figure 1).

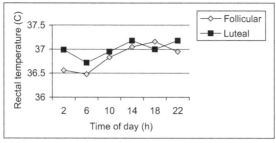

**Figure 1**. Circadian variation in rectal temperature in the follicular and luteal phases.

The acrophase of rectal temperature occurred marginally later in the luteal phase (18:18 h) than in the follicular phase (17:26 h), but these differences were not significant (p > 0.05). However, there was a significant difference in the circadian amplitude of the rectal temperature rhythm between the follicular (0.33 °C) and the luteal (0.16 °C) phases (p < 0.05).

### 3.3 Dynamic strength: Quadriceps

Repeated measures ANOVA did not reveal any significant differences in the mean quadriceps muscle strength at 1.05 rad.s$^{-1}$ between follicular and luteal phases ($\overline{X}$ = 128.7 ± 9.9 vs 130 ± 9.2 N.m, $F_{1,7}$ = 0.75, p > 0.05). There was a difference in quadriceps muscle strength at 1.05 rad.s$^{-1}$ between different times of day ($F_{5,7}$ = 4.3, p < 0.05). Bonferroni's test indicated the difference was significant between 02:00 h and 18:00 h, with greater values at 18:00 h than 02:00 h (Figure 2a). There were no interaction effects between time of day and menstrual phases on knee extensors peak torque at 1.05 rad.s$^{-1}$ ($F_{5,7}$ = 0.24, p > 0.05).

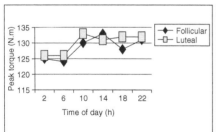
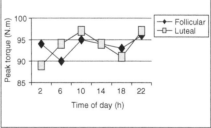

**Figure 2**. Circadian variation in peak torque of quadriceps at 1.05 (a) and 3.14 (b) rad.s$^{-1}$ in the follicular and luteal phases.

Further analysis to decrease the error due to individual differences compared the percentage change from the lowest peak torque of knee extensors at 1.05 rad.s$^{-1}$ across times of the day. There was a difference between 02:00 h and 10:00 h, 14:00 h, 18:00 h, 22:00 h, between 06:00 h and 10:00 h, 18:00 h, 22:00 h ($F_{5,7} = 4.1$, p < 0.05).

According to cosinor analysis, there was a significant circadian rhythm in quadriceps muscle strength at 1.05 rad.s$^{-1}$. The acrophases of the rhythm were located at 15:00 h and 15:28 h in the follicular and luteal phases, respectively. The circadian amplitudes of the peak torque of knee extensors were 3.9 and 2.7 N.m in the follicular and luteal phases, respectively.

There was no time of day ($F_{5,7} = 1.89$, p >0.05), cycle phase ($\overline{X}$ = 93.5 ± 9 vs 93.7 ± 9.4 N.m) ($F_{1,7} = 0.002$, p > 0.05) or interaction effects ($F_{5,7} = 1.12$, p > 0.05) at the angular velocity of 3.14 rad.s$^{-1}$ (Figure 2b).

### 3.4 Dynamic strength: Hamstrings

Dynamic muscle strength of the knee flexors (at 1.05 rad.s$^{-1}$) was lower in the follicular phase than in the luteal phase ($\overline{X}$ = 84 ± 10 vs 90 ± 11 N.m), ($F_{1,7} = 6.3$, p < 0.05). Repeated measures ANOVA did not show any time of day effect in hamstring muscle strength at the angular velocity of 1.05 rad.s$^{-1}$ ($F_{5,7} = 0.85$, p > 0.05) (Figure 3a). Also, cosinor analysis did not show a significant circadian rhythm in knee flexors strength at 1.05 rad.s$^{-1}$ (p > 0.05).

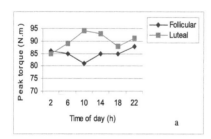 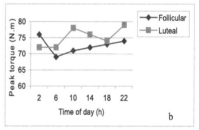

**Figure 3**. Circadian variation in hamstrings peak torque at 1.05 (a) and 3.14 rad.s$^{-1}$(b) in the follicular and luteal phases.

At 3.14 rad.s$^{-1}$, there was no difference ($F_{1,7} = 0.96$, p > 0.05) in hamstrings muscle strength between the follicular and luteal phases ($\overline{X}$ = 72.6 ± 8.2 vs 75.0 ± 8.5 N.m) and the difference was non significant between times of day ($F_{5,7} = 1.37$, p > 0.05). No interaction effect of daily rhythms and cycle phases was detected ($F_{5,7} = 1.76$, p > 0.05) (Figure 3b). Further analysis comparing the percentage change from the minimum peak torque of knee flexors at 3.14 rad.s$^{-1}$ during the day indicated that there was a significant circadian variation with a difference between 06:00 h and both 14:00 h and 22:00 h (p < 0.05).

### 3.5 Isometric muscle strength of quadriceps and hamstring

There were no significant differences in isometric torque of the knee extensors between times of day ($F_{5,7} = 0.74$, $p > 0.05$), cycle phases ($\overline{x} = 176.6 \pm 14.8$ vs $177.2 \pm 14.8$ N.m; $F_{1,7} = 0.02$, $p > 0.05$) nor any significant interaction effects ($F_{5,7} = 0.92$, $p > 0.05$) (Figure 4a). There was no time of day effect ($F_{5,7} = 3.02$, $p > 0.05$) and no circamensal rhythm ($\overline{x} = 77.5 \pm 10.5$ vs $78.4 \pm 9.9$ N.m; $F_{1,7} = 0.17$, $p > 0.05$) for maximal voluntary isometric contraction of knee flexors.

Significant interaction effects of time of day and cycle phases were observed on isometric contraction of knee flexors ($F_{5,7} = 3.43$, $p < 0.05$). The profile shows that, in the follicular phase, peak torque of knee flexors under isometric mode increased by 4% at 06:00 h compared to 02:00 h, then gradually decreased until 14:00 h, to increase again (%10) until 18:00. Further analysis on the percentage variations from the lowest isometric contraction (the relative change in the six values across the solar day) across times of day showed significant differences between 18:00 h and 02:00 h, 06:00 h, 10:00 h ($p < 0.05$) (Figure 4b).

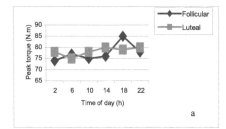 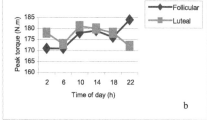

**Figure 4**. Circadian variation in maximal voluntary isometric contraction of knee extensors (a) and flexors (b) in the follicular and luteal phases.

### 3.6 Quadriceps isometric strength with superimposed electrical twitches

Isometric peak torque of electrically stimulated knee extensors showed no significant difference between follicular and luteal phases ($\overline{x} = 184.6 \pm 16$ vs $185.7 \pm 16.7$ N.m) ($F_{1,7} = 0.03$, $p > 0.05$), between times of day ($F_{5,7} = 1.4$, $p > 0.05$) nor any interaction effects ($F_{5,7} = 1.2$, $p > 0.05$) (Figure 5).

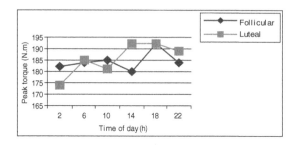

**Figure 5**. Circadian variation in maximal isometric contraction of electrically stimulated knee extensors in the luteal and follicular phases.

Further analysis showed that there was a significant circadian rhythm in isometric contraction of electrically stimulated quadriceps with a difference between 02:00 h and 18:00 h (p < 0.05). The acrophase of isometric contraction of electrically stimulated knee extensors was observed at 18:32 h and 16:55 h in the follicular and luteal phases, respectively.

## 3.7 Circadian rhythm in the difference between maximal voluntary contraction with and without electrical stimulation of knee extensors

There was a significant time of day effect in the difference between voluntary and involuntary (voluntary + percutaneous electrical stimulation) isometric contraction of knee extensors ($F_{5,7}$ = 3.6, p < 0.05). There was a significant difference between 02:00 h and 06:00 h, 02:00 and 18:00 h, between 10:00 h and 18:00 h, between 14:00 h and 18:00 and between 18:00 h and 22:00 h (Figure 6).

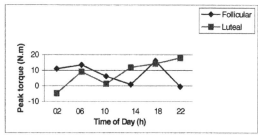

**Figure 6**. Circadian variation in the difference between isometric peak torque of knee extensors performed with and without superimposed electrical twitches.

Further analysis, using percentage change from the lowest circadian value, indicated a circadian variation in the percentage difference between voluntary and involuntary isometric contraction of knee extensors ($F_{5,7}$ = 4.2, p < 0.05). Repeated measures ANOVA showed that these differences existed between 02:00 h and both 06:00 h and 18:00 h, between 06:00 h and 10:00 h and between 14:00 h and 18:00 h) (Figure 7).

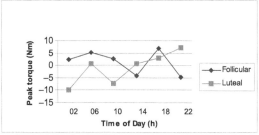

**Figure 7**. Circadian variation in the difference between voluntary and involuntary (voluntary + stimulation) isometric strength of knee extensors expressed as the percentage of variations from the lowest value.

## 4. DISCUSSION AND CONCLUSION

In the circadian and circamensal studies, measurement of core temperature provides a base for interpreting rhythmical patterns particularly when focussing on muscle strength measurements. In the present study, a circamensal variation was found for rectal temperature. The mean daily temperature was about 0.2°C higher in the luteal than in the follicular phase which is in agreement with previous reports (Vollman, 1977; Reilly, 1990). The circamensal rhythm in body temperature has been shown to be related to the thermogenic effect of progesterone (Cagnacci *et al.*, 1996).

In the present study, rectal temperature showed a significant circadian rhythm characterised by a mean value around 37°C, an acrophase around 18:00 h and a bathyphase around 06:00 h which is similar to previous findings observed in men (Minors and Waterhouse, 1981; Brooks and Reilly, 1984). A circadian rhythm for rectal temperature was found in both the follicular and the luteal phases, and there was no significant difference between phases for the occurrence of the acrophase and the bathyphase. Although there were no significant differences in the acrophase or the bathyphase of rectal temperature between follicular and luteal phases, there was a significant interaction effect (time of day × cycle phase). Rectal temperature was higher during the night points (02:00 h and 06:00 h) in the luteal compared to the follicular phase which led to a reduction of about 0.2°C in the circadian amplitude during the luteal phase. These observations are in agreement with Cagnacci *et al.* (1996) and Kattapong *et al.* (1995) who also demonstrated a decrease in the circadian amplitude of the rectal temperature rhythm partly related to the inhibitory effect of progesterone on the hypothermic role of melatonin at night (Cagnacci *et al.*, 1996).

A circamensal rhythm was observed in the peak torque of knee flexors at 1.05 rad.s$^{-1}$ in the current study. This finding partly confirms results of Greeves (1997) who also reported an increase in muscle strength of the knee flexors in the luteal compared to the follicular phase. However, in the present study, in spite of the fact that indices of dynamic muscle performance were often slightly higher in the luteal compared to the follicular phase, no significant change in peak torque was demonstrated in most cases. These results are in agreement with Gur (1997) and more recently Janse de Jonge *et al.* (2001). In the present study, the statistical power for the effect of the menstrual cycle phase was low (< 0.8). Therefore, the present results would indicate that a type II error could have occurred (Thomas and Nelson, 1990).

No effect of the cycle phase was found for isometric force of quadriceps and hamstrings muscles in the current study. These findings agree with Janse de Jonge *et al.* (2001) who reported no variation in isometric strength of knee extensors throughout the menstrual cycle (muscle function was measured on menstruation, late follicular phase and luteal phase). Sarwar *et al.* (1996) investigated isometric leg strength and handgrip five times throughout the cycle in regularly menstruating females (cycle phases were estimated from the first day of menstrual bleeding). These authors reported a peak in isometric force of quadriceps and handgrip strength at mid-cycle (ovulation). Greeves (1997) also reported a circamensal rhythm in isometric contraction of knee extensors (90° knee flexion) but greater strength was observed in the mid-luteal phase. In the present study, muscle strength was not measured at mid-cycle, which is a very awkward period characterised by an unsteady hormonal milieu. It has been frequently suggested that determination of ovulation by BBT, LH or hormonal measurements and frequent assessment during the menstrual cycle are essential factors in the study of the circamensal rhythm in muscle performance. However, as for the present study, protocols are often constraining for the subjects. It means that assessment of maximal muscle performance is often unrepresentative in the context of sport performance during the menstrual cycle. Furthermore, a circamensal rhythm was not observed in the present study for maximal isometric strength of quadriceps with superimposed electrical stimulation which confirms previous observations of Janse de Jonge *et al.* (2001).

In the present study, circadian rhythms were found for peak torque of quadriceps (at 1.05 rad.s$^{-1}$), peak torque of hamstrings (at 3.14 rad.s$^{-1}$), isometric peak torque of hamstrings, isometric peak torque of quadriceps performed with superimposed electrical twitches and in the difference between voluntary and involuntary(voluntary + stimulation)conditions. These findings partly agree with previous results observed in males (Atkinson and Reilly, 1996; Deschenes *et al.*, 1998) and females (Giacomoni and Garnett, 2002).

A circadian rhythm in isometric contraction of knee extensors was not found in the present study. In contrast, Taylor *et al.* (1994) reported a circadian rhythm in isometric contraction of knee extensors and Giacomoni and Garnett (2002) reported a time of day effect on maximal voluntary isometric contraction of knee extensors. The sex difference, knee angle, sample size and level of physical activity of subjects could explain in part discrepancies with Taylor *et al.* (1994). The frequency of measurements might be also a cause of differences between the present results and those of Giacomoni and Garnett (2002). In the present study isometric contractions of knee flexors and extensors were measured on the dominant leg in sedentary or moderately active females in the follicular and the luteal phases and at 6 times of day whilst Giacomoni and Garnett (2002) assessed isometric contraction of knee extensors in active females but only at two times of day. Taylor *et al.* (1994) measured isometric contraction of knee extensors of the right leg at 90° of knee flexion, with a strain-gauge assembly. In addition, the statistical power for detecting a circadian rhythm in muscle strength was low in the present study. Therefore further research should incorporate a larger sample size. The most interesting result was the circadian rhythm in maximal isometric strength of electrically stimulated knee extensors.

In a voluntary contraction, central and peripheral factors control maximal performance of muscles. In a maximal contraction with superimposed twitches, central factors such as motivation are offset. In the present study, we measured muscle force generated by the subject with and without electrical stimulation. In that way, we obtained information regarding the capacity to generate force by peripheral mechanisms (with stimulation) compared to central plus peripheral factors (without stimulation). Our results suggest that peripheral factors are implicated in the circadian rhythm in muscle strength of females. This is in agreement with recent studies on males (Davenne and Gauthier, 1997; Martin *et al.*, 1999). Circadian changes in muscle temperature could be in part responsible for the circadian rhythm in maximal muscle performance through an effect on muscle viscosity (reduction) and enzymatic activity (increase) leading to a better efficiency of contractile components. However, to date, no study has demonstrated a causal link between changes in muscle temperature during the day and circadian changes in muscle function. Circadian changes in substrate availability and turnover (ATP, PCr) as well as ionic changes could also be involved in the circadian rhythm in muscle strength. The present study also showed a time of day effect in the differences between maximal muscle strength performed with and without stimulation. This result suggests that the part played by central factors on circadian rhythms in muscle performance, and particularly by motivation, could mask at some points and in some subjects the circadian variations in muscle function. Significant interaction effects of time of day and menstrual cycle phase were observed in the present study on maximal isometric strength of knee flexors. However, due to the lack of consistency regarding interaction effects on muscle function, this result remains difficult to interpret. As chronobiological variations are greatly dependent of individual sensitivity, further research on a larger sample would be needed to ascertain the true interaction effects between time of day and menstrual cycle on muscle strength.

It is concluded there is a circadian rhythm in muscle strength of females at a slow angular velocity. Failure to show consistent circadian variations in all aspects of muscle function could be the result of a masking effect of individual differences, motivational effects, or reproducibility of some measurements (e.g. high velocities, hamstring strength assessment). Further studies on a larger sample would be needed to minimize inter-individual variability, particularly in the effect of the menstrual cycle on circadian variations. The present study suggests that peripheral, more than central mechanisms are implicated in the circadian variations in maximal isometric strength of women but that central factors could be preferentially involved at some times of day compared to others.

## Acknowledgements

Effat Bambaeichi is supported by a research grant from the Ministry of Sciences, Research and Technology of Iran and also by Isfahan University. The help of Dr Ben Edwards and Dr Jim Waterhouse with data analysis is gratefully appreciated.

## REFERENCES

Atkinson, G. and Reilly, T., 1996, Circadian variation in sports performance. *Sports Medicine*, **21**, 292-312.

Brooks, G.A. and Reilly, T., 1984, Thermoregulatory responses to exercise at different times of day. *Journal of Physiology*, **354**, 99P.

Cagnacci, A., Soldani, R., Laughlin, G.A. and Yen, S.C., 1996, Modification of circadian body temperature rhythm during the luteal menstrual phase: role of melatonin. *Journal of Applied Physiology*, **80**, 25-29.

Davenne, D. and Gauthier, A., 1997, Location of the mechanisms involved in the circadian rhythm of muscle strength. In *Proceedings of the International Congress on Chronobiology*, Paris, France, 7-11, September.

Deschenes, M.R., Kraemer, W.J., Bush, J.A., Doughty, T.A., Kim, D., Mullen, K. M. and Ramsey, K., 1998, Biorhythmic influences on functional capacity of human muscle and physiological responses. *Medicine and Science in Sports and Exercise*, **30**, 1399-1407.

Edwards, B., Atkinson, G., Waterhouse, J., Reilly, T., Godfrey, R. and Budgett, R., 2002, Use of melatonin in recovery from jet-lag following an eastward flight across 10 time-zones. In *Advances in Sport, Leisure and Ergonomics*, edited by Reilly T. and Greeves J., (London: Routledge), pp. 67-79.

Giacomoni, M. and Garnett, C., 2002, Interaction of time of day and menstrual cycle phase on muscle function in physically active women. *Journal of Sports Sciences*, **20**, 36-37.

Greeves, J.P., 1997, The effect of reproductive hormones on muscle function in young and middle-aged females. *Ph.D. thesis, Liverpool John Moores University*.

Greeves, J.P., Cable, N.T., Luckas, M.J.M., Reilly, T. and Biljan, M.M., 1997, Effects of acute changes in oestrogen on muscle function of the first dorsal interosseus muscle in humans. *Journal of Physiology*, **500**, 266-270.

Gur, H., 1997, Concentric and eccentric isokinetic measurements in knee muscles during the menstrual cycle: A special reference to reciprocal moment ratios. *Archives of Physical Medicine and Rehabilitation*, **78**, 501-505.

Janse de Jonge, X.A.K., Boot, C.R.L., Thom, J.M. and Ruell, P.A., 2001, The influence of menstrual cycle phase on skeletal muscle contractile characteristics in humans. *Journal of Physiology*, **530**, 161-166.

Kattapong, K.R., Fogg, L.F. and Eastman, C.I., 1995, Effect of sex, menstrual cycle phase and oral contraceptive use on circadian temperature rhythms. *Chronobiology International*, **12**, 257-266.

Martin, A., Carpentier, A., Guissard, N., Van Hoecke, J. and Duchateau, J., 1999, Effect of time of day on force variation in a human muscle. *Muscle and Nerve*, **22**, 1380-1387.

Minors, D.S. and Waterhouse, J.M., 1981, *Circadian Rhythms and the Human*, Bristol: Wright, J. and Sons Ltd.

Moos, R., 1985, *Perimenstrual symptoms*: a manual and overview of research with the menstrual distress questionnaire. Social Ecology Laboratory, Department of Psychiatry and Behavioural Sciences, Stanford University and Veterans Administration Medical Centre, Palo Alto, California.

Nelson, W., Tong, T.L., Lee, J.K. and Halberg, F., 1979, Methods for cosinor rhythmometry. *Chronobiologia*, **6**, 305-323.

Phillips, S.K., Sanderson, A.G., Birch, K., Bruce, S.A. and Woledge, R.C., 1996, Changes in maximal voluntary force of human adductor pollicis muscle during the menstrual cycle. *Journal of Physiology*, **496**, 551-557.

Reilly, T., 1990, Human circadian rhythms and exercise. Critical Reviews in *Biomedical Engineering*, **18,** 165-180.

Reilly, T., Atkinson, G. and Waterhouse, J., 1997, Biological Rhythms and Exercise. Oxford: Oxford University Press. pp. 41-43.

Sarwar, R., Beltran Niclos, B. and Rutherford, O.M., 1996, Change in muscle strength, relaxation rate and fatigability during the human menstrual cycle. *Journal of Physiology*, **493**, 267-272.

Smith, C.S., Reilly, C. and Midkiff, K., 1989, Evaluation of three circadian rhythm questionnaires with suggestions for an improved measure of morningness. *Journal of Applied Psychology*, **74**, 728-738.

Taylor, D., Gibson., H., Edwards, R.H.T. and Reilly, T., 1994, Correction of isometric leg strength test for time of day. *European Journal of Experimental Musculoskeletal Research*, **3**, 25-27.

Thomas, J.R. and Nelson, J.K., 1990, *Research Methods in Physiological Activity*, Champaign: Human Kinetics.

Vollman, R.F., 1977, The menstrual cycle. In *Major Problems in Obstetrics and Gynaecology*, edited by Freidman, E.A. (Philadelphia: W.B. Saunders Company), Vol 7, pp. 171-193.

# 23 The Anthropometric Concomitants of Women's Hammer Throwing: The Implications for Talent Identification

Allan Staerck
Department of Sport Health and Exercise Science,
St Mary's College, Twickenham, TW1, 4SX, UK

## 1. INTRODUCTION

In a number of studies, top athletes in various sports have been measured and 'characteristic' physiques have been suggested for different sports. One implication of such studies is that this information might serve as a guideline to early prediction of athletic performance (Bar-Or, 1975). In Great Britain over the past few years standards of women's hammer competition have risen and distances thrown have generally improved, but there is little known about the anthropometric and physical status of women hammer throwers.

Successful selection of future international class performers is dependent on identification of a complex set of qualities. There is a need therefore for coaches to be able to identify the qualities that appear to have a bearing on performance, are extremely difficult to develop through training and which mainly have a strong genetic component. According to research, anthropometric measurements, movement speed and some psychological factors are classified in this category. This study will therefore measure a number of these components with particular reference to basic rotational speed and the athlete's reach. Rotational speed and reach are both important as measures of potential talent selection in women's hammer throwing due to the speed which needs to be achieved by the hammer head at release. The mechanics of hammer throwing indicate that both of these areas are reported to have an effect on the release velocity of the hammer and any increase in release velocity will bring about an increase in distance thrown. The measurement of the athlete's ability to rotate quickly has been identified as a factor in talent identification by coaches (Bondarchuk, 1987) and although improvements in turning speed can be made through training, observations have shown that not all athletes have the natural ability to turn fast. However, no data have been reported on any measurement methods used or any records of the measurement of rotational speed in relation to women's hammer throwing. A knowledge of an athlete's reach by the coach is pertinent as the athlete's reach will affect the radius of the path of the hammer; the larger the radius the greater the angular velocity and the faster the hammer head would be travelling during each rotation. The reach test only concentrates on static reach as this can easily be measured by the coach in a field testing situation. However, it is acknowledged that change in the athlete's body position caused by centripetal and centrifugal forces acting on the body during the execution of a throw can affect the athlete's reach.

Symmetry is an important consideration in the structural appraisal of hammer throwing, due to the bilateral nature of the event. In this study limb lengths were measured, from previously identified landmarks on both sides of the body in the sagittal plane, with the participants standing erect looking straight ahead with their arms hanging by their sides. The mean of the values of the limb length obtained from both sides was calculated and used in this study.

## 2. METHODS

### 2.1 Participants

Thirty-two women hammer throwers, aged 14 to 39 years, were selected on performance criteria based on information available in the National Senior and Junior women's performance ranking lists from the previous season, published by The National Union of Track Statisticians, and in consultation with the British Athletic Federation National Event coaches and Women's Hammer Development Officer. The testing and data collection were undertaken at various venues in conjunction with selected national and area coaching clinics, league meetings, area and national championships. The subjects were divided into two sub-groups, fourteen elite throwers (>50 m), mean age 25.79 (SD 6.18) years, and eighteen non-elite throwers (<50 m), mean age 19.72 (SD 6.14), years based on their distances thrown in the previous athletics season.

The variables selected for measurement in this study were based on recommendations from previous research on female track and field athletes (Malina *et al.*, 1971; Freedson, 1988; Wells, 1991; Barclay, 1997). No specific reference has been made to these variables in relation to women's hammer throwing. The inclusion of reach and rotational speed was based on the mechanical theory associated with the release speed of the hammer.

Each participant was advised of the requirements of the research prior to her participation which included a thorough explanation of the intention, methods and procedures of each test. The participant was also informed that any information obtained for the purpose of this research would be kept confidential.

## 2.2 Anthropometic measurements

*Body mass* was measured using Slater weighing scales to the nearest 0.1 kg with the subjects in minimal clothing, without shoes. The measurement was taken with the participant standing erect looking straight ahead.

*Standing height* (free-standing stature) was determined using a Harpenden stadiometer to the nearest 0.5 cm, with the participants standing erect, looking straight ahead without shoes, and feet flat on the floor with their heels together and their arms hanging naturally by their sides. The measurement was taken as the maximum distance from the floor to the vertex of the head.

*Sitting height* (free-seated stature) was determined using a Harpenden stadiometer to the nearest 0.5 cm, with the participant sitting with her back vertical. The measurement was taken as the maximum distance from the base of the sitting surface to the vertex of the head when the head is held in the Frankfort plane.

*Arm span* was determined using a Holtain flexible steel measuring tape to the nearest 0.1 cm. The arm span measurement was taken with the participants standing erect, looking straight ahead with their arms outstretched to the side at 90 degrees abduction in the sagittal plane and hands facing forward. The arm span measurement was taken as the maximum distance posteriorly running across the participant's back (through the 7th cervical vertebrae) from the tip of the second finger on the left hand to the tip of the second finger on the right hand.

*Limb lengths* were determined using a Holtain flexible steel measuring tape to the nearest 0.1 cm following basic guidelines on measurement protocol outlined by MacDougall, Wenger and Green (1991).

*Landmarks*: The following landmarks were identified in the sagittal plane and marked on both sides of the participant. The participant was standing erect looking straight ahead with her arms hanging by her sides.

Shoulder:   Lateral point on the superior and external border of the acromion process when the participant is standing erect with relaxed arms.

Elbow:   On a line through the humeral epicondyles 1 cm proximal to the head of the radius.

Wrist:   A point midway along a line joining the ulnar and radial styloid processes on the dorsal surface of wrist.

Hip:   Superior aspect of anterior iliac spine.

Knee:     Mid-point of line through centres of posterior convexities of femoral condyles.

Ankle:    The most distal tip of the lateral malleolus.

*Arm reach* was determined using a Reach Vernier, to the nearest 0.1 cm. The arm reach measurement was taken with the athlete in a semi-standing position with the buttocks and lower back supported against a wall and the feet approximately half a metre away from the wall. This position was adopted to eliminate any forward lean by the participant. The 'Tee' end on the beam of the 'reach vernier' was positioned on the suprasternal notch, the athlete held the handle of the vernier slider with both hands, the handle located between the two interphalangeal joints on the fingers of the left hand using a hammer throwing style grip. The participant was instructed to reach out as far as possible pushing the slider along the beam keeping the vernier at 90° to the vertical in front of the body. The measurement was taken as the maximum distance from the suprasternal notch to the grip between the two interphalangeal joints of the fingers on the handle of the slider. The reach of each participant can be used as an indicator of the maximum radius that could be obtained on the hammer head.

*Toe/Turning Velocity*: A 2D video recording in the frontal plane was made of the participant performing three consecutive toe turns about the longitudinal axis to carry out a quantitative analysis of the action. The video camera was mounted on a stationary tripod and set up following British Association of Sport and Exercise Sciences guidelines (Bartlett, 1996). The participant was instructed to stand erect with her feet shoulder width apart and her hands on her hips. The participants performed a series of three continuous turns on the toe/ball of their left foot (right handed throwers). The data collected were analysed using a Panasonic slow-motion play-back system with frame counter and timer. Each series of turns was analysed and the time taken to the nearest 0.02 s, from first pick up of the right foot at the start of the series of turns, to its final touch down at the end of the third turn. This test is used to obtain an indication of the participant's ability to turn quickly, without any specific hammer throwing technique.

*Body Mass Index*: The Body Mass Index was determined to 0.01% using the following formula: Body Mass Index = Body mass/Height squared where body mass is expressed in kilograms and height in metres.


### 2.3 Reliability

Intratester and Intertester Reliability: Reliability was established for the toe turning velocity and the anthropometric measurement of reach tests. The reliability sample consisted of 10 female sport science students. An Intratester test-retest method with a two-day period between administrations and an Intertester testing method as outlined by Thomas and Nelson (1990) were adopted to test the reliability of the test procedures and equipment used.

The Bland and Altman (1986) boundaries of agreement method for assessing reliability was used to establish the extent of reliability of the results obtained from both the intratester and intertester methods and equipment used.

## 2.4 Data collection

Statistical tests were used to collect, analyse and assess information about the performance levels of each athlete, based on the guidelines laid down by Thomas and Nelson (1990).

An independent t-test was performed upon the data collected for each variable using SPSS for Windows computer data analysis package. The t value obtained for each set of data was compared with 5% levels of significance.

Table 1. The data collected for each of the variables measured in this study, including the mean and standard deviation for each sub-group.

| Variables | Elite (n = 14) | | Non-elite (n = 18) | | p |
|---|---|---|---|---|---|
| | Mean | SD | Mean | SD | |
| Age (years) | 25.79 | 6.18 | 19.72 | 6.14 | <0.01 |
| Height (m) | 1.700 | 0.064 | 1.719 | 0.047 | 0.352 |
| Body mass (kg) | 85.82 | 11.74 | 82.64 | 14.14 | 0.508 |
| B.M.I. | 30.22 | 4.03 | 27.62 | 5.18 | 0.133 |
| Span (m) | 1.7196 | 0.0 768 | 1.7283 | 0.0756 | 0.366 |
| Reach (m) | 0.6461 | 0.0344 | 0.6592 | 0.0335 | 0.287 |
| Sitting height (m) | 0.9043 | 0.0360 | 0.9136 | 0.0211 | 0.366 |
| Shoulder-Elbow (m) | 0.3243 | 0.0159 | 0.3228 | 0.0199 | 0.819 |
| Elbow-Wrist (m) | 0.2661 | 0.0161 | 0.2697 | 0.0158 | 0.524 |
| Hip-Knee (m) | 0.5196 | 0.0357 | 0.5289 | 0.0288 | 0.424 |
| Knee-Ankle (m) | 0.4336 | 0.0168 | 0.4319 | 0.0204 | 0.811 |
| Distance thrown (m) | 0.5493 | 0.0395 | 0.4136 | 0.0639 | < 0.0001 |
| Turn time (s) | 1.66 | 0.20 | 2.02 | 0.32 | < 0.0001 |

## 3. RESULTS

The results given in Table 1 show that there is a significant difference ($p < 0.0001$) between the distances thrown by the elite group of throwers and the non-elite group of throwers. A significant difference was also found between the turn time recorded for the elite group of throwers compared to the non-elite group of throwers ($p = 0.001$). Similarly a significant difference was found between the age recorded for the elite throwers and the non-elite throwers ($p = 0.010$).

No significant differences were found between the elite women hammer throwers and the non-elite women hammer throwers in height, body mass, body mass index, arm span, reach and sitting height.  The elite women throwers were found to be slightly heavier with a higher body mass index score (p = 0.133). However, the non-elite throwers were taller, had a slightly larger measured arm span and slightly larger reach.  Sitting height was also greater for the non-elite athletes.

There were no significant differences between the upper body limb lengths shoulder to elbow (p = 0.819) and elbow to wrist (p = 0.524).  Similarly no significant differences were found between the limb length measurements of the legs, hip to knee (p = 0.424) and knee to ankle (p = 0.811).

## 4. DISCUSSION

The main aims of this study were to analyse the demands of women's hammer throwing through the measurement of a number of anthropometric and physical parameters and to develop a specific test battery to provide guidelines for coaches regarding the event and for talent identification.  It was found that the following parameters should be considered by the coach when identifying young female athletes who have the potential to become elite hammer throwers; the young athlete should possess good basic rotational speed, have a standing height  of at least 1.71 metres and a span at least 2 centimetres greater than her standing height with a reach in a range from 64-66 centimetres.  It should be noted that there was a difference in mean age between the two groups (elite mean = 25.79 years, non-elite mean = 19.72 years) although there was an overlap in the range of ages (elite 18-37 years, non-elite 14-39 years). The anthropometric and physical measures used in this study should not be significantly affected by the difference in age between the two groups and therefore this will have little bearing on the results.

The athletes' physical and physiological capacities must be carefully assessed in order that the coach will be able to ascertain the level of their talent.  A talent identification programme for a particular sport must be concerned with every part of that particular sport or event. The physical capacity of the individual athlete can be an important self-selector for many sports and events. Bompa (1985) suggested that anthropometric measurements of an individual must be considered among the main criteria for talent identification and that height and body mass, or the length of limbs, often play a dominant role in certain sports.  Bloomfield et al. (1995) noted that many accurate forecasts with relation to individual and team performances have been made during the last two decades on the measurements of height and body mass alone.

Stature can play an important part in the selection of an athlete for a particular sport or event and with respect to hammer throwing the athlete needs to be reasonably tall (Bartonietz et al., 1988). This study revealed no significant difference between the mean height of the two groups (1.70 m–1.72 m). Track and Field News (2000) reported that the height of the women's world record holder for hammer was 1.72 m. The results of both groups in this study compare well with this value.

The results from this study indicate that there were no significant differences in the body mass of the elite women throwers and the non-elite women throwers. The elite throwers were, however, slightly heavier with a mean body mass of 85.82 (SD11.74) kg compared to a mean body mass of 82.64 (SD14.41) kg for the non-elite throwers. The mean body mass measurements recorded for each of the groups (85.28 and 82.65 kg) are heavier than the body mass noted by Track and Field News (2000) of 78 kg for Mihaela Melinte, the holder of the world record for women's hammer throwing.

The body mass figures observed in this study for both the elite and non-elite groups of throwers could be attributed to a higher level of muscle mass developed through the amount of strength training they have undertaken. One athlete in the elite group and two athletes in the non-elite group had a body mass in excess of 105 kg; this slightly skewed the body mass recordings and may not give a true reflection of the mean body mass of the majority of throwers in either group. Fahey, Akka and Rolph (1975) identified that body mass is important in hammer throwing and noted that if speed can be maintained, a larger body mass is of a considerable advantage in throwing events. If the body mass is too large the athlete may have difficulty in building up the required speed.

Anspaugh *et al.* (1993) noted that a body mass index of 21-23 kg.m² is desirable for women in their twenties (these figures may rise slightly with age); however, these values were based on research on the general population and made no specific reference to female athletes. In this study the elite group of athletes had a mean body mass index of 30.72 compared to a mean body mass index of 27.62 for the non-elite group. Both groups of athletes recorded a body mass index higher than the normal reported values for women in their respective age ranges. However, the body mass index does not make any allowance for an increase in body mass of the athlete due to the build-up of muscle mass caused through regular training and it can be considered that the higher values obtained in this study are a result of the subjects having a higher muscle mass. As training methods for athletes continue to become more sophisticated, techniques for assessing physiological and body composition correlates of performance will become increasingly more important (Puhl *et al.*, 1988).

There was a significant difference recorded between the ages of the two groups of throwers (elite group mean 25.79, non-elite group mean 19.72 years). A large number of the athletes in the elite group of throwers were over 22 years old. A possible explanation for this is that hammer throwing is a highly technical and strength-related event and generally the athlete will need to take a number of years to develop these fully. In contrast a large number of the non-elite group of athletes in this study were under 19, had reported not having been involved in any form of specific strength training and were at the beginning of the development of their hammer throwing techniques.

The results of this study indicate that there were no significant differences found in the limb lengths measured (shoulder–elbow, elbow–wrist, hip–knee, knee–ankle) for the elite and non-elite groups of throwers. The mean distances recorded for the span of the two groups showed that there was no significant difference between them but in both cases they were greater than the mean height recorded. In hammer throwing the length of the upper extremities of the body can have an important overall bearing on the hammer radius. The larger the span of the athlete the greater the potential radius that could be attained on the path of the hammer during the turns. Bartonietz *et al.* (1988) recommended that when identifying potentially talented young athletes, an arm span greater than 5 cm above their standing height is desirable. Barclay (1996) noted that the women's hammer world record holder had an arm span 1 cm greater than her standing height. This compares well with the results from this study where the mean arm span recorded for both groups measured greater than 1 cm more than their stature.

There was no significant difference between the mean scores obtained in the reach test. There is no record of this type of test being carried out before. However, information about the length of an athlete's reach can play an important part in establishing the radius of the hammer's path during the turning phase of the throw. The further the hammer head is away from the centre of rotation, the faster it will be travelling for a given turning speed of the body. An examination of the relation between the athlete's reach and her sitting height was developed by dividing the mean reach value obtained for each group of throwers by the mean value obtained for the sitting height. In the case of this study the mean reach was found to be 72% of the mean sitting height. The size of the sample and absence of a control group mean that it would not be pertinent to infer too much from this figure. However, this area has scope for future study to determine if an optimal ratio exists.

A significant difference was found between the turning speed of the elite group of throwers compared to the non-elite group of throwers. This is felt to be a key area in the identification of talented athletes with respect to throwing the hammer a long distance, as the ability to rotate fast is an important aspect in the acceleration of the hammer. The simple toe-turning test was used as it was not part of the standard hammer throwing technique and therefore not affected by any learned ability by the more skilful hammer throwers. It is important in hammer throwing that the athlete shows acceleration as the throw progresses (Jabs, 1979; Dick, 1997). Morriss and Bartlett (1995) studied the angular velocity of women hammer throwers and found that the top international thrower in their study who recorded a throw in excess of 60 m had total turn time of 1.51 s; this was achieved using three conventional heel–toe turns.

A comparison between the mean sitting heights recorded for both groups, indicated that there was no significant difference between the values. The ratio of sitting height to stature provides an estimate of relative trunk length and conversely, relative leg length of the athlete. For both groups in this study the mean ratio of trunk length was calculated to be 53% of their stature. Maud and Foster (1995) reported that this ratio can be useful in identifying athletes in different sports or even events within a given sport. Klafs and Lyon (1978) suggested that the longer upper body is seen as a basic asset in throwing events. The shorter legs are associated with fast initial movement and speed, while long arms are associated with a longer upper body and are relative to reach and the radius of the hammer.

Future work in this area might use and develop these tests to produce some strong performance predictors, thereby enabling the early identification of future elite female hammer throwers. Future recommendations would be to increase the number of athletes being tested to a sample size of 50 based on the results of statistical power calculations and incorporate laboratory based tests as opposed to field tests.

To complement this study, which primarily looked at the physical attributes of the female hammer thrower, a psychological study of elite and non-elite women hammer throwers' performance characteristics and a full biomechanical comparison of their technical turning ability, with and without the hammer, would be of interest.

## 5. CONCLUSIONS

The results of this study indicate that there is a relationship between rotational speed and the level of performance, as the elite women hammer throwers in this study recorded significantly faster turning times than the non-elite women hammer throwers. In contrast, the results indicate that there was no significant difference between the results obtained for reach of the throwers in the two groups.

The aim of this study was to identify anthropometric and physical characteristics unique to elite female hammer throwers compared to non-elite female hammer throwers and examine these with respect to talent identification. Within the limitations of this study the following conclusions have been reached regarding talent identification and the elite female hammer thrower. The elite female hammer thrower should be at least 1.71 m tall with an arm span a minimum of 2 cm greater than her standing height and a reach measured in a range from 64 to 66 cm. She should have a longer upper body with a sitting height measurement of 53% of her stature.  The mean body mass and mean body mass index ratios obtained in this study are slightly high due to one thrower in each group having a body mass in excess of 110 kg. However, based on the recorded body mass of the world record holder at 75 kg and the mean body mass of the two groups, it is suggested that a body mass in a range of 75 to 83.5 kg would be desirable. This would give a body mass index in the range of 24 to 28 kg.m². The most significant variable was found to be the ability of the elite athlete to turn quickly. Here the coach should look for an athlete who records a time in the region of 1.66 s for the three consecutive toe–turn test.

As training methods for athletes continue to become more sophisticated, techniques for assessment of physiological and body composition correlates of performance, will be increasingly important. This scientific information will be invaluable to coaches in their quest to identify athletic potential and maximise athletic performance in their specific event. There is no doubt that the essential ingredients for development of elite female hammer throwers are expert coaches, supported by sport scientists. It is hoped that this study will serve not only to inform coaches and athletes as to what can be regarded as a starting point, in relation to the anthropometric and physiological requirement of elite female hammer throwers, but also has identified and shown new directions for further research in this field.

## REFERENCES

Anspaugh, D., Hamrick, M. and Rosato, F., 1993, *Wellness Concepts and Application*, (London: Mosby).

Bar-Or, O., 1975, Predicting athletic performance. *Physician and Sportsmedicine*, 3(2), 81-85.

Barclay, L., 1997, Round table: Hammer throw. *New Studies in Athletics*, 12(2/3), 13-27.

Bartlett, R., 1996, *Biomechanical Analysis of Movement in Sport and Exercise*. (Leeds: British Association of Sport and Exercise Sciences).

Bartonietz, K., Hinz, L., Lorenz, D. and Lunau, G., 1988, The hammer. *New Studies in Athletics*, 3(1), 39-56.

Bland, J.M. and Altman, D.G., 1986, Statistical methods for assessing agreement between two methods of clinical measurement. *Lancet,* Feb 8th, 307-310.

Bloomfield, J., Fricker, P.A. and Fitch, K.D. 1995, *Science and Medicine in Sport.* (London: Blackwell Scientific Publications).

Bompa, T.O., 1985, Talent identification. *Sports Science Periodical on Research and Technology in Sport,* 5(2), 1-11.

Bondarchuk, A. 1987, *Selection and training of youth and junior hammer throwers.* Communication to IXVth Congress of European Coaches Association. Aix-lLes-Bains France, January.

Dick, F., 1997, *Sports Training Principles*. (London: Lepus Books).

Fahey, T., Akka, L. and Rolph, R., 1975, Body composition and $VO_{2\,max}$ of exceptional weight-trained athletes. *Journal of Applied Physiology*, 39, 559-561.

Freedson, P., 1988, Body composition and performance, In *Sportscience Perspectives for Women*, edited by Puhl, J. Brown, C.H. and Voy, R.O. (Champaign, Illinois: Human Kinetics Books).

Jabs, R.G., 1979, Velocity in hammer throwing. *Track and Field Technique,* 77, 2449-2450.

Klafs, C. and Lyon, J., 1978, *The Female Athlete*. (Saint-Louis: C.V. Morsby Co).

MacDougall, J.D. Wenger, H. and Green, H., 1991, *Physiological Testing of the High Performance Athlete*. (Champaign, Illinios: Human Kinetics Books).

Malina, R. Harper, A. Avent, H. and Campbell, D., 1971, Physique of female Track and Field athletes. *Medicine and Science in Sport,* 3, 32-38.

Maud, P.J. and Foster, C., 1995, *Physiological Assessment of Human Fitness.* (Champaign, Illinois: Human Kinetics).

Morriss, C. and Bartlett, R., 1995, *Biomechanical Analysis of Hammer Throw*. Vol 2, Manchester Metropolitan University.

Puhl, J., Brown, C.H. and Voy, R.O., 1988, *Sport Science Perspectives for Women*. (Champaign Illinois: Human Kinetics Books).

Thomas, J. and Nelson, J., 1990, *Research Methods in Physical Activity*. (Champaign, Illinois: Human Kinetics Books).

Track and Field News, 2000, Women's World Rankings, **53**(2), 52-65.

Wells, C., 1991, *Women Sport and Performance*. (Champaign, Illinois: Human Kinetics Books).

# Part V
# HEALTH-RELATED STUDIES

# 24    The Effects of a Walking Programme on Body Composition and Serum Lipids and Lipoproteins in Sedentary Men Aged 42-52 Years

Farhad Rahmani-Nia
University of Guilan, Rasht, Iran

## 1. INTRODUCTION

Cardiovascular disease (CVD) is the leading cause of death in Iran for both men and women. The risk factors for CVD include age, family history, current cigarette smoking, hypertension, hypercholesterolemia, diabetes mellitus, and a sedentary lifestyle (White *et al.*, 2001). While some of these risk factors are non-modifiable (e.g. age and family history), the majority of risk factors are modifiable by means of lifestyle changes in diet and physical activity level. Physical activity may positively influence the risk factors associated with CVD in both men and women (Hespel *et al.*, 1987; Parkkari *et al.*, 2000).

Specifically, physical activity may help lower blood pressure, cholesterol, and may facilitate positive changes in body composition (Hinkleman *et al.*, 1993). There is some evidence that walking may reduce serum lipids and lipoproteins (Plank and Hargreaves, 1990; Stensel *et al.*, 1994) although the frequency, intensity, and duration of training necessary to elicit changes in risk factors have not been clearly established. Walking is a rhythmic, dynamic, and aerobic activity of large muscles that confers many benefits with minimal adverse effects. Stensel *et al.* (1994) have reported that walking regimens have been effective in reducing skinfold thickness in middle-aged men (42-59 years). Also Plank and Hargreaves (1990) demonstrated that regular walking on a golf course is a feasible and safe form of recreational physical activity that has favourable effects on the health and fitness of previously sedentary subjects. They stated that cholesterol and LDL decreased with walking. Their results agree with Whitehurst and Menendez (1991) and Toriola (1984) but there are a few studies indicating that walking may not change body composition, lidips and lipoproteins positively and together. Therefore, the purpose of this study was to identify the effects of 4 weeks of walking (3 times per week) on body composition and serum lipids and lipoproteins in sedentary men 42-52 years.

## 2. METHODS

Thirteen sedentary men, 42-52 years of age (mean age = 47± 5 years), volunteered to participate in this study. All subjects attended an orientation session and completed a medical history questionnaire, a physical activity readiness questionnaire and an informed consent form. Prior to and at the end of the walking programme, weight and height were measured; then skinfolds of chest, abdomen and thigh were assessed (Laffayete Caliper) according to Pollock *et al.* (1972). Fat percent and fat free mass were estimated from these measures. Blood samples were obtained by venepuncture of the anterior forearm using a vacutainer following a 12-hour fast. Total cholesterol and HDL-C levels were measured using a Vitros DT II chemistry system (Ortho-Clinical Diagnostic-Johnson & Johnson, Rochester, NY). Values for LDL were estimated using an equation that considered measured concentrations of total cholesterol, HDL-C, and triglycerides.

All subjects were asked to refrain from physical activity, drugs and smoking. Also, they were asked to continue their ordinary nutrition programme through the study. The walking programme consisted of 3 times per week for 4 weeks and the duration of each session was 30 minutes.

The intensity of walking in the first and second sessions was 50% $HR_{max}$. In sessions 3–10 it was 60% $HR_{max}$ and for sessions 11 and 12 was 70% $HR_{max}$.

## 3. RESULTS

The characteristics and means and standard deviations of pre-training and post-training tests are summarized in Table 1. Statistical analysis of the data with t-tests demonstrated that there were significant differences ($p \leq 0.05$) in body mass, body fat percent, cholesterol and LDL between pre-training and post-training tests. There were no significant changes in skinfolds of chest, abdomen and thigh regions, fat free mass, triglycerides and HDL.

**Table 1.** Mean and SD of the characteristics and results of pre- and post-training tests.

| | | Pre-test | Post-test |
|---|---|---|---|
| Mass (kg) | | 75.55 ± 9.95 | 74.58 ± 10.02 |
| Skinfold fat (mm) | Chest | 22.15 ± 8.07 | 20 ± 6.68 |
| | Abdomen | 34.15 ± 8.69 | 31.77 ± 8.64 |
| | Thigh | 21.54 ± 7.90 | 20.46 ± 7.21 |
| Body fat percent | | 23.88 ± 5.52 | 22.12 ± 4.12 |
| Fat free mass (kg) | | 56.73 ± 4.24 | 57.58 ± 6.44 |
| Chol (mg.dl$^{-1}$) | | 206.92 ± 30.02 | 197.08 ± 28.80 |
| HDL (mg.dl$^{-1}$) | | 37.46 ± 4.74 | 37.23 ± 5.76 |
| LDL (mg.dl$^{-1}$) | | 139.62 ± 29.78 | 119.22 ± 28.32 |
| Triglycerides (mg.dl$^{-1}$) | | 193.08 ± 96.47 | 177.54 ± 70.88 |

## 4. DISCUSSION

We explored the effects of walking on several indicators of health (cholesterol and HDL) and observed favourable effects on body composition (body fat percent) in middle-aged men. The study had some limitations. First, randomization could not be done and second, our walking programme was only 4 weeks long and 30 minutes in duration for each session.

Several recent studies suggest that the fitness and health of sedentary middle-aged people can be improved through adoption of low levels of leisure activity (Nakamura *et al.*, 1985; Hespel *et al.*, 1987). The largest health gains are achieved when someone progresses from the lowest to a slightly greater level of physical activity or physical fitness, walking is a low- to moderate-intensity exercise that can be engaged in regularly and thus fulfils criteria for health-enhancing physical activity (Parkkari *et al.*, 2000). Current recommendations propose a programme more than 30 minutes and about 5 METs or 6.5 kcal.min$^{-1}$ for 3-5 times per week (Savage *et al.*, 1986). The walking programme in the present study was about this level and it seems was sufficient to improve health-related fitness in sedentary middle-aged men.

In conclusion, we showed that a short programme of walking could be favourable for health (cholesterol and LDL) and body fat percent in middle-aged men. Consequently, walking is an appropriate form of exercise with some benefits and can be recommended as a form of health-enhancing physical activity.

## REFERENCES

Hespel, P., Lijnen, P., Fagord, R., Vanhoof, R. and Amery, A., 1987, The effect of endurance training on blood pressure and serum lipoprotein profiles in middle aged sedentary men. *Hermes Tijdschriftvanhet Instituut voor Lichamelijke Opleiding*, **19**, 153-166.

Hinkleman, L.L. and Nieman, D.C., 1993, The effects of a walking program on body composition and serum lipids and lipoproteins in overweight women. *Journal of Sports Medicine and Physical Fitness*, **33**, 49-58.

Nakamura, N., Kobori, S., Vawa, H. and Maeda, H., 1985, The effect of regular jogging on the time course of serum high density lipoprotein cholesterol level. *International Journal of Sports Cardiology*, **2**, 55-60.

Parkkari, J., Natri, A., Kannus, P., Manttari, A., Laukkanen, R., Haapasalo, H., Nenonen, A., Pasanen, M., Oja, P.O. and Vuori, I., 2000, A controlled trial of the health benefits of regular walking on a golf course. *American Journal of Medicine*, **109**, 102-108.

Plank, E.A. and Hargreaves, E.H., 1990, The benefits of walking the golf course: effects on lipoprotein levels and risk ratios. *Physician and Sportsmedicine*, **18** (10), 77-80.

Pollock, M.L., Broida, J., Kendrick, Z., Miller, H.S. and Janeway, R., 1972, Effects of training two days per week at different intensities on middle-aged men. *Medicine and Science in Sports*, **4**, 192-197.

Savage, M.P., Petratis, M.M., Thomson, W.H., Berg, K., Smith, J.L. and Sady, S.P., 1986, Exercise training effects on serum lipids of prepubescent boys and adult men. *Medicine and Science in Sports and Exercise*, **16**, 197-204.

Stensel, D.J., Brooke-Wavell, K., Hardman, A.E., Jones, P.R.M. and Morgan, N. G., 1994, The influence of a 1 year programme of brisk walking on endurance fitness and body composition in previously sedentary men aged 42-59 years. *European Journal of Applied Physiology and Occupational Physiology*, **68**, 531-537.

Toriola, A.L., 1984, Influence of 12 week jogging on body fat and serum lipids. *British Journal of Sports Medicine*, **18**, 13-17.

White, J.L., Flohr, J., Ransdell, L. and Saunders, M.J., 2001, Time sequence of measurable changes in cardiovascular diseases risk factors as a results of physical activity in women. *International Electronic Journal of Health Education*, **4**, 361-367.

Whitehurst, M. and Menendez, Z.E., 1991, Endurance training in older women: lipid and lipoprotein responses. *Physician and Sportsmedicine*, **19** (6), 95-98.

# 25 The Investigation of Thoracic Kyphosis in Cyclists and Non-cyclists

R. Rajabi[1], A.J. Freemont[1] and P. Doherty[2]
[1]Musculoskeletal Research Group, University of Manchester, UK
[2]Manchester School of Physiotherapy, Manchester Royal Infirmary, UK

## 1. INTRODUCTION

The popularity of cycling as a recreational, competitive and transportation activity, especially in developing countries, continues to grow. In 1990 more than 56 million persons rode their bicycles six or more times within the year in the United States (Burke, 1996). In Germany about 700,000 people participate in indoor-cycling each week (Rudack et al., 2001). In the Netherlands and China around 50% of daily trips for all purposes are made by bicycle (Director-General of Transport South Australia, 1995). In Britain, there are an estimated 20 million owners of bicycles which people use for various purposes (Lumsdon, 1994). In York, 20% of all journeys to work are by bicycle (Bhopal and Unwin, 1995). Health promotion, cheap transport, leisure and competition are some reasons for cycling. The negative effects, if any, of the cycling position on the spine (posture) of the cyclist, especially while using a racing bike, remains to be properly evaluated.

The position of the spinal column during cycling differs greatly from its anatomical standing position. The position adopted by racing cyclists is a deviation from the normal alignment of the vertebral column in the standing position, which is sustained for up to eight hours per day and repeated daily for many years (Ashcroft, 1992). Theoretically this position could have an adverse effect on the spine, especially the thoracic spine, increasing the degree of kyphosis possibly by adaptive changes in some elements of the spine. The sagittal thoracic posture of cyclists and the interrelationships between posture and cycling have received little or no attention in the research literature.

Data on cycling and its direct association with the topic of this study (kyphosis) are rare. Nevertheless there are a few studies indicating increased thoracic curvature problems and concern particularly regarding cycling in adolescence. Elegem (1983) reported that 46% of a group of bicycle racers under the age of 20 presented with signs of Scheuermann's kyphosis. There are also some unpublished reports since the 19th century, which indicate some concern about cyclists' kyphosis. The most important concern, however, was about the negative effects of the riding posture in cyclists, which implicated the development of a bicycle-related kyphosis "kyphosis bicyclistarum" (Smith, 1972). In agreement, Junghanns (1990) stated that total kyphosis is an inevitable status symbol of bicycle racers. The previous studies, however, were mostly based on the experiences of physicians, coaches or cyclists. These studies did not include a control group and their sample numbers of cyclists X-rayed (or available X-rays from hospital) were also small. Therefore the current study was undertaken to investigate whether the alignment of the thoracic spine differs between cyclists and non-cyclists.

## 2. MATERIALS AND METHODS

### 2.1 Participants and materials

A sample comprising 120 British male cyclists (generally road cyclists) and 120 British male non-cyclists within four age groups (20-29, 30-39, 40-49 and 50-59 years), each group consisting of 30 subjects, was recruited for the present study. Three classes of cyclists were considered: 1) Professional-British National Team members; 2) Amateur club cyclists; and 3) Recreational cyclists. The criterion for non-cyclists in this study was not being engaged in cycling as a favourite sport, while the criterion for the cyclist group was cycling at for least 5 years.

The main research materials used in this study were:- Questionnaire (designed by the researcher) for demographic, metre rule and weight scale for anthropometirc data (Table 1) and a modified electrogoniometer (EGO) to measure kyphosis. This device is a simple non-invasive instrument that traditionally has been used to determine range of motion (ROM). The researcher modified this device to measure static thoracic spine angle in the erect standing position. After modifying original EGO for the purpose of the current study and before collecting the main data, a familiarization pilot study (n=30) was undertaken. This was carried out because the modified EGO was a new assessment tool and as such had not been validated for postural measurement. The pilot study afforded an opportunity to practice how to set the EGO on the spine in order to secure an accurate measurement and to speed up the measurement process to minimize any inconvenience to the volunteers.

Prior to commencing the main study, the intra-rater (n=30) and inter-rater agreement (n=3) reliability of the modified EGO was assessed. Validity analysis used old X-rays (n=11) from the institution's radiology department where the spinous processes of T3 to T11 (T= thoracic vertebrae) were clearly visible. Kyphosis was measured with the EGO and the Cobb's method on four separate occasions over four different days by a colleague. In both reliability and validity studies, the angle between T3 to T11 was determined as kyphosis degree.

## 2.2 Measurement procedure

The measuring procedure utilized during this study was developed with reference to current literature, and to the findings from measurement tool development and a pilot study. The general measurement procedure was similar in both groups (cyclist and non-cyclist), that is to say; 1) Each potential volunteer was provided with an introductory leaflet, which outlined the procedure and the modified EGO to be used. Verbal explanations were supplied when necessary. 2) Once the consent form was signed, subjects were given the appropriate questionnaire to complete and their weight and height were measured. 3) Subjects were asked to remove their upper-body clothing and their T3-T4 and T10-T11 spinous processes were identified. 4) The angle of kyphosis was measured as the degree between spinous processes of the third and fourth (T3 and T4) and the tenth and eleventh (T10 and T11) thoracic vertebrae. The points of measurement were localized by palpation by the researcher.

In order to define the spinous processes of T3 and T4, first the C7 spinous process was located by having the subject bend the head down and palpating the first prominence at the lower end of the neck. This method has been described by Ensrud *et al.* (1997). Then spinous processes were counted down from C7 to T3 and T4 where the positions of these two processes were marked lightly on the skin using a non-permanent marker pen. In order to define T10 and T11 spinous processes, the procedure described by Youdas *et al.* (1995) was followed. When the desired spinal processes were identified and marked, the degree of kyphosis was measured in the sagittal standing position described by Youdas *et al.* (1995). The ability of the researcher in accurately identifying bony landmarks in the spinal region (palpating the spinous processes) was considered competent and reliable by a specialist physiotherapist as he completed a tutorial course at the Manchester School of Physiotherapy, Central Manchester Health Care Trust.

The zero starting position (on display unit) was set at the start of each measurement session. Then, with the examiner standing facing the side of the subject (Figure1), the two endblocks of the modified EGO were grasped lightly between the thumb and first finger of each hand (the middle fingers were on top of the endblocks). First, the fixed endblock was placed on the spine (T10-T11), and then the telescopic endblock was pushed gently to contact on the marked spinous processes (T3 and T4). This enabled the telescopic endblock to cover the spinous processes of T3 and T4 and the fixed endblock to cover the spinous processes of T10 and T11. When the length between two marked points (T3-T4 to T10-T11) was bigger than the length of the sensor (EGO), the telescopic endblock could extend to reach the proper point to cover the spinous processes of T3-T4.

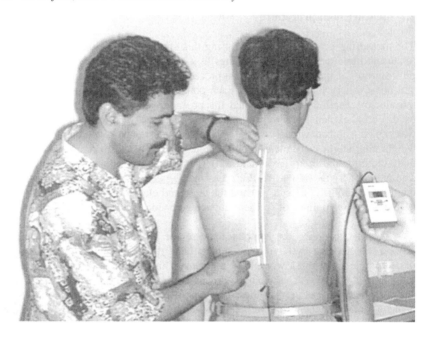

**Figure 1.** Measurement of kyphosis.

The angle of kyphosis in degrees on the angle display unit represented by the angle between the upper endblock (T3 and T4) and lower endblock (the T-10 and T-11) was recorded. To ensure there was no bias from the subjects and the investigator, subjects were kept unaware of the hypotheses of the study. The investigator was unaware of the kyphosis degree during the procedure as a colleague recorded the measurement.

In order to prevent subjects' bias influencing the result, all measurements were performed when subjects were in their usual upright posture without attempting to stand unusually straight, weight evenly on both feet, with upper clothing removed. During this time they were looking straight ahead and breathing normally with their arms hanging gently at their sides.


## 3.  RESULTS

### 3.1 Instrumentation

Intraclass correlation coefficient (ICC) established the intra-rater and inter-rater reliability of the modified EGO and found ICC=0.99 and 0.97 respectively. An additional method, limits of agreement (LOA) as described by Bland and Altman (1986) was used to show the significance of differences that ICC could not indicate. Overall the mean differences between trials was 0.31° and 0.73° with

95% confidence intervals (CI) of −1.28° to +1.88° and −3.15° to +3.53 for intra-rater and inter-rater reliability respectively. In the validity study, Pearson product moment coefficients (r) showed that the two measurement tools (Cobb's and EGO methods) were correlated (r=+0.88) in measuring the degree of kyphosis. The LOA showed an agreement between the two methods with the mean difference of 0.9° and 95% (confidence limits) of −8.3° to +10.1°.

## 3.2 Study results

Results of t-test showed that the degree of kyphosis was significantly higher among cyclists (mean 30.7°; SD 5.8°) compared with non-cyclists as a whole (mean 25.5°; SD 6.0°) (p<0.001) (Figure 2).

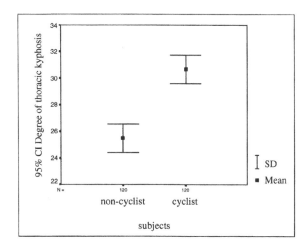

**Figure 2.** Mean values of kyphosis among the study participants (n=240).

To investigate whether any statistically significant difference existed in kyphosis between the subjects (non-cyclist versus cyclist groups) in different age groups, a one-way analysis of variance (ANOVA) was performed. The result of ANOVA was significant ($F_{7,232} = 7.40$, p<0.001). Post hoc analysis (Tukey's procedure) indicated that all the four cyclist groups had a significantly higher degree of kyphosis (p<0.05) than their non-cyclist pairs (Table 2). The anthropometirc data for the non-cyclists and cyclists are incorporated in Table 1.

**Table 1**. Demographic and anthropometric data characteristics of the study participants (n=240).

| | Age group | N | Non-cyclist Mean | SD | Min | Max | Cyclist Mean | SD | Min | Max |
|---|---|---|---|---|---|---|---|---|---|---|
| **Age** | 20-29 | 30 | 24.3 | 2.9 | 20 | 29 | 23.4 | 3.2 | 20 | 29 |
| | 30-39 | 30 | 34.8 | 2.9 | 30 | 38 | 33.7 | 2.9 | 30 | 39 |
| | 40-49 | 30 | 44.0 | 2.7 | 40 | 49 | 44.2 | 2.6 | 40 | 49 |
| | 50-59 | 30 | 53.3 | 2.9 | 50 | 59 | 54.8 | 3.3 | 50 | 59 |
| Total | 20-59 | 120 | 39.1 | 11.2 | 20 | 59 | 38.9 | 12.1 | 20 | 59 |
| **Height (m)** | 20-29 | 30 | 1.82 | 0.66 | 1.63 | 1.95 | 1.78 | 0.07 | 1.71 | 2.04 |
| | 30-39 | 30 | 1.80 | 0.79 | 1.69 | 1.93 | 1.80 | 0.05 | 1.60 | .1.99 |
| | 40-49 | 30 | 1.79 | 0.71 | 1.56 | 1.95 | 1.67 | 0.076 | 1.71 | 1.96 |
| | 50-59 | 30 | 1.80 | 0.07 | 1.65 | 1.83 | 1.76 | 0.045 | 1.60 | 1.90 |
| Total | 20-59 | 120 | 180.2 | 7.1 | 150 | 195 | 177.6 | 6.6 | 160 | 204 |
| **Mass (kg)** | 20-29 | 30 | 78.6 | 9.9 | 60 | 87 | 73.6 | 9.9 | 59 | 102 |
| | 30-39 | 30 | 87.3 | 12.2 | 59 | 90 | 75.5 | 12.2 | 54 | 131 |
| | 40-49 | 30 | 87.0 | 12.2 | 65 | 110 | 78.5 | 12.2 | 51 | 111 |
| | 50-59 | 30 | 85.2 | 12.3 | 61 | 99 | 74.4 | 12.3 | 61 | 107 |
| Total | 20-59 | 120 | 83.8 | 12.7 | 59 | 110 | 75.5 | 9.3 | 51 | 131 |
| **BMI** | 20-29 | 30 | 23.7 | 2.9 | 19.3 | 32.4 | 23.4 | 3.1 | 19.5 | 31.6 |
| | 30-39 | 30 | 26.0 | 3.9 | 20.1 | 39.5 | 23.4 | 2.6 | 18.2 | 29.4 |
| | 40-49 | 30 | 27.1 | 3.5 | 16.3 | 36.1 | 25.4 | 2.8 | 22.0 | 34.1 |
| | 50-59 | 30 | 26.3 | 3.8 | 18.6 | 34.4 | 24.0 | 3.3 | 19.8 | 32.7 |
| Total | 20-59 | 120 | 25.8 | 3.7 | 16.3 | 39.5 | 24.1 | 3.1 | 18.2 | 34.1 |

**Table 2**. Values of kyphosis in different age groups (n=240).

| Age Range | Non-cyclist Mean | SD | Cyclist Mean | SD | F | p |
|---|---|---|---|---|---|---|
| 20-29 | 24.2 | 6.3 | 29.2 | 6.3 | 4.92 | 0.02 |
| 30-39 | 25.4 | 4.3 | 30.9 | 5.9 | 5.49 | 0.001 |
| 40-49 | 25.4 | 5 | 30.9 | 5.5 | 5.48 | 0.001 |
| 50-59 | 26.6 | 7.2 | 31.6 | 5.6 | 4.83 | 0.03 |

Analysis of data by category of cycling (leisure; amateur and professional), and preferred type of handlebar (aerobar, racing and straight handlebar) showed no significant difference in kyphosis among these variables (p>0.05). Hence, within group comparison of kyphosis amongst different age categories was not significant (p>0.05). Multiple regression (Step-wise) did not show a significant association between kyphosis and predictive variables (age; average time spent on saddle in each training session; average mileage cycled per week; frequency of training and length of career in cycling). Although the result for the predictor variables of body mass index and age at starting serious cycling was statistically significant (r=0.26; p=0.046), $R^2$ was 0.07, which suggests that 93% of the variance can not be explained by these variables.

## 4. DISCUSSION

The results of this study showed that the mean degree of kyphosis of cyclists was higher than in non-cyclists as a whole. This study also showed that the mean degree of kyphosis in all four age ranges in cyclists was higher than in non-cyclists. One of the reasons for this finding amongst cyclists might be the mechanical stress on the anterior portion of the spinal column whilst adopting the cycling position. This seems to be more likely when the cyclist is younger. This is emphasised by a theory that suggests a "remodelling" or "reforming" of the vertebral bone in the presence of anterior compression as a result of the flexed kyphotic posture in cycling (Elegem, 1983). This theory suggests that less compressive stress in the posterior part of the vertebral column leads to increased growth of this area compared with the anterior portion of the vertebral body, which is under more compressive stress.

In comparison with the usual (anatomical) posture of the spine in the standing position, competitive cycling puts this part of the body (spine) in an unusual position. Theoretically this position seems to have an adverse effect on the spine and might be an important factor associated with increased kyphosis. When the spine is exposed to flexion stress, e.g. in the cycling position, the anterior portion of the vertebral body in the affected region experiences a compressive load that is greater than the tensile load on the posterior portion of the vertebral body (Mellion, 1994). This situation could lead to an increased kyphosis of the thoracic spine. Possible explanations of increased kyphosis amongst the cyclists revolve around two theories.

One theory is that the pressure on the anterior portion of the vertebra as a result of flexed kyphotic posture in cycling produces a "remodelling" or "reforming" of the bone resulting in the appearance of anterior compression. Due to little compressive stress in the posterior part of the vertebral column there is an increase in growth of this area compared with the anterior portion of the vertebral body (Mellion, 1994). Another theory is that the heavily flexed position in cyclists causes fractures of the anterior portion of the vertebral end plate, resulting in vertebral wedging (Micheli, 1985; Sward *et al.*, 1990).

Although there is no experimental evidence to support either view, predictions can be made by Wolff's law in respect of bone (generally) and by Volkmann's law in respect of vertebrae (specifically). Volkmann's law indicates that pressure on an epiphysis delays the speed of growth in an affected area whilst tension in the posterior portion of the vertebral column increases the amount of growth. The similar situation (the flexed position of the spine) during cycling puts more pressure on the anterior portion in comparison with the posterior portion of the vertebrae. If the cyclist is young, this pressure could compress the anterior vertebral epiphysis, which can delay the speed of growth in this area. Therefore this might lead to increased kyphosis amongst cyclists. According to Junghanns (1990), the above situation may even lead to a further increase of kyphosis in cyclists if they produce a traction force by pulling on the handlebars.

Regarding the above-mentioned theories and laws, it can be postulated that there is an association between the normal development of the sagittal curvatures of the spine and the mechanical environment (excessive compressive loading of the anterior and tensile loading of the posterior portion of the thoracic vertebrae) in cyclists. This may affect the vertebral shape in the affected region (thoracic) and thereby, potentially the thoracic curvature as a whole.

The influence of mechanical loading (stress) on the thoracic vertebrae in the flexed position and its association with morphological adaptation of the thoracic elements and an accompanying increase in thoracic kyphosis are well established (Nordin and Frankel, 1980; Goh *et al.*, 1999 and Watkins, 1999). There was no attempt to analyze the cause and effect relationship between cycling and kyphosis in this study. According to the literature the increased kyphosis in cyclists may be attributed to; 1-Change in the vertebral body, especially in young cyclists as a result of compressive force in the anterior part (Volkmann's law). 2- Change in the intervertebral discs as a result of anterior compressive forces. 3- Degenerative change in the two above elements (vertebral body and intervertebral discs). 4- Adaptation in posterior spinal musculature (muscles and ligaments) (Goh *et al.*, 1999 and Sizer *et al.*, 2001).

This study suggests a strong relationship between cycling posture and kyphosis, the reasons for which will only be adequately determined by an experimental study and possibly with some invasive device e.g. use of X-ray method on vertebral bodies.

It is concluded that kyphosis differs between cyclists and non-cyclists in all age categories. The mechanism for this increase in kyphosis is theoretically supported and implicates the cycling posture as a contributor to kyphosis.

## REFERENCES

Ashcroft, H., 1992, Standing sagittal spinal curvature in cyclists and non-cyclists. B.App.Sc. Physiotherapy project (Honours), University of South Australia.

Bhopal, R. and Unwin, N. 1995, Cycling, physical exercise, and the millennium fund. *British Medical Journal* [5 August], 311-344.

Bland, J.M. and Altman, D.G., 1986, Statistical methods for assessing agreement between two methods of clinical measurement. Lancet Feb;1(8476):307-10.

Burke E.R., 1996, Cycling. In *The Spine in Sports*, edited by Watkins, R.G. (St. Louis, London: Mosby), pp. 593-560.

Director-General of Transport South Australia, 1995. A Review of Bicycle Policy and Planning Developments in Western Europe and North America – *A Literature Search*. Director-General of Transport South Australia .

Elegem, P., 1983, Bicycling and chronic pathology. *Acta Orthopedica Belgica*, **49**, 88-100.

Ensrud, K.E., Black, D.M., Harris, F., Ettinger, B. and Cummings, S.R., 1997, Correlates of kyphosis in older women. The Fracture Intervention Trial Research Group. *Journal of the American Geriatric Society*, **45**, 682-687.

Goh, S., Price, R.I., Leedman, P.J. and Singer, K.P., 1999, The relative influence of vertebral body and intervertebral disc shape on thoracic kyphosis. *Clinical Biomechanics (Bristol., Avon.)*, **14**, 439-448.

Junghanns, H., 1990, *Clinical Implications of Normal Biomechanical Stresses on Spinal Function,* English Language Edition, edited by Hager, H.J., (Aspen, Rockvile, Maryland).

Lumsdon, L., 1994, *Cycle UK!: The Essential Guide to Leisure Cycling,* (Wilmslow: Sigma Leisure).

Mellion, M.B., 1994, Neck and back pain in bicycling. *Clinics in Sports Medicine*, **13**, 137-164.

Micheli, L.J., 1985, Back injuries in gymnastics. *Clinics in Sports Medicine*, **4**, 85-93.

Nordin, M. and Frankel, V.H., 1980, *Basic Biomechanics of the Musculoskeletal Systems,* First Edition, (Philadelphia: Lea & Febiger).

Rudack, P., Kilch, K., Formme, A., Mooren, F., Thorwesten, L. and Volker, K., 2001, *Characteristic parameters of physical exercise in indoor-cycling as a (typical) fitness sport*. German Society of Sport Science, Koln.

Sizer, P.S., Phelps, V. and Azevedo, E. 2001, Disc related and non-disc related disorders of the thoracic spine. *Pain Practice*, **1**[2], 136-149.

Smith, R.A., 1972, *A Social History of the Bicycle, Its Early Life and Times in America,* (New York: American Heritage Press).

Sward, L., Hellstrom, M., Jacobsson, B. and Peterson, L., 1990, Back pain and radiologic changes in the thoraco-lumbar spine of athletes. *Spine*, **15**, 124-129.

Watkins, J., 1999, *Structure and Function of the Musculoskeletal System,* Champaign, IL.: Human Kinetics).

Youdas, J.W., Suman, V.J. and Garrett, T.R., 1995, Reliability of measurements of lumbar spine sagittal mobility obtained with the flexible curve. *Journal of Orthopaedic and Sports Physical Therapy*, **21**, 13-20.

# 26 Health-related Fitness Trends in 6-12 Year-old New Zealand Children from 1984-85 to 2000

Michael Hamlin[1], Jenny Ross[1] and Sang-Wan Hong[2]
[1]Human Sciences Division, Lincoln University,
Canterbury, New Zealand
[2]Daegu National University of Education, Daegu, Korea

## 1. INTRODUCTION

Adults in most developed countries have undergone a significant change in body size and composition over the last century. If population data are generalised for developed countries over the 20th century, such trends typically indicate an increase in height of about 1 cm per decade and an increase in body mass of about 1 kg per decade (Meredith, 1976; Pheasant, 1996). However, since the mid-1980s body mass has increased disproportionately to height in adults. Between 1989 and 1997 the average New Zealand adult increased in weight by 3.2 kg but demonstrated no significant change in height, resulting in an overall increase in BMI of 1.1 $kg.m^{-2}$ over this 8-year period (Russell and Wilson, 1991; Russell et al., 1999). Unfortunately the increase in body mass and BMI values found in adults are also starting to appear in the younger generation. Recent data on 10-14 year old New Zealand children indicate that height did not change during the 1990s but body mass increased by 2.5 kg and BMI by 1.23 $kg.m^{-2}$ over this decade.

An increase in body mass without changes in height can be attributed to either higher energy intakes or lower energy outputs, or some combination of the two. Overseas studies report children's weight as progressively increasing despite consuming similar or lower total calories (Muecke et al., 1992; James, 1995). While there is little research on the caloric intake of New Zealand children's diets, there is growing evidence that older New Zealand children and adolescents are becoming less physically active (Calvert et al., 2001) and that fitness levels in these older children are declining (Dawson et al., 2001) at a similar rate to trends found overseas (Dollman et al., 1999; Luepker, 1999). Such changes are a cause for concern as increased body fat and reduced fitness levels are associated with health problems such as lower bone mass (Goulding et al., 2000), hyperlipidaemia (Freedman et al., 1992), hypertension (Hill and Trowbridge, 1998) and increased prevalence of diabetes (Hypponen et al., 2000). It is currently unknown whether the changes in body shape and health-related fitness parameters found in 10-14 year-old New Zealand Intermediate school children are also occurring in younger primary school children. The aim of this study was to investigate changes in health-related fitness parameters of young New Zealand primary school-aged children over a 15-16 year period. This study found that despite the recognised health benefits of regular physical activity, New Zealand children as young as 10 years old have poorer aerobic fitness levels and higher BMI values than children of a similar age 15-16 years ago. Such trends may result in a deterioration of children's health and increase the risk of obesity and other associated morbidities later in life.

## 2. METHODS

Fitness variables that are related to health were measured on 228 boys and 195 girls (aged 5-12 years) from five randomly selected Christchurch primary schools. The schools covered a range of socio-economic areas. The test parameters and procedures completed in 2000 were identical to tests completed on children in earlier surveys (Department of Education, 1984; Russell *et al.*, 1989). Informed consent was obtained from each child and the parent/guardian and the study carried the approval of the Canterbury Ethics Committee. Children were tested at their own school, during school hours. Children were tested in light clothing with shoes removed for height (stretch stature method with a Seca stadiometer, Hamburg, Germany) and weight with calibrated portable scales (Seca, Hamburg, Germany). One researcher with the aid of an assistant, measured children's skinfolds at two sites (triceps and subscapular) with Harpenden skinfold calipers (West Sussex, England). Measurement was taken to the nearest 0.1 mm and an average of three readings was obtained. Children's sit-and-reach, broad jump and 550-m run performance were also measured and a full description of these tests may be found in Russell *et al.* (1989) and Department of Education (1984).

An unpaired t-test assuming unequal variance was used to analyse the differences in the health-related fitness measures between the 6, 8, 10 and 12 year-old children in 2000 and similar data published in 1984 (Department of Education, 1984) and 1985 (Russell *et al.*, 1989). The data for 5, 7, 9 and 11 year olds were not used in this analysis because the earlier surveys did not sample these age groups. Measurements of broad jump and 550-m run, were not taken in the 1984-85 studies on the younger children (6 and 8 year-olds), therefore comparisons on these parameters between the 1984-85 and 2000 cohorts are for the 10 and 12 year old children only. A p value of 5% was chosen for declaration of statistical significance; precision of estimates were represented by the 95% confidence interval.

## 3. RESULTS

Younger boys (6 and 8 year olds) and girls (6 year olds) from the 2000 cohort were significantly taller (Tables 1 and 2) than their 1984-85 peers (p < 0.05), but no significant difference in height was observed in the older children. Girls aged 12 years and boys aged 8 years and older in the 2000 cohort tended to be heavier than their 1984-85 peers but these increases in weight were not significant (Tables 1 and 2). However, the sum of skinfolds for 12-year-old girls was significantly higher in the 2000 cohort compared to the 1984-85 cohort (Table 2).

**Table 1**. Comparison of health-related fitness levels in 6-12 year old boys between 1984-85 and 2000.

| | Height (m) | Mass (kg) | BMI (kg.m⁻²) | Sit & Reach (cm) | Skinfolds (mm) | Broad Jump (cm) | 550-m Run (s) |
|---|---|---|---|---|---|---|---|
| 6 year olds | | | | | | | |
| 1984-85 | 1.21 ± 0.05 | 23.8 ± 3 | 16.2 ± 2* | 27 ± 6 | 15.5 ± 4 | | |
| 2000 | 1.25 ± 0.04* | 23.2 ± 2 | 14.8 ± 1 | 27 ± 4 | 15.6 ± 4 | 134 ± 19 | 200 ± 27 |
| 8 year olds | | | | | | | |
| 1984-85 | 1.32 ± 0.05 | 28.8 ± 5 | 16.8 ± 3 | 25 ± 7 | 16.7 ± 6 | | |
| 2000 | 1.34 ± 0.03* | 29.4 ± 4 | 16.3 ± 2 | 23 ± 5* | 16.9 ± 6 | 161 ± 15 | 165 ± 30 |
| 10 year olds | | | | | | | |
| 1984-85 | 1.43 ± 0.06 | 36.5 ± 6 | 17.7 ± 3 | 24 ± 7 | 19.9 ± 10 | 165 ± 29 | 134 ± 25 |
| 2000 | 1.43 ± 0.06 | 38.2 ± 7 | 18.4 ± 3* | 22 ± 5* | 22.4 ± 12 | 172 ± 20* | 154 ± 21* |
| 12 year olds | | | | | | | |
| 1984-85 | 1.54 ± 0.08 | 44.7 ± 8 | 18.6 ± 3 | 23 ± 8 | 20.3 ± 10 | 182 ± 34 | 126 ± 26 |
| 2000 | 1.52 ± 0.08 | 45.5 ± 10 | 19.3 ± 3* | 20 ± 8* | 19.1 ± 8 | 180 ± 29 | 157 ± 36* |

Data are mean ± SD. * Indicates significantly different means.

**Table 2.** Comparison of health-related fitness levels in 6-12 year old girls between 1984-85 and 2000.

| | Height (m) | Mass (kg) | BMI (kg.m$^{-2}$) | Sit & Reach (cm) | Skinfolds (mm) | Broad Jump (cm) | 550-m Run (s) |
|---|---|---|---|---|---|---|---|
| **6 year olds** | | | | | | | |
| 1984-85 | 1.20 ± 0.05 | 23.7 ± 3 | 16.3 ± 2* | 29 ± 6 | 19.2 ± 5 | | |
| 2000 | 1.23 ± 0.04* | 23.0 ± 4 | 15.0 ± 2 | 27 ± 4 | 20.5 ± 8 | 128 ± 14 | 208 ± 28 |
| **8 year olds** | | | | | | | |
| 1984-85 | 1.32 ± 0.05 | 30.0 ± 5 | 17.0 ± 3 | 28 ± 7 | 21.9 ± 8 | | |
| 2000 | 1.32 ± 0.04 | 29.7 ± 6 | 16.8 ± 3 | 27 ± 4* | 22.2 ± 8 | 145 ± 13 | 182 ± 29 |
| **10 year olds** | | | | | | | |
| 1984-85 | 1.43 ± 0.06 | 37.7 ± 7 | 18.1 ± 4 | 28 ± 5 | 25.7 ± 11 | 160 ± 29 | 150 ± 27 |
| 2000 | 1.44 ± 0.07 | 36.8 ± 8 | 17.6 ± 2 | 25 ± 6* | 23.9 ± 8 | 157 ± 22 | 166 ± 17* |
| **12 year olds** | | | | | | | |
| 1984-85 | 1.56 ± 0.06 | 47.6 ± 9 | 19.5 ± 3 | 29 ± 8 | 26.1 ± 10 | 176 ± 32 | 142 ± 29 |
| 2000 | 1.55 ± 0.07 | 49.3 ± 11 | 20.6 ± 4* | 26 ± 8* | 30.6 ± 13* | 160 ± 28* | 171 ± 37* |

Data are mean ± SD. * Indicates significantly different means.

Although the 1984-85 surveys did not supply BMI information, we were able to calculate mean BMI from the height and mass data. Unexpectedly the BMI was significantly higher in the 1984-85, 6-year-old children compared to their 2000 cohort peers; this increase was not due to increased body mass but a significantly lower overall height (Table 1 and 2). The BMI was significantly higher in the older 2000 cohort children (10-12 year old boys and 12 year old girls) compared to their 1984-85 cohort peers.

Boys and girls aged 8 years old and over had significantly poorer sit-and-reach scores in 2000 compared to the children in 1984-85. While 10-year-old boys' broad jumping ability was significantly better in 2000 than in the 1984-85 cohort, 12-year-old girls' broad jump performance had significantly declined since 1984-85. Ten-year-old girls' 550-m run performance in 2000 was 16 s (95% CI = 10-22, $p < 0.05$) and boys' 20 s (CI = 14-26, $p < 0.05$) slower than their peers in 1984-85. Similarly, 12-year-old girls were 29 s (CI = 20-38, $p < 0.05$) and boys were 31 s

(CI = 24-38, p < 0.05) slower than children of similar age in 1984-85 (Table 1 and 2).

## 4. DISCUSSION

It was interesting to find that younger, but not older children were significantly taller in 2000 than their counterparts back in 1984-85. In a recent study investigating trends in health-related fitness of 5579, 10-14 year-old New Zealand children, no significant difference was found in height over a nine-year period (Dawson *et al.*, 2001). The increased height in the young children in the 2000 cohort of this study may be explained by differences in the genetic makeup between the two cohorts or by differences in the mean ages of the two cohorts. Since five and six-year olds can increase height by about 5-6 cm per year (Whitehouse and Takaishi, 1966), the mean age of the two cohorts will significantly influence results. The 2000 cohort six-year-olds had a mean age of 6.2 years but unfortunately the mean age of the 1984-85 six-year-old cohort is unavailable. It would also be interesting to see whether the difference in height in these younger children remained if sample sizes were increased.

The 2000 cohort was sampled from a range of socio-economic areas, which may have been considerably different to the socio-economic make-up of the 1984-85 cohort sample. Changes in the socio-economic make-up of cohorts may influence parameters such as physical activity levels (Yang *et al.*, 1996) and body weight (Bray, 1999). New Zealand has a multicultural society, which is dominated by people from a European background, but Maori and Pacific Islanders, as well as Asians also make up the total population. Approximately 85% of the children sampled in the 2000 cohort were European, 10% were Maori or Pacific Islanders, and 5% were of Asian descent, which is similar to the ethnic make-up of New Zealand as a whole, but may be considerably different from the ethnic make-up of the 1984-85 cohort sample which was not published. Any change in the ethnic make-up of the two samples may affect the results of this study. For example, the number of Pacific Island people living in New Zealand has doubled between 1981 and 1996 (Statistics New Zealand, 2001) and it is well known that Pacific Island children are significantly taller, heavier and have higher BMI values than European children (Salesa *et al.*, 1997). In addition, due to problems of different measurement techniques used in the two population samples, some technique-related variability may have occurred particularly in relation to measuring skinfolds. The relatively large samples involved will help to balance out such distortions.

Whereas no significant change in body mass was witnessed in this study, it was noticeable that the older children's mean mass was in most cases higher in 2000 than in 1984-85. As body mass had increased but height remained unchanged, the BMI increased significantly for these older 2000 cohort children. In addition, the 12-year-old 2000 cohort girls had a significantly higher skinfold thickness than similarly-aged girls in 1984-85. It is well documented that older children in New Zealand (Dawson *et al.*, 2001), and overseas (Tremblay and

Willms, 2000) are becoming heavier and fatter and that the proportion of children classified as overweight or obese is increasing dramatically (Chinn and Rona, 2001; Dawson *et al.*, 2001). The present study shows that New Zealanders as young as 10 years of age are starting to be affected by the overweight epidemic.

An increase in body weight can be attributed to an increase in energy intake, a decrease in energy output or some combination of both. International studies indicate that children are eating the same (Troiano *et al.*, 2000) or less overall calories (Cavadini *et al.*, 2000) than previously, which suggests that the increased prevalence of obesity found in today's children results from decreased energy expenditure rather than increased energy intake.

In a study that used heart rate data to estimate daily physical activity levels, only 53% of 10-13 year-old New Zealand children met the Ministry of Health's Physical Activity Guideline, which is to accumulate 30-60 min of moderate intensity physical activity per day (Calvert *et al.*, 2001). It also seems that New Zealand children's involvement in physical activity at school may also be decreasing. A recent study indicated that allocated physical education time in New Zealand primary and intermediate schools had dropped significantly between 1984 and 1993 (Ross *et al.*, 1995). While decreased energy expenditure may well be one of the mechanisms behind the increased weight of children, more research is required to substantiate the magnitude of change in energy expenditure levels of New Zealand children both at home and at school.

A clear sign of deteriorating physical activity levels is a decrease in physical fitness scores. The children in this study were found to have a significantly poorer 550-m run performance than the children in 1984-85. The size of the decrement in performance was considerable and matched reports of decreased aerobic fitness in previous studies on school-aged children in New Zealand (Dawson *et al.*, 2001), Australia (Dollman *et al.*, 1999) and the United States (Luepker, 1999). While the trend is not so clear for anaerobic power (estimated by the broad jump test), children's flexibility also deteriorated. Inactive lifestyles in children result in low physical fitness levels (Pate *et al.*, 1990), which are related to increased health problems such as low bone mineral density (Turner *et al.*, 1992) and increased levels of obesity and type 1 diabetes (Hypponen *et al.*, 2000). Poor aerobic fitness has been linked to increased cardiovascular disease risk and total mortality (Boreham *et al.*, 2001; Erickssen, 2001).

The recent increase in passive electronic entertainment has been blamed for much of the deterioration in children's fitness and the increase in children's weight (Grund *et al.*, 2001). Passive entertainment draws children away from physical recreation and active leisure into more passive forms of leisure, which is thought to impact on childhood obesity in three ways. Firstly, television viewing displaces physical activity; secondly, it further reduces resting metabolic rate and thirdly, children often increase calorie consumption while watching television (Robinson, 2001). In a recent study, a significant relationship was reported between television viewing and obesity prevalence in 9 to 16-year old children (Hernandez *et al.*, 1999). Moreover, when electronic entertainment including television viewing was reduced children's body fat levels decreased (Robinson, 1999).

Promotion of active recreation is one way to help ease the problem of deteriorating fitness and body fat levels. Suitable and appropriate activities for children need to incorporate fun, be inexpensive, uncomplicated and burn energy. Many agencies including schools, local and central governments, parents and health-care workers have a mandate to facilitate and promote such activities. Parents can also promote more habitual physical activity in children by encouraging and promoting manual tasks around the home like washing the car, mowing the lawn and digging the garden. Walking or cycling to schools can also consume a significant amount of energy and provide exercise for the working muscles of children. In a recent survey of Christchurch schools just over half of the children were transported to school in cars despite the majority of them (66%) actually preferring to walk and cycle (Christchurch City Council City Streets Unit, 1999).

While the home is probably the ideal environment for promoting physical activity, it has become difficult to encourage such behaviour in the busy modern two-income family. As an alternative, school settings can provide a structured and safe environment where interventions may be more successful. Physical activity intervention programmes in the New Zealand (Dragicevick *et al.*, 1987) and Australian school settings (Dwyer *et al.*, 1983) have shown limited short-term success. If we are to make any significant change to children's health and physical activity patterns then a more long-term, holistic, co-ordinated and structured national approach is warranted including the family, sports and physical recreation clubs, local and central government.

## REFERENCES

Boreham, C., Twisk, J., Murray, L., Savage, M., Strain, J.J. and Cran, G., 2001, Fitness, fatness, and coronary heart disease risk in adolescents: the Northern Ireland Young Hearts Project. *Medicine and Science in Sports and Exercise*, **33**, 270-274.

Bray, G.A., 1999, Nutrition and obesity: prevention and treatment. *Nutrition Metabolism Cardiovascular Diseases*, **9**, 21-32.

Calvert, S.A., Ross, J.J. and Hamlin, M.J., 2001, Levels of physical activity of a sample of 10-13 year old New Zealand children. *New Zealand Medical Journal*, **114**, 496-498.

Cavadini, C., Siega-Riz, A.M. and Popkin, B.M., 2000, US adolescent food intake trends from 1965 to 1996. *Western Journal of Medicine*, **173**, 378-383.

Chinn, S. and Rona, R.J., 2001, Prevalence and trends in overweight and obesity in three cross sectional studies of British children, 1974-94. *British Medical Journal*, **322**, 24-26.

Christchurch City Council City Streets Unit. 1999, Safe Routes To School. *(New Zealand: Christchurch City Council, 2001). Retrieved August 8, 2001 from the World Wide Web: http://www.ccc.govt.nz/SafeRoutes.*

Dawson, K.A., Hamlin, M.J., Ross, J.J. and Duffy, D.F., 2001, Trends in the health-related physical fitness of 10-14 year old New Zealand children. *Journal of Physical Education New Zealand*, **34**, 26-39.

Department of Education, 1984, *Trial Revision Fitness Activities – Physical Education – 2-F2*. (Wellington: Government Printer).

Dollman, J., Olds, T., Norton, K. and Stuart, D., 1999, The evolution of fitness and fatness in 10-11-year-old Australian schoolchildren: Changes in distributional characteristics between 1985 and 1997. *Pediatric Exercise Science*, **11**, 108-121.

Dragicevick, A.R., Hill, P.M., Hopkins, W.G. and Walker, N.P., 1987, The effects of a year of physical education on physical fitness in two Auckland schools. *New Zealand Journal of Health, Physical Education and Recreation*, **20**, 7-11.

Dwyer, T., Coonan, W.E., Leitch, D.R., Hertzel, B.S. and Baghurst, R.A., 1983, An investigation of the effects of daily physical activity on the health of primary school students in South Australia. *International Journal of Epidemiology*, **12**, 308-313.

Erickssen, G., 2001, Physical fitness and changes in mortality: the survival of the fittest. *Sports Medicine*, **31**, 571-576.

Freedman, D.S., Lee, S.L., Byers, T., Kuester, S. and Sell, K.I., 1992, Serum cholesterol levels in a multiracial sample of 7439 preschool children from Arizona. *Preventive Medicine*, **21**, 162-176.

Goulding, A., Taylor, R.W., Jones, I.E., McAuley, K.A., Manning, P.J. and Williams, S.M., 2000, Overweight and obese children have low bone mass and area for their weight. *International Journal of Obesity Related Metabolic Disorders*, **24**, 627-632.

Grund, A., Krause, H., Siewers, M., Rieckert, H. and Muller, M.J., 2001, Is TV viewing an index of physical activity and fitness in overweight and normal weight children? *Public Health Nutrition*, **4**, 1245-1251.

Hernandez, B., Gortmaker, S.L., Colditz, G.A., Peterson, K.E., Laird, N.M. and Parra-Cabrera, S., 1999, Association of obesity with physical activity, television programs and other forms of video viewing among children in Mexico city. *International Journal of Obesity Related Metabolic Disorders*, **23**, 845-854.

Hill, J.O. and Trowbridge, F.L., 1998, Childhood obesity: future directions and research priorities. *Pediatrics*, **101**, 570-574.

Hypponen, E., Virtanen, S.M., Kenward, M.G., Knip, M. and Akerblom, H.K., 2000, Obesity, increased linear growth, and risk of type 1 diabetes in children. *Diabetes Care*, **23**, 1755-1760.

James, W.P., 1995, A public health approach to the problem of obesity. *International Journal of Obesity*, **19**, S37-S45.

Luepker, R.V., 1999, How physically active are American children and what can we do about it? *International Journal of Obesity*, **23**, S12-S17.

Meredith, H.V., 1976, Findings from Asia, Australia, Europe and North America on secular change in mean height of children, youth and young adults. *American Journal of Physical Anthropology*, **44**, 315-326.

Muecke, L., Simons-Morton, B., Huang, I.W. and Parcel, G., 1992, Is childhood obesity associated with high-fat foods and low physical activity? *Journal of School Health*, **62**, 19-23.

Pate, R.R., Dowda, M. and Ross, J.G., 1990, Associations between physical activity and physical fitness in American children. *American Journal of Diseases of Children*, **144**, 1123-1129.

Pheasant, S.T., 1996, *Bodyspace: Anthropometry, Ergonomics and the Design of Work*. (London: Taylor & Francis).

Robinson, T.N., 1999, Reducing children's television viewing to prevent obesity: a randomised controlled trial. *Journal of American Medical Association*, **282**, 1561-1567.

Robinson, T.N., 2001, Television viewing and childhood obesity. *Pediatric Clinics of North America*, **48**, 1017-1025.

Ross, J., Hargreaves, J. and Cowley, V., 1995, The demise of school physical education with deregulation. In *Proceedings of the ANZALS Conference*, Canterbury, edited by Simpson, C. and Gidlow, B. (Canturbury: Lincoln University), pp. 242-247.

Russell, D.G., Isaac, A. and Wilson, P.G., 1989, *The New Zealand Fitness Test Handbook: A test of health related fitness*. (Wellington: Hillary Court Print Ltd).

Russell, D.G., Parnell, W. and Wilson, N., 1999, *NZ Food: NZ People. Key results of the 1997 National Nutrition Survey*. (Wellington: Ministry of Health).

Russell, D.G. and Wilson, N.C., 1991, *Life in New Zealand Commission Report Volume 1: Executive Overview*. (Dunedin, N.Z.: University of Otago).

Salesa, J.S., Bell, A.C. and Swinburn, B.A., 1997, Body size of New Zealand Pacific Islands children and teenagers. *New Zealand Medical Journal*, **110**, 227-229.

Statistics New Zealand. 2001, Pacific Peoples. *(New Zealand: Statistics New Zealand, 2001, December 06). Retrieved May 28, 2002 from the World Wide Web:http://www.stats.govt.nz/domino/external/web/prod_serv.nsf/htmldocs/ Pacific+peoples*.

Tremblay, M.S. and Willms, J.D., 2000, Secular trends in the body mass index of Canadian children. *Canadian Medical Association Journal*, **163**, 1429-1433.

Troiano, R.P., Briefel, R.R., Carroll, M.D. and Bialostosky, K., 2000, Energy and fat intakes of children and adolescents in the united states: data from the national health and nutrition examination surveys. *American Journal of Clinical Nutrition*, **72**, 1343S-1353S.

Turner, J.G., Gilchrist, N.L., Ayling, E.M., Hassall, A.J., Hooke, E.A. and Sadler, W.A., 1992, Factors affecting bone mineral density in high school girls. *New Zealand Medical Journal*, **25**, 95-96.

Whitehouse, R.J. and Takaishi, M., 1966, Standards from birth to maturity for height, weight, height velocity and weight velocity: British children, 1965. I. *Archives of Disease in Childhood*, **41**, 454-471.

Yang, X., Telamo, R. and Laakso, L., 1996, Parents' physical activity, socioeconomic status and education as predictors of physical activity and sport among children and youths – a 12 year follow up study. *International Review of Sociology of Sport*, **31**, 273-294.

# 27  Anthropometric and Somatotype Characteristics of HIV+ Lipodystrophic Individuals Undergoing 'Haart' Therapy

Dominic A. Doran[1], Paul Chantler[1], Simon Jones [2] and Peter Leatt[1]
[1]Research Institute for Sport and Exercise Sciences, Liverpool John Moores University, UK
[2]HIV Research Group, The University of Liverpool, UK

## 1. INTRODUCTION

Current treatment regimens for HIV infection are based on pharmacological intervention with nucleoside reverse transcriptase inhibitors (NRTI) and protease inhibitors (PI), which act to constrain HIV viral replication and reduce systemic viral load (Hammer et al., 1997). To enhance their potency these medications are generally prescribed in combination under the term 'Highly Active Anti-Retroviral Therapy' (HAART). Adherence to these therapies has been causally linked with the development of various metabolic disorders and alterations in body morphology in both paediatric and adult populations (Hengel et al., 1997; Carr et al., 1998; Babl et al., 2002; Tsiodras et al., 2000; van de Valk et al., 2001; Amaya et al., 1999).   Some questioned the validity of this causal relationship given reported lipodystrophy in the absence of HAART therapy (Kotler, 2000; Saint-Marc et al., 2000). Irrespective of the controversy, patients on 'HAART' typically present with a combination of symptoms including hyperlipidaemia, insulin resistance, osteopenia and adipose tissue wasting and/or redistribution, collectively termed lipodystrophy syndrome (Carr et al., 1998; Carr et al., 1999). Rather than be seen a single entity, at least several lipodystrophic phenotypes are expressed, e.g. lipodystrophy with subcutaneous lipoathrophy from the periphery (arms, legs) and fat pads of the face (Ho et al., 1999). A mixed lipodystrophy with lipoathrophy and adipose tissue redistribution is evidenced by enlargement of the dorsocervical fat pad (buffalo hump) and visceral abdominal adiposity development (Miller et al., 1998; Lo et al., 1998; Saint-Marc et al., 2000; Martínez et al., 2001a). These morphological phenotypes are empirically associated with the aetiological progression of accompanying metabolic disturbances (Saint-Marc et al., 2000; Heath et al., 2001; Kosmiski et al., 2001; Estrada et al., 2002), although this association between lipodystrophy-related body morphology changes and metabolic abnormalities has not always been supported by research (Mulligan *et al.*, 2000; Rakotambinina *et al.*, 2001).

Assuming this association, morphological changes have been utilised as a surrogate for lipodystrophy syndrome presence and progression (Hadigan *et al.*, 2000; Heath *et al.*, 2001; Kosmiski *et al.*, 2001; Estrada *et al.*, 2002; Meininger *et al.*, 2002). In clinical practice monitoring, lipodystrophy has generally relied on self-report assessments of syndrome progression with the application of more objective measures such as bioelectrical impedance or anthropometry to characterise the expressed phenotype (Parisien *et al.*, 1993; Shikuma *et al.*, 1999; Schwenk *et al.*, 1999; Gerrior *et al.*, 2001; Schwenk *et al.*, 2001; Dreezeen *et al.*, 2002; Schwenk, 2002). However, a number of problems arise with these techniques. Firstly the diagnosis and surveillance of lipodystrophy is generally confounded by a lack of objective and quantitative diagnostic measures of the condition (Carter *et al.*, 2001). Secondly, the assumptions fundamental to the anthropometric methods may be invalidated given the diverse nature of the lipodystrophy syndrome and dearth of similar reference populations in producing suitable equations (Corcoran *et al.*, 2000; Schwenk *et al.*, 2002). Where a BIA equation has been generated for HIV wasting, its applicability to assess and track body compositional change in HIV syndromes may be limited (Paton *et al.*, 1998; Wanke *et al.*, 2002). Kinanthropometric techniques that report simple ordinal or ratio measurement such as waist-hip ratios and muscle circumferences scales have been used to characterise the population and monitor body morphology alterations with varying degrees of sensitivity to lipodystrophy diagnosis and progression (Parisien *et al.*, 1993; Wanke *et al.*, 2002). Technological solutions (Computerised Tomography, Magnetic Resonance imaging, Dual X-ray absorptiometry) can overcome these problems, but are generally expensive, time consuming and fall outside methods that can easily be applied in a 'clinical outpatient' setting. Rather they have been confined to research-based monitoring.

The need exists for a method that allows the 'bedside' quantification of lipodystrophy syndrome and facilitates the tracking of body morphology change over time to assesses its progression (Gilquin and Marchandise, 1997). Somatotype may fulfil this role. It is a rating scale independent of body size that reports body morphology based on a series of objective associations between simple anthropometric measurements, facilitating a morphological representation of the relative fatness (endomorphy), muscularity (mesomorphy) and linearity (ectomorphy) of an individual. As such, it presents a snapshot of the individual's current phenotype, independent of the need for specific validation equations. It has been applied in a variety of clinical conditions to monitor associations between phenotype and various disease processes and clinical outcomes (Koleva *et al.*, 2002). Given that HIV infection and adherence to HAART therapy influence adiposity and muscle mass, such a technique may provide an effective tool for quantifying and monitoring body morphology alterations that occurs with lipodystrophy syndrome. The aim of this study, therefore, was to establish anthropometric and somatotype profiles of HIV[+] individuals diagnosed with lipodystrophy syndrome.

## 2. METHODS

### 2.1 Subjects

Eleven HIV⁺ individuals with physician-diagnosed lipodystrophy (10 males and 1 female) and 9 sero-negative controls (8 males and 1 female) volunteered to participate. After being informed of the nature and methodology of the study, written informed consent was obtained in accordance with the institutional ethical procedures. All lipodystrophy individuals were recruited from a local HIV support network. The control sero-negative subjects were recruited from within the university population. Eligibility criteria for inclusion in the sero-positive cohort were defined as (a) the presence of documented HIV infection evidenced by HIV viral RNA copies, presenting a CD4 count above 200-cells/mm$^3$ and the absence of opportunist infections; (b) currently following an NRTI/PI regimen; (c) not adhering to testosterone replacement therapy; and (d) not engaged in a current exercise regimen. Lipodystrophy was diagnosed on the basis of physician's confirmation of patient self-report of facial lipoathrophy in the face, arms and/or legs, presence of abdominal adiposity and/or symmetrical lipomatosis (buffalo hump) development (Lo *et al.*, 1998; Engleson *et al.*, 1999). The duration of time patients had adhered to the NRTI/PI combination therapy was between 1-5 years. Population characteristics are presented in Table 1.

### 2.2 Anthropometric measurements

Anthropometric characteristics were determined from standard anthropometric techniques as described by Lohman *et al.* (1991). The technical error of measurement was calculated for all measurements and was less than 2%. In addition to age, a total of 11 anthropometric measures was determined on the right hand side of the body. Each participant height (m) was measured in the Frankfort plane to the nearest 0.001 (m) with a portable stadiometer (Seca, Menheimn, Germany), body mass (kg) was determined to the nearest 0.1 kg on balance beam scales (Seca, Menheimn, Germany). Subcutaneous adipose tissue was measured at six skinfold sites (mm) (biceps, triceps, subscapular, suprailiac, anterior thigh and medical calf) utilising Harpenden calipers (British Indicators LTD, Luton). Further, two diameters (cm) biepicondylar humerus and biepicondylar femur and three circumferences (cm) mid-thigh, maximal calf and upper arm circumference were recorded. These directly-determined anthropometric variables were utilised to permit the calculation of a series of derived measurements. These included somatotype ratings for ectomorphy, mesomorphy, and endomorphy (n=5) according to the technique of Carter and Honeyman-Heath (1990), body mass index (BMI) (kg/m$^2$), Fat Free Mass Index (FFMI) (kg/m$^2$) (Gonzalez-Cadavid *et al.*, 1998), and waist:hip ratio (WHR). Body density was determined utilising the sum of four skinfold sites: biceps, triceps, subscapular and suprailiac (Durnin and Womersley, 1974). Body fat % was calculated based upon the equation of Siri (1956).

## 2.3 Data analysis

Data were expressed as mean (± SD). Data were checked for normal distribution using the Anderson-Darling technique. Data for all variables were analysed using independent student t-tests. The $p < 0.05$ level of confidence was determined as the minimal level for acceptance of statistical significance.

## 3. RESULTS

All HIV[+] subjects presented with a combination of physician-diagnosed lipodystrophy symptoms that varied in rating from none through to severe, particularly in relation to facial lipoathrophy, peripheral lipoathrophy, and abdominal adiposity (Table 1).

**Table 1.** Categorical definitions of lipodystrophy-defining symptoms in the five subjects undergoing somatotyping.

|  | Peripheral wasting of arms | Periphera l wasting of legs | Facial wasting | Central adiposity | Buffalo hump | Somatotype Rating |
|---|---|---|---|---|---|---|
| 1 | Moderate | Moderate | Moderate | Moderate | No | 1.9-4.3-1.9 |
| 2 | Severe | Severe | Severe | Moderate | No | 1.0-4.1-4.4 |
| 3 | Moderate | Moderate | Moderate | Severe | Yes | 4.9-6.1-1.4 |
| 4* | Mild | No | No | No | No | 4.5-4.0-1.7 |
| 5 | Severe | Severe | Severe | Moderate | No | 2.8-2.8-3.6 |

* Female.

All of the subjects had been treated with 'HAART' for a mean time of 5.3 ± 1.9 years. The mean time for the progression of lipodystrophy symptoms from the introduction of HAART with PIs was 23.8 ± 11.3 months. All sero-positive subjects presented a mixed viral RNA status; 6 participants viral RNA load was less than <50 copies/ml while others viral RNA status was much higher (Table 2). Immune status expressed in terms of CD4 (T-Helper) count indicated that at the time of assessment all participants were currently asymptomatic (Table 2).

**Table 2.** Biographical and selected anthropometric and performance characteristics of the populations
Data are mean (± SD).

|  | HIV⁺ lipodystrophy | Sero-negative controls | P Value |
|---|---|---|---|
| **Skinfolds** | | | |
| Biceps | 4.6 ± 2.2 | 4.7 ± 2.3 | P>0.05 |
| Triceps | 7.2 ± 5.1 | 7.7 ± 5.2 | P>0.05 |
| Subscapular | 11.7 ± 3.0 | 15.4 ± 3.7 | P<0.05 |
| Suprailliac | 9.0 ± 3.3 | 17.9 ± 5.3 | P<0.05 |
| Anterior Thigh | 5.0 ± 1.4 | 13.1 ± 8.8 | P<0.05 |
| Medial calf | 6.2 ± 6.7 | 7.3 ± 3.7 | P>0.05 |
| Σ 4 skinfolds | 34.9 ± 14.0 | 45.7 ± 9.5 | P<0.05 |
| Σ 6 skinfolds | 37.2 ± 14.6 | 54.5 ± 16.6 | P<0.05 |
| % Body Fat | 14.7 ± 5.4 | 18.4 ± 2.7 | P<0.05 |
| **Circumferences** | | | |
| Mid-thigh | 44.8 ± 4.5 | 54.3 ± 3.74 | P<0.05 |
| Mid-calf | 25.9 ± 3.4 | 31.4 ± 3.4 | P<0.05 |
| Upper arm flexed | 33.7 ± 3.5 | 38.3 ± 1.8 | P<0.05 |

The lipodystrophy group presented with a lower absolute body mass and BMI (p<0.05) together with a higher waist: hip ratio than the sero-negative group (p>0.05) (Table 2). Fat free mass index was also significantly lower in the lipodystrophy group (p<0.006). Mid-thigh, calf and upper arm circumferences were also significantly less in the lipodystrophy group than in the sero-negative controls (p<0.05) (Table 3). Skinfold thickness as expressed by the sum of four and six measurement sites were also lower in the lipodystrophy group (p<0.05) (Table 3). The average somatotype ratings were 3.0-4.3-2.6 vs 3.9-5.5-0.9 in the lipodystrophy and seronegative group respectively (Figure 1). This difference was significant (p<0.05).

**Table 3.** Adipose tissue distribution and muscle circumferences in HIV⁺ lipodystrophy and seronegative controls. Data are mean (± SD).

|  | HIV⁺ lipodystrophy | Seronegative controls | P value |
|---|---|---|---|
| Age (years) | 49.0 ± 13.0 | 40.7 ± 7.0 | P>0.05 |
| CD4 Count (mm³) | 447.8 ± 143 | Not taken | - |
| Viral load (mm³) | 7756 ± 18357 | Not taken | - |
| Height (m) | 1.73 ± 0.07 | 1.71 ± 0.08 | P>0.05 |
| Body Mass (kg) | 67.8 ± 14.1 | 79.2 ± 10.6 | P<0.02 |
| BMI kg/m² | 23.5 ± 5.01 | 27.1 ± 2.31 | P<0.02 |
| FFMI (kg/m²) | 18.3 ± 3.18 | 22.2 ± 1.5 | P<0.006 |
| WHR | 1.01 ± 0.166 | 0.97 ± 7.01 | P>0.05 |

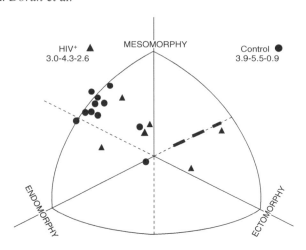

**Figure 1.** Somatoplot of HIV and Control groups with mean somatotype ratings in the centre and individuals' somatotypes distributed around it.

## 4. DISCUSSION

The diagnosis of lipodystrophy syndrome and the monitoring of its progression has relied on subjective physician and patient-based assessments of body morphology changes using predefined criteria (Carr *et al.*, 1999). The diversity of morphological conditions associated with lipodystrophy syndrome has made this process difficult, and the emergence of several distinct lipodystrophy phenotypes reflects this difficulty (Carter *et al.*, 2001). The problem is further confounded in that different lipodystrophy phenotypes can either be independently or co-expressed making the categorisation of the syndrome, and the classification of it severity, problematic. It is against this background that the referencing of various anthropometric and technological methods for assessing lipodystrophy syndrome has taken and is taking place. In the present study, the use of somatotype to characterise the morphological phenotype of HIV lipodystrophic individuals was examined. Historically, somatotype has been used to examine associations between body morphology and the occurrence of various clinical conditions (Carter and Honeyman-Heath, 1990). The usefulness of somatotype in fulfilling this role resides, in its three-component rating system. It provides a mechanism of expressing lipodystrophy-related morphology within a single-rating system, by acting as a proxy for the lipoathrophy-related adipose tissue change (endomorphy), the potential cachexic tendencies in muscle mass (mesomorphy) and increased linearity (ectomorphy) associated with the presence and progression of the syndrome. The lipodystrophy and seronegative groups both present an endo-mesomorphic profile, which, while similar in classification, masks the marked differences in somatotype ratings and, consequently, morphology expressed by the groups. A significant degree of heterogeneity around the mean somatotype in the lipodystrophy group contrasts with the homogeneity displayed in the seronegative group (Figure 1). Presentation by the lipodystrophy group of an endo-mesomorphic profile orientated toward the central portion of the somatoplot may reflect the contribution lipoathrophy and covert muscle wasting may have in altering body morphology. Calculation of endomorphy is based on the assessment of subcutaneous adipose tissue at three sites, one of which, triceps, is peripherally, and two of which, subscapular and supra-iliac are centrally located. The aetiology of lipoathrophy suggests that subcutaneous adipose tissue removed from the periphery (arms/legs) is not always redistributed subcutaneously to the truncal region. Abdominal adiposity commonly described in lipodystrophy syndrome is more strongly related to visceral rather than subcutaneous adipose tissue redistribution (Miller *et al.,* 1998). Where adipose tissue is lost or redistributed viscerally, endomorphy ratings will decline with subsequent alterations in ectomorphy ratings. The variance in somatotype ratings displayed amongst the lipodystrophy group was unsurprising given the diversity and severity of lipodystrophy symptoms exhibited (Table 1). Somatotype ratings successfully discriminated between those with severe (1.1-4.2-4.4) and mild (4.5-4.0-1.7) lipodystrophy. However, where a more homogenous diagnosis of lipodystrophy was established using the categorical rating system of Carr *et al.* (1999)(subjects 2 and 5; Table 1), the differences in somatotype ratings were still significantly different. While both subjects were defined as having severe lipodystrophy, the widely-differing somatotype ratings presented highlights the breadth of the current classification system in accommodating divergent body morphologies. As highlighted by Carter *et al.* (2001), where thresholds and criteria for lipodystrophy are not clearly delineated then confirmation of lipodystrophy syndrome presence and the categorisation of phenotype expressed will be difficult.

Given the categorical nature of the lipodystrophy rating scales utilised in clinical practice, and the variance expressed in somatotype within these categories, further assessment of the usefulness of somatotype in quantifying lipodystrophy-related body morphology and its potential to track syndrome progression is required.

The other findings of this study suggest that, despite both cohorts being of a similar age and stature, body composition and somatotype were significantly different between the lipodystrophy and sero-negative groups. Body mass, BMI, adiposity rating (sum of four and six skinfolds) and muscle circumferences in the lipodystrophy group were all reduced emphasising the clinical impact of HIV infection on body composition. The duration of exposure to HIV infection, the medication used to control it, the adverse nutritional and lifestyle effects that are associated with its presence contribute to the expression of the current phenotype. These body composition estimates are comparable to figures presented in other persons with lipodystrophy syndrome who have adhered to 'HAART' over a similar time period (Schwenk *et al.,* 1999).

Muscle wasting is a defining characteristic of HIV infection. Previously, HIV viremia was associated with the presence of a general catabolic state and loss of body cell mass (Kotler, 2000). Evaluation of the viral load present in the lipodystrophy group, demonstrated that six subjects had extremely low levels of viral RNA that were classified as borderline, undetectable. The remainder of the cohort presented with elevated viral load as evidenced by the large standard deviation in the data (Table 2). The cause of this variance was undetermined; clinical practice has suggested it can relate to individuals either not having taken or missed the precise window of opportunity to consume their medication. Where viral loads are elevated there is the possibility of loss in body cell mass continuing. The presence of lipodystrophy syndrome can mask underlying body cell mass loss (Kotler, 2000; Wanke *et al.*, 2002). Increased resting energy expenditure and loss of body cell mass have been reported in lipodystrophy patients (Hadigan *et al.*, 2002; Sekhar *et al.*, 2002). Such factors may contribute to the differences in the mesomorphy and muscularity ratings noted between the lipodystrophy and seronegative group as well as within the lipodystrophy group. Fat Free Mass Index has also been used to provide an indication of muscularity in HIV-infected individuals with muscle wasting (Gonzalez-Cadavid *et al.*, 1998). Normative values of 18 $kg.m^2$ or below for FFMI indicate a low muscularity rating while values above 22 $kg.m^2$ indicates a high level of muscularity. In the lipodystrophy group FFMI was approximately 18.3 $kg.m^2$ which exceeds the FFMI rating of 15.5 $kg.m^2$ presented for HIV positive males with 10% body mass loss and 17.6 $kg.m^2$ for those with between 0-10% body mass loss (Gonzalez-Cadavid *et al.*, 1998). While a FFMI of ~18 $kg.m^2$ is sub-optimal in relation to seronegative controls, it compares favourably to other HIV [+] persons, although subjects presented a wide range of FMMI values that spanned this normative data range.

## 5. CONCLUSIONS

In the present study, the use of somatotype as an objective means of defining lipodystrophy syndrome presence was investigated. Initial diagnosis of the lipodystrophy phenotype and its severity were based on a consensual physician and patient derived diagnosis in relation to predefined criteria (Carr *et al.*, 1999). The lipodystrophy group presented several phenotypes with combinations of facial and peripheral lipoathrophy, visceral abdominal adiposity and dorso-cervical fat pad (buffalo hump) enlargement that were categorically rated as 'none present' through to 'severe'. The corresponding somatotype ratings while objectively rating the lipodystrophy phenotype and discriminating between subjects with mild to severe lipodystrophy, also showed significant variation in ratings where subjects were given the same categorical rating of lipodystrophy presence. Somatotype, clearly provides a more sensitive means of quantifying the body morphology associated with a lipodystrophy phenotype. However, relating it to present clinical criteria is not advised due to the lack of consensus on defining criteria for lipodystrophy and criterion thresholds for the severity of lipodystrophy abnormalities. At present the strength of somatotyping lies not in providing a categorisation of lipodystrophy phenotype, but in providing the clinician with a simple 'bedside' means of tracking body morphology over time.

# REFERENCES

Amaya, R.A., Kozinetz, C.A., McMeans, A., Schwarzwald, H. and Kline, M.W., 2002, Lipodystrophy syndrome in human immunodeficiency virus-infected children. *Paediatric Infectious Disease Journal*, **21**, 405-10.

Babl, F.E., Regan, A.M. and Pelton, S.I., 1999, Abnormal body-fat distribution in HIV-1-infected children on antiretrovirals. *Lancet*, **353**, 1243-1244.

Carr, A., Samaras, K., Chrisholm, D.J. and Cooper, D.A., 1998, Pathogenesis of HIV-1 protease inhibitor associated peripheral lipodystrophy, hyperlipidemia and insulin resistance. *Lancet*, **351**, 1881-1883.

Carr, A., Samaras, K., Thorisdottir, A., Kaufmann, G.R., Chrisholm, D.J. and Cooper, D.A., 1999, Diagnosis, prediction, and natural course of HIV-1 protease inhibitors associated lipodystrophy, hyperlipidemia, and diabetes mellitus: a cohort study. *Lancet*, **353**, 2093-2099.

Carter, J.E.L. and Honeyman-Heath, B., 1990, *Somatotyping: Developments and Applications*, (Cambridge: Cambridge University Press).

Carter, V.M., Hoy, J.F., Bailey, M., Colman, P.G., Nyulasi, I. and Mijch, A.M., 2001, The prevalence of lipodystrophy in an ambulant HIV-infected population: it all depends on the definition. *HIV Medicine,* **2**, 174-180.

Corcoran, C., Anderson, E.J., Burrows, B., Stanley, T., Walsh, M., Poulos, A.M. and Grinspoon, S., 2000, Comparison of total body potassium with other techniques for measuring lean body mass in men and women with AIDS wasting. *American Journal of Clinical Nutrition*, **72**, 1053-1058.

Dreezen, C., Schrooten, W., de Mey, I., Goebel, F.D., Dedes, N., Florence, E. and Colebunders, R., 2002, Self-reported signs of lipodystrophy by persons living with HIV infection. *International Journal of Sexually Transmitted Diseases and AIDS*, **13**, 93-98.

Durnin, J.V.G.A. and Womersley, J., 1974, Body fat assessed from total body density and its estimation from skinfold thickness: measurements on 481 men and women aged from 16 to 72 years. *British Journal of Nutrition*, **32**, 77-97.

Engelson, E.S., Kotler, D.P., Tan, Y.X., Agin, D., Wang, J., Pierson, R.N. and Heymsfield, S.B., 1999, Fat distribution in HIV infected patients reporting truncal enlargement quantified by whole-body magnetic resonance imaging. *American Journal of Clinical Nutrition*, **69**, 1162-1169.

Estrada, V., Serrano-Ríos, M., Martínez-Larrad, M.T., Villar, N.G., Gonzalez-Lopez, A., Tellez, M.J. and Fernandez, C., 2002, Leptin and adipose tissue maldistribution in HIV-infected male patients with predominant fat loss treated with antiretroviral therapy. *Journal of Acquired Immune Deficiency Syndrome*, **29**, 32-40.

Gerrior, J., Kantaros, J., Coakley, E., Albrecht, M. and Wanke, C., 2001, The fat redistribution syndrome in patients infected with HIV: measurements of body shape abnormalities. *Journal of American Dietetic Association*, **101**, 1175-80.

Gilquin, B. and Marchandise, X., 1997, Body composition during HIV infection: physiopathology, methods of measurement, and review of results. *Review of Internal Medicine*, **18**, 786-794.

Gonzalez-Cadavid, N.F., Taylor, W.E., Yarasheski, K., Sinha-Hikim, I., Ma, K., Ezzat, S., Shen, R., Lalani, R., Asa, S., Mamita, M., Nair, G., Arver, S. and Bhasin, S., 1998, Organization of the human myostatin gene and expression in healthy men and HIV-infected men with muscle wasting. *Proceeding of the National Academy of Sciences*, **95**, 14938-14943.

Hadigan, C., Corcoran, C., Stanley, T., Piecuch, S., Klibanski, A., and Grinspoon, S., 2000, Fasting hyperinsulinemia in human immunodeficiency virus-infected men: relationship to body composition, gonadal function, and protease inhibitor use. *Journal of Clinical Endocrinology and Metabolism*, **85**, 35-41.

Hadigan, C., Borgonha, S., Rabe, J., Young, V. and Grinspoon, S., 2002, Increased rates of lipolysis among human immunodeficiency virus-infected men receiving highly active antiretroviral therapy. *Metabolism*, **51**, 1143-1147.

Hammer, S.M., Squires, K.E., Hughes, M.D., Grimes, J.M., Demeter, L.M., Currier, J.S., Eron, J.J., Feinberg, J.E., Balfour, H.H., Deyton, L.R., Chodakewitz, J.A. and Fischl, M.A., 1997, A controlled trial of two nucleoside analogues plus indinavir in persons with human immunodeficiency virus infection and CD4 cell counts of 200 per cubic millimetre or less. AIDS Clinical Trials Group 320 Study Team. *New England Journal of Medicine*, **337**, 725-733A.

Heath, K.V., Hogg, R.S., Chan, K.J., Harris, M., Montessori, V., O'Shaughnessy, M.V. and Montanera, J.S., 2001, Lipodystrophy-associated morphological, cholesterol and triglyceride abnormalities in a population-based HIV/AIDS treatment database. *AIDS*, **15**, 231-239.

Hengel, R.L., Watts, N.B. and Lennox, J.L. 1997, Benign symmetric lipomatosis associated with protease inhibitors. *Lancet*, **350**, 1596.

Ho, T.T., Chan, K.C., Wong, K.H. and Lee, S.S., 1999, Indinavir-associated facial lipodystrophy in HIV-infected patients. *AIDS Patient Care and Sexually Transmitted Diseases*, **13**, 11-16.

Koleva, M., Nacheva, A. and Boev, M., 2002, Somatotype and disease prevalence in adults. *Review of Environmental Health*, **17**, 65-84.

Kosmiski, L.A., Kuritzkes, D.R., Lichtenstein, K.A., Glueck, D.H., Gourley, P.J., Stamm, E.R., Scherzinger, A.L. and Eckel, R.H., 2001, Fat distribution and metabolic changes are strongly correlated and energy expenditure is increased in the HIV lipodystrophy syndrome. *AIDS*, **15**, 1993-2000.

Kotler, D.P., 2000, Body Composition studies in HIV-infected individuals. *Annals of the New York Academy of Sciences*, **904**, 546-552.

Lohman, T.G., Roche, A.F. and Martorell, R., 1991, *Anthropometric Standardisation Reference Manual*, (Champaign, Il: Human Kinetic Books).

Lo, J.C., Mulligan, K., Tai, V.W., Algreen, H. and Schambelan, M., 1998, Buffalo hump in men with HI-1 infection. *Lancet*, **351**, 867-870.

Martinez, E., Mocroft, A., Garcia-Viejo, M.A., Perez-Cuevas, J.B., Blanco, J.L., Mallolas, J., Bianchi, L., Conget, I., Blanch, J., Phillips, A. and Gatell, J.M., 2001a, Risk of lipodystrophy in HIV-1-infected patients treated with protease inhibitors: a prospective cohort study. *Lancet*, **357**, 592-598.

Martinez, E., Garcia-Viejo, M.A., Blanch, L. and Gatell, J.M., 2001b, Lipodystrophy syndrome in patients with HIV infection: quality of life issues. *Drug Safety*, **24**, 157-66.

Meininger, G., Hadigan, C., Laposata, M., Brown, J., Rabe, J., Louca, J., Aliabadi, N. and Grinspoon, S., 2002b, Elevated concentrations of free fatty acids are associated with increased insulin response to standard glucose challenge in human immunodeficiency virus-infected subjects with fat redistribution. *Metabolism*, **51**, 260-266.

Miller, K.D. Jones, E., Yanovski, J.A., Shankar, R., Feuerstein, I. and Fallon, J. 1998. Visceral abdominal fat accumulation with the use of indinavir. *Lancet*, **351**, 871-875.

Mulligan, K., Grunfield, C., Tai, V.W., Algren, H., Pang, M., Chernoff, D.N., Lo, J.C. and Schambelan, M., 2000, Hyperlipedemia and insulin resistance are induced by protease inhibitors independent of changes in body composition in patients with HIV infection. *Journal of Acquired Immune Deficiency Syndrome*, **23**, 35-43.

Parisien, C., Gaclinas, M.D. and Cossette, M., 1993, Comparison of anthropometric measures of men with HIV infection: asymptomatic, symptomatic, and AIDS. *Journal of American Dietetic Association*, **93**, 1404-1408.

Paton, N.I., Elia, M., Jennings, G., Ward, L.C. and Griffin, G.E., 1998, Bioelectrical Impedance analysis in human immunodeficiency virus-infected patients: comparison of single frequency with multifrequency, spectroscopy, and other novel approaches. *Nutrition*, **14**, 658-666.

Rakotoambinina, B., Médioni, J., Rabian, C., Jubault, V., Jais, J.P. and Viard, J.P., 2001, Lipodystrophic syndromes and hyperlipidemia in a cohort of HIV-1-infected patients receiving triple combination antiretroviral therapy with a protease inhibitor. *Journal of Acquired Immune Deficiency Syndrome*, **27**, 443-449.

Saint-Marc, T., Partisani, M., Poizot-Martin, I., Rouviere, O., Brouno, F., Avellaneda, R., Lang, J.M., Gastaut, J.A. and Touraine, J.L., 2000, Fat redistribution evaluated by computed tomography and metabolic abnormalities in patients undergoing antiretroviral therapy: preliminary results of the LIPCO study. *AIDS*, **14**, 37-49.

Schwenk, A., 2002, Methods of assessing body shape and composition in HIV-associated lipodystrophy. *Current Opinions in Infectious Disorders*, **15**, 9-16.

Schwenk, A., Breuer, P., Kremer, G. and Ward, L., 2001, Clinical assessment of HIV-associated lipodystrophy syndrome: bioelectrical impedance analysis, anthropometry and clinical scores. *Clinical Nutrition*, **20**, 243-249.

Schwenk, A., Beisenherz, A., Kremer, G., Diehl, V., Salzberger, B. and Fätkenheuer, G., 1999, Bioelectrical Impedance Analysis in HIV-infected patients treated with triple antiretroviral treatment. *American Journal of Clinical Nutrition*, **70**, 867-873.

Sekhar, R.V., Jahoor, F., White, A.C., Pownall, H.J., Visnegarwala, F., Rodriguez-Barradas, M.C., Sharma, M., Reeds, P.J., and Balasubramanyam, A., 2002, Metabolic basis of HIV-lipodystrophy syndrome. *American Journal of Physiology Endocrinology and Metabolism*, **283**, 332-337.

Shikuma, C.M., Waslien, C., McKeague, J. Barker, N., Arakaki, M., Cui, X.W., Souza, S., Imrie, A. and Arakaki, R., 1999, Fasting hyperinsulinemia, and increased waist-hip ratios in non wasting individuals with AIDS. *AIDS*, **13**, 1359-65.

Siri, W.E., 1956, Gross composition of the body. In *Advances in Biological and Medical Physics*, edited by Lawerence, J.H. and Tobais, C.A., (New York: Academic Press, Inc).

Tsiodras, S., Mantzoros, C., Hammer, S. and Samore, M., 2000, Effects of Protease Inhibitors on Hyperglycemia, hyperlipidemia and lipodystrophy: A 5-year Cohort Study. *Archives of Internal Medicine*, **160**, 2050-2056.

van der Valk, M., Gisolf, E.H., Reiss, P., Wit, F.W., Japour, A., Weverling, G.J. and Danner, S.A., 2001, Increased risk of lipodystrophy when nucleoside analogue reverse transcriptase inhibitors are included with protease inhibitors in the treatment of HIV-1 infection. *AIDS*, **15**, 847-55.

Wanke, C., Polsky, B. and Kotler, D., 2002, Guidelines for using body composition measurement in patients with human immunodeficiency virus infection. *AIDS Patient Care and Sexually Transmitted Diseases*, **16**, 375-388.

# Index